CURRENT TOPICS IN

EXPERIMENTAL ENDOCRINOLOGY

Volume 1

CONTRIBUTORS

T. Chard
L. J. Deftos
Eugene R. DeSombre
R. P. Ekins
John D. Flack
Béla Flerkó
Allan L. Goldstein

Elwood V. Jensen
D. S. Munro
H. D. Niall
J. T. Potts, Jr.
Peter W. Ramwell
Jane E. Shaw
Abraham White

EDITORIAL BOARD

J. C. Beck
E. Diczfalusy
B. Flerkó
R. O. Greep
M. M. Grumbach
G. W. Harris
I. MacIntyre

A. Jost
C. H. Li
G. W. Liddle
S. Lieberman
J. E. Rall
A. Renold
C. H. Sawyer

S. J. Segal

Current Topics in
EXPERIMENTAL ENDOCRINOLOGY

Edited by

L. MARTINI

DEPARTMENT OF PHARMACOLOGY
UNIVERSITY OF MILAN
MILANO, ITALY

V. H. T. JAMES

ST. MARY'S HOSPITAL
MEDICAL SCHOOL
UNIVERSITY OF LONDON
LONDON, ENGLAND

VOLUME 1

ACADEMIC PRESS   New York and London   1971

Copyright © 1971, by Academic Press, Inc.
ALL RIGHTS RESERVED
NO PART OF THIS BOOK MAY BE REPRODUCED IN ANY FORM,
BY PHOTOSTAT, MICROFILM, RETRIEVAL SYSTEM, OR ANY
OTHER MEANS, WITHOUT WRITTEN PERMISSION FROM
THE PUBLISHERS.

ACADEMIC PRESS, INC.
111 Fifth Avenue, New York, New York 10003

United Kingdom Edition published by
ACADEMIC PRESS, INC. (LONDON) LTD.
24/28 Oval Road, London NW1 7DD

LIBRARY OF CONGRESS CATALOG CARD NUMBER: 70-187922

PRINTED IN THE UNITED STATES OF AMERICA

CONTENTS

LIST OF CONTRIBUTORS	ix
PREFACE	xi

Basic Concepts of Saturation Analysis Techniques
R. P. Ekins

I. Introduction	1
II. Saturation Assay	3
III. Some Practical Aspects of Saturation Assay Procedures	31
IV. Conclusions	37
References	38

Steroid Hormones and the Differentiation of the Central Nervous System
Béla Flerkó

I. General Introduction	42
II. The Androgen-Sterilized Rat	42
III. The Possible Site of Action of Androgen	48
IV. The Possible Mechanism of Action of Androgen	62
V. Effects of Neonatal Treatment with Steroid Hormones Other Than Androgen on Subsequent Fertility	67
VI. Protection Against Steroid-Induced Sterility	70
VII. Summary and Conclusions	74
References	75

Recent Trends in the Physiology of the Posterior Pituitary
T. Chard

I. Introduction	82
II. Neurosecretion	83

III. Neurophysin	86
IV. Vasopressin	93
V. Oxytocin	98
VI. The Natriuretic Hormone	114
VII. Summary and Conclusions	114
References	115

Role of Thymosin and Other Thymic Factors in the Development, Maturation, and Functions of Lymphoid Tissue
Allan L. Goldstein and Abraham White

I. Introduction	122
II. Embryonic Development and Differentiation of the Thymus Gland	123
III. Role of the Thymus in the Development, Maturation, and Function of the Lymphoid System	125
IV. Thymic Malfunction; Clinical Disorders	128
V. Mechanism of Action of the Thymus	130
VI. Concluding Comments	142
References	145

Calcitonin
J. T. Potts, Jr., H. D. Niall, and L. J. Deftos

I. Introduction	151
II. The Chemistry of Calcitonins	152
III. Control of Secretion of Calcitonin	161
IV. Therapeutic Uses of Calcitonin	169
References	172

The Long-Acting Thyroid Stimulator
D. S. Munro

I. Introduction	176
II. Clinical Importance of LATS	183
III. Chemical Nature of LATS	186
IV. Effects of LATS and Its Active Fragments in Relation to Actions of TSH	189
V. Absorption of LATS by Thyroid Extracts	191
References	195

Endocrinological Implications of Prostaglandins
John D. Flack, Peter W. Ramwell, and Jane E. Shaw

I. Introduction	200
II. Tropic Hormone Effects	202

III. Neuroendocrinological Considerations	210
IV. Posterior Pituitary	212
V. Exocrine Hormone Interaction	218
VI. Actions on Lipid and Carbohydrate Metabolism	220
VII. Conclusions	222
References	223

Effects of Ovarian Hormones at the Subcellular Level
Elwood V. Jensen and Eugene R. DeSombre

I. Introduction	229
II. Estrogens	231
III. Progestins	250
IV. Hormone–Receptor Interaction Pattern and Its Biochemical Significance	259
References	263

AUTHOR INDEX	271
SUBJECT INDEX	290

LIST OF CONTRIBUTORS

Numbers in parentheses indicate the pages on which the authors' contributions begin.

T. CHARD (81), Department of Chemical Pathology, St. Bartholomew's Hospital Medical College, London, England

L. J. DEFTOS (151), Endocrine Unit, Massachusetts General Hospital, Boston, Massachusetts

EUGENE R. DESOMBRE (229), The Ben May Laboratory for Cancer Research, The University of Chicago, Chicago, Illinois

R. P. EKINS (1), Institute of Nuclear Medicine, Middlesex Hospital Medical School, London, England

JOHN D. FLACK (199), Worcester Foundation for Experimental Biology, Shrewsbury, Massachusetts

BÉLA FLERKÓ (41), Department of Anatomy, University Medical School, Pécs, Hungary

ALLAN L. GOLDSTEIN (121), Department of Biochemistry, Albert Einstein College of Medicine, Yeshiva University, Bronx, New York

ELWOOD V. JENSEN (229), The Ben May Laboratory for Cancer Research, The University of Chicago, Chicago, Illinois

D. S. MUNRO (175), Department of Pharmacology and Therapeutics, The University of Sheffield, Sheffield, England

H. D. NIALL (151), Endocrine Unit, Massachusetts General Hospital, Boston, Massachusetts

J. T. POTTS, JR. (151), Endocrine Unit, Massachusetts General Hospital, Boston, Massachusetts

PETER W. RAMWELL (199), Alza Corporation, Palo Alto, California

JANE E. SHAW (199), Alza Corporation, Palo Alto, California

ABRAHAM WHITE (121), Department of Biochemistry, Albert Einstein College of Medicine, Yeshiva University, Bronx, New York

PREFACE

Endocrinology is now one of the most rapidly advancing of the biological sciences, and both novel experimental procedures and the development and exploitation of new concepts have radically altered endocrinological views over the last few years. The ever-extending use of new experimental procedures, such as isotopic methods for tracing molecular events or defining minute hormonal concentrations, has substantially extended our knowledge, and these and other techniques are now making it possible to study endocrine events in considerable detail. The purpose of this series is to provide readers with a continuing and critical review of the field. For this purpose, the editorial board has attempted to select certain aspects of experimental endocrinology which appear particularly dominant or fundamental and which are also of sufficient general interest to justify reviewing in detail. The invited authors have been offered the opportunity to discuss their field critically from a personal standpoint rather than to provide an extensive reference list to the area under discussion. In this way it is hoped that the reader will be able to derive from this survey a closer understanding of contempory problems and advances in these particular areas.

L. MARTINI
V. H. T. JAMES

CURRENT TOPICS IN
EXPERIMENTAL ENDOCRINOLOGY

Volume 1

BASIC CONCEPTS OF SATURATION ANALYSIS TECHNIQUES

R. P. Ekins

INSTITUTE OF NUCLEAR MEDICINE
MIDDLESEX HOSPITAL MEDICAL SCHOOL
LONDON, ENGLAND

- I. Introduction 1
- II. Saturation Assay 3
    - A. Basic Principle 3
    - B. Definitions 6
    - C. Assay Design: Optimization with Respect to Sensitivity . . 11
    - D. Sensitivity in "Competitive" Assays (i.e., Tracer Differing Chemically from the Test Compound) 22
    - E. Assay Precision 23
    - F. Assay Specificity 27
    - G. "Linearization" of Assay Response Curves 30
- III. Some Practical Aspects of Saturation Assay Procedures . . . 31
- IV. Conclusions 37
    - References 38

I. Introduction

One of the major factors which has led to the advance of endocrinology in the last few years has been the emergence of analytical methods with sensitivities encompassing the range of concentration at which many hormones exert their effects in biological systems. Many of these methods have relied essentially upon the use of radioactive reagents—a dependence which reflects the delicacy of radioactive measurement as compared with many other physical detection methods. These radioanalytical methods may in turn be broadly subdivided into two classes: labeled derivative techniques, and those termed by the author "saturation assay" methods. This article will deal almost exclusively with the latter group; nevertheless a brief review of the labeled derivative method is not out of place since some of the reagents and techniques employed are common to both assay techniques notwithstanding the fundamental difference in principles on which they each rely.

The derivative method was originally introduced by Keston and his colleagues in 1946 (Keston et al., 1946) and subsequently exploited in the measurements of the steroid hormones by various groups, notably those of Tait and co-workers in England (Avivi et al., 1954) and Peterson (1959) in the United States. The method was likewise adopted for the measurement of the thyroid hormones by Whitehead and Beale (1959).

Fundamentally the technique is akin to "activation analysis" (commonly employed in the measurement of trace elements) in that it depends upon the radioactivation of the compound under test. However, in contrast with conventional activation analysis, activation is achieved by chemical reaction with a labeled reagent rather than by physical methods. The initial amount or concentration of the test compound can be deduced from a measurement of the labeled derivative formed, the latter being quantitated (after its isolation from labeled contaminants) by a measurement of the radioactivity appearing in the purified product. "Indicator" compounds, either the original test compound or its derivative, labeled with a second isotope, are usually added at an appropriate point in the procedure to monitor recovery of the labeled derivative through the necessary extraction and purification stages.

In this simple form, the technique suffers from a major disadvantage: that is, the nonspecificity of the primary chemical reaction on which the method depends. Most labeled reagents used in these procedures (acetic anhydride, thiosemicarbazide, fluorodinitrobenzene, etc.) react with a considerable range of compounds, with the consequence that the specificity of the method depends critically on the efficiency of the procedures whereby the particular reaction product is separated from all other derivatives, from residual unused reagent, and from other radioactive contaminants. Such procedures are frequently time consuming, and they severely limit the number of samples that may be processed.

Moreover, they are never completely successful, and labeled contaminants persisting through successive purification stages almost invariably restrict the ultimate assay detection limits achieved to values far greater than those dictated by the final radioactive measurements (Brodie and Tait, 1969).

Although laborious, the labeled derivative method has formed the basis of major advances in endocrinology in the last decade, particularly in the steroid field. Nevertheless the more recently introduced saturation assay techniques, because of their greater simplicity and, frequently, sensitivity, are tending to displace the original derivative methods.

A recent development, however, has circumvented the basic objection to the derivative technique by imparting a much higher degree of chemical specificity to the initial reaction. This is the immunoradiometric technique, initiated by Miles and Hales (1968), wherein labeled antibody, specific in its reaction with the test compound, is employed as the labeled reagent. This approach has, at the present time, been employed in the assay only of protein hormones. Nevertheless, there seems to be little doubt that its use will be extended to other compounds, such as the thyroid and steroid hormones, against which antisera can be raised by appropriate methods. Ultimately also, it is probable that other specific binding proteins may be isolated in a sufficiently purified form to enable their use as labeled reagents to be contemplated.

II. Saturation Assay

A. *Basic Principle*

The fundamental principle of the saturation assay method is shown in Fig. 1. (In practice there are many variants of the basic sequence of steps, and those shown in this figure are representative rather than obligatory.) The first step consists of the addition of radioactive P to the biological medium under test. After equilibration of exogenous labeled and endogenous unlabeled compounds, P may, if necessary, be extracted from its biological milieu and purified, extraction recovery being monitored by the radioactivity present in the final extract. Subsequently the extracted compound is mixed with a specific reagent, shown in Fig. 1 as Q, in such relative concentration that part of P reacts with Q (bound, or reacted, P) and part remains in the unreacted form (free P). The distribution of reacted and unreacted P, as revealed by the ratio of radioactivity appearing in the two fractions, is dependent upon the total concentration of P present, so that, provided certain conditions

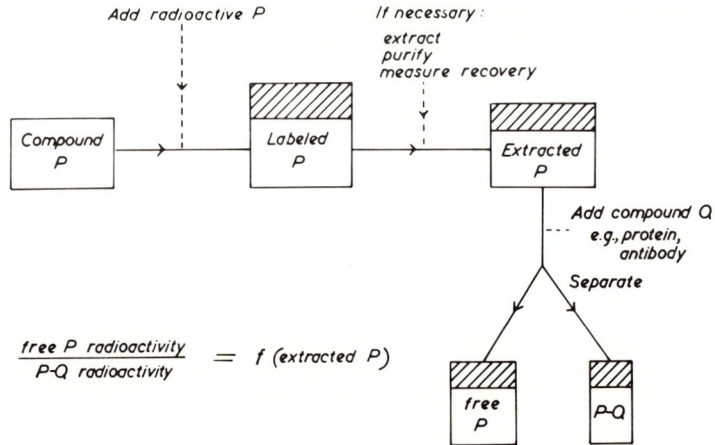

Fig. 1. Fundamental principle of saturation analysis.

are fulfilled, the distribution can be used to deduce the concentration of an unknown amount of P introduced into the system.

To emphasize the generality of this analytical principle, its broad areas of application are set out in Table I. The list is by no means

Table I
Saturation Analysis
(*Displacement Analysis, Radiostereoassay, Competitive Radioassay*)

Class of reagent	Common name	Compounds to which applied
Specific antibodies	Radioimmunoassay	Polypeptide hormones Proteins Steroid hormones Thyroid hormones Cyclic nucleotides Tumor antigens Viral antigens
Specific serum and tissue proteins, and other binders (e.g., intrinsic factor, milk)	Competitive protein-binding assay	Thyroid hormones Steroid hormones Vitamins Trace elements Cyclic nucleotides Polypeptide hormones
Specific enzymes	Radioenzymatic assay	Folic acid Cyclic nucleotides
Microorganisms	Radiomicrobiological assay	Folic acid
Inorganic reagents	Substoichiometric assay	Metals

comprehensive, and almost any attempt to make it so would be futile by virtue of the rapidity of current developments in the field. Conversely, certain categories of compound have been included under particular headings because their assay using a particular type of specific reagent is *potentially* possible, or desirable, although the experimental procedures may not as yet have been described.

Several terms have been proposed—other than saturation analysis—which encompass the several classes of specific, saturable, reagents which have been exploited in methods of this general type. There are, however, in the author's view, conceptual objections to many of these terms. For example, the adjective "competitive" misrepresents the fundamental principle, since the method does not essentially depend upon competition with or "displacement" of, a labeled competitor compound. Indeed, *any* physicochemical measurement of the distribution of the test compound can serve as the response parameter enabling unknown amounts of that compound to be estimated. Only when measurements are confined to exceedingly low values does the addition of radioactive tracer provide a convenient means of quantitating the distribution. The word "competitive" should perhaps be restricted to the description of those techniques which rely on a genuine competition between two chemically distinct compounds for identical reaction sites.

The single basic requirement common to all forms of exploitation of the principle is that the specific reagent (Q) should be present in the assay system at such concentration that the amount of P that can react is limited, so that the distribution of the latter is a rapidly changing function of the total weight or concentration present. This implies that the reactive sites associated with Q must be saturated or approaching saturation (although it is evident from a consideration of the law of mass action that reaction sites can never be *fully* saturated). Clearly the concentration of Q must be selected so that the distribution of P changes most rapidly in the particular concentration range of interest; hence, for the measurement of high values of P, a larger concentration of Q is appropriate than for measurements falling in the lower ranges. In general, therefore, the concentration of Q must be of the same order of magnitude as the range of values of P that it is desired to assay.

The purpose of this presentation is essentially to enumerate and discuss the fundamental principles contributing to an accurate measurement of P. This necessitates consideration of the theoretical relationships between the concentrations of reagents, and their optimization to yield assay systems displaying maximal precision. Some of the factors affecting specificity (and, hence, accuracy) can likewise be considered from a theoretical point of view. Other factors of a more practical nature, not amenable to detailed mathematical analysis, will be briefly considered in Section III. First, however, we must define exactly what constitutes an "accurate" measurement.

B. Definitions

An "accurate" measurement can be defined as one that yields a value close to the "true" value of the measured quantity. This implies that the measurement must be both precise (as defined below) and specific, i.e., unaffected by systematic extraneous factors. A particular requirement is that the response of the measuring system must be identical (or related by a known constant factor) to both the "standard" and "unknown."

A "precise" measurement is one that is reproducible, although this statement does not imply that the measured value is necessarily "true" or "correct." Usually "precision" is defined by the standard deviation of replicate estimates of the measured quantity if these are normally distributed about the mean or, alternatively, by confidence limits that likewise reflect the probability that any single measurement will fall within the given range, but which do not depend upon the assumption of a normal frequency distribution of the replicate values. Figure 2a illustrates the relationship between the precision of measurement of a concentration denoted by h, that of the response metameter (R), and the slope of the response curve (dR/dh) at the corresponding point.

In the special circumstances in which both the standard error of the

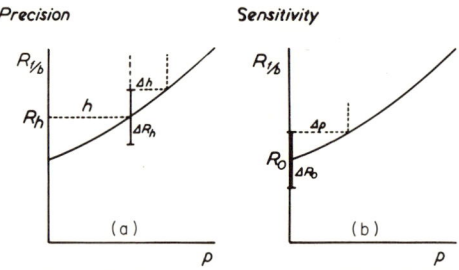

Fig. 2. (a) Definition of precision. The precision of measurement of h (i.e., Δh) is given, approximately, by the precision of the response metameter (ΔR_h) divided by the slope of the response curve at R_h. (b) Definition of sensitivity. The sensitivity of an analytical technique may be defined as that quantity (Δp) which yields a response which can just be distinguished from the zero, or blank response (R_0). It is given (approximately) by the precision of measurement of the zero response (ΔR_0) divided by the slope of the response curve at R_0.

response, and the slope of the response curve (with "dose" plotted on a log scale) are constant, the precision of measurement of all values of the "dose" (expressed as the coefficient of variation of the measurement) is the same. This has led to the concept of the so-called "index of precision," the constant given by dividing the standard error of the response by the response curve slope (Gaddum, 1933). In these circumstances it is legitimate to speak of the "precision of the assay," since this is not a function of the measured quantity. In the more usual situation, in which the quotient is *not* constant at all points along the response curve, then it is permissible to refer only to the precision with which a particular "dose" is estimated.

The term "sensitivity" as applied to measurement techniques commonly refers to the ability of a system to measure "small" amounts with acceptable precision.† Thus a technique is regarded as more "sensitive" if it enables smaller amounts to be measured with the same precision, or the same small amount with a greater precision. This concept may be formalized by defining the sensitivity of an assay as the precision of measurement of a zero quantity (see Fig. 2b), and it is clearly related to the precision of measurement of the response when no test compound is present (other, in a saturation assay system, than the standard amount of labeled compound used to quantitate the response), and the slope of the response curve at this point. In short, this concept of assay sensitivity represents a limiting case of the general concept of precision in the particular circumstance where h, the measured quantity, equals zero. This definition essentially corresponds to the limit of detection of the system as defined by Kaiser and Specker‡ [1956] and other authors (Borth, 1957; Jones, 1959; Wilson, 1961).

In designing an assay system, the assayist is primarily concerned with measuring an "unknown" with maximal precision. In practice he is usu-

---

† Many authorities explicitly (Morrison and Skogerboe, 1965) or implicitly would disagree with this definition. Their objections are discussed below.

‡ Kaiser and Specker have defined the detection limit of an assay as $\bar{x} - \bar{x}_b = k\sqrt{2}\,S_b$ where S_b = standard deviation of the blank reading, $\bar{x}$ = average analytical reading, $\bar{x}_b$ = average blank reading, k = a constant related to the confidence level demanded by the experimenter. This expression may be rewritten in terms of the response metameter y as: $\bar{x} - \bar{x}_b = k\sqrt{2}S_b{}^1/(dy/dx)_b$, where $S_b{}^1$ = standard deviation of the response metameter y, and $(dy/dx)_b$ is the slope of the response curve at the zero, or blank, point. The factor $\sqrt{2}$ in these expressions reflect the fact that the determination of the detection limit requires *two* measurements: that of the "zero" response (y_b) and that of the response when the minimum detectable amount of the test substance is present.

ally confronted with a range of unknowns, and he must therefore attempt to maximize precision with respect to a single representative value, bearing in mind the relative importance of other values in the anticipated range. Thus a diagnostician may be concerned in distinguishing patients suffering from vitamin B_{12} deficiency. Although the bulk of his measurements of serum B_{12} might fall in the region of 300–600 pg/ml, he will nevertheless usually wish to optimize the precision of his method with respect to values in the order of 150 pg/ml, which represents the borderline value between normal and deficient subjects. In many circumstances, however, the anticipated values fall close to the ultimate detection limit obtainable with the method (as defined by Kaiser and Specker), and the experimenter is then forced to "maximize precision with respect to values close to zero"—that is, to maximize the "sensitivity" of his assay system.

These concepts may, at first reading, appear so widely accepted and incontrovertible as not to merit extended discussion in this article. They are, however, misunderstood, disregarded, or even challenged by many workers, and it is therefore essential, before proceeding to the question of optimal assay design, that the disagreements that exist in this area be fully understood and dissipated.

The confusion surrounding the concepts of "sensitivity" and (to a lesser extent) "precision" is reflected in the many definitions which currently exist for these terms, and the misunderstanding of the relationship that exists between the two. "Sensitivity" has been formally defined by the American Chemical Society as the "rate of displacement of the indicating element with respect to the change of the measured quantity" (Macurdy et al., 1954). Finney (1964) defines a "sensitive subject" as one having a high value of the regression coefficient of y on x, where y is the response metameter and x the dose metameter. Morrison and Skogerboe (1965) likewise define sensitivity as the slope of the response curve, and they specifically recommend that the term be distinguished from, and not applied to, the lower limit of detection. A brief review of radioimmunoassay or "protein-binding assay" literature will reveal many instances of the use of the term in this sense. Thus Yalow and Berson (1968a) frequently use the term in the sense $d(B/F)/d[H]$ though, in contrast, they also regard "sensitivity" as a maximum when $db/d[H]$ is a maximum, where B/F = "bound to free" radioactivity ratio and b = fraction of activity bound. Rodbard et al. (1968) consider the "50% intercept" (i.e., the point where B/T is one half of $(B/T)_o$, T representing total radioactivity in the system) as a measure of the "sensitivity" of an assay. On the other hand, the term is also almost universally employed, implicitly, as the detection limit of the measuring system, as is reflected by its frequent expression in units of weight or concentration.

The indeterminacy regarding the concept of sensitivity is particularly serious since it is the necessary objective of many assayists (particularly in the field of endocrinology) to render their techniques as "sensitive" as possible. Since the choice of assay conditions yielding maximum sensitivity depends upon which concept of sensitivity is involved, it is not surprising that workers employing "saturation" assay techniques frequently differ in their approach to the setting up of optimal systems. Moreover, it is often impossible to deduce with certainty (from published reports) which of two assay methods yields a lower detection limit, or to be certain of the true implications of a recommended change in experimental procedure which is claimed to increase "sensitivity."

Finally, the confusion surrounding these concepts has been particularly highlighted by the spirited controversy regarding the theoretical principles relating to assay design as enunciated by Yalow and Berson and the present author (see discussions following Yalow and Berson, 1970a,b; Ekins, 1968, p. 612 *et seq.*).

As implied above, definitions of sensitivity basically fall into one of two groups: those which relate to the detection limit of an assay, and therefore necessarily involve an estimate of the error in the determination of the "blank" or zero response (concept A), and those which merely reflect the change in the response metameter for a given change in the "dose" (concept B). It is, of course, arguable that *any* definition is, *ipso facto*, necessarily "correct." Difficulties primarily arise, therefore, because the same word is indiscriminately used for fundamentally different concepts. However, beyond this essentially semantic problem, it is readily demonstrable that concept B is meaningless and inconsistent, and frequently leads to fallacy and misunderstanding.

The irrelevance of high sensitivity as represented by concept B has, of course, been demonstrated in many fields. A rough balance is not transformed into an instrument suitable for use in a high grade analytical laboratory merely by extending the length of the pointer, though such action increases sensitivity in terms of concept B. Likewise distant radio signals are not necessarily better detected (by a simple receiver) simply by increasing the gain of the amplifier. As both of these examples illustrate, steps taken to increase the slope of the response curve may be without practical benefit if they simultaneously increase the magnitude of (and the variation in) the blank, zero, "noise," or "background" measurement.

Other fallacies stemming from concept B are readily illustrated. A plot of a saturation assay standard curve in terms of $R_{b/f}$ (the bound to free ratio) against hormone concentration (see Fig. 3) yields a curve with the steepest slope when the hormone concentration is zero. This has been adduced as the principal argument for using a "vanishingly small concentration of tracer" to maximize "sensitivity" (Yalow and Berson, 1968a; Berson and Yalow, 1968). However, identical data plotted in terms of $R_{f/b}$ (the free to bound ratio) frequently yield a curve with a *minimum* slope at zero hormone concentration, and application of the same argument would suggest that maximum sensitivity is attained by employing infinitely large concentrations of tracer. In short, the form of the response curve and the region of maximum slope (i.e., of maximum "sensitivity"—concept B) is determined essentially by the choice of the response metameter. Likewise, it can be shown that reduction in the concentration of Q in the system *reduces* the slope of the response curve plotted in terms of $R_{b/f}$, but *increases* its slope when data are expressed in terms of $R_{f/b}$. Thus the "sensitivity" (concept B) of the assay system can be said to have decreased or to have increased depending upon the personal conventions adopted by the experimenter. Nevertheless, illusions that particular experimental stratagems increase or decrease "sensitivity" but which merely reflect the experimenter's choice of response metameter are particularly well represented in the literature relating to saturation assay.

These observations exemplify some of the fundamental absurdities stemming from the uncritical and unqualified acceptance of the slope of the dose response curve (or related parameters) as indices of assay sensitivity, and underline the futility of many experimental maneuvers designed to increase the slopes of assay response curves without regard to their effect on other assay parameters. However, these inconsistencies are entirely circumvented if the "sensitivity" of an assay is specifically defined as the detection limit of the system as illustrated in Fig. 2b. Clearly the detection limit of an assay is not affected by the manner in which the response metameter is expressed since it is defined solely in terms of a weight or concentration (though, naturally, it may be affected by the manner in which the response is measured). Moreover, reduction of the detection limit, since it implies an increase in the precision of measurement of small amounts, is normally the principle aim of practical relevance to the assayist; indeed, the "responsiveness" of his system per se is totally irrelevant in this context, though, as will be shown later, it becomes a matter of concern when the *specificity* of the system is under consideration.

Scientific literature is in general more restrained in its use of the term "precision"; however, because their theoretical analysis of optimal design of radioimmunoassays is central to the theme of this chapter, it is necessary to consider the definition initiated by Yalow and Berson (1968a,b). This they give as $db/(d[H]/[H])$. This expression is equivalent to $db/(d \log[H])$: thus, it may be phrased as "the slope of the response curve on a log dose plot." This definition is open to essentially similar objections to those that have already been raised here against definitions of sensitivity which merely reflect the slope of the response curve, whatever the dose and response metameters selected. Because it contains no term related to the error of measurement of the response, it is entirely unrelated to the accepted concept of precision. Consequently, it is difficult to accept as relevant the conclusions that these authors draw to the experimenter intent on maximizing "precision" in the sense in which the word is normally used.

C. Assay Design: Optimization with Respect to Sensitivity

As emphasized earlier, an assay designed for maximum sensitivity represents merely a special case of the general requirement to optimize the system with respect to precision, with the restriction that h, the hormone† concentration to be measured, "target" concentration is equal, or close to, zero.

The general approach to the problem is, however, perhaps best illustrated by this particular case since the equations and conclusions that emerge from the analysis are somewhat easier to manipulate and understand. As we have seen, the fundamental issue is the selection of reagent concentrations which yield a minimum value of the detection limit. Because the latter depends both upon the slope of the response curve at R_0 and on the error (ΔR_0) in determination of the zero response‡ (R_0), it is necessary to consider the effects of change in reagent concentrations on both these parameters.

As a first step in the analysis, equations must be derived describing the relationship between the response metameter and the total concentration of P (p) and of specific reagent in the system. Let us postulate that the reagent comprises a number of reaction sites (Q_1, Q_2, ..., Q_i, ..., Q_n) each characterized by equilibrium constants $K_1, K_2, \ldots, K_i, \ldots, K_n$ at concentrations $q_1, q_2, \ldots, q_i, \ldots, q_n$, and let us assume that the law of mass action governs their reactions with P. Then, taking $R_{b/f}$ to represent the distribution of radioactivity between

---

† The compound under assay will henceforth be referred to as a "hormone," although the application of the saturation assay technique to other classes of compound of interest to the endocrinologist [such as cyclic AMP (Brown et al., 1970)] underlines the inadequacy of this terminological choice.

‡ The "zero" response is that observed in the standard assay tube containing only tracer (together with specific reagent), but no unlabeled P.

bound and free moieties at equilibrium, and assuming that radioactive P *exactly* represents the distribution of the unlabeled P in the system (i.e., that tracer and inactive compounds react with all sites with identical energies), it may be shown (Ekins et al., 1968) that:

$$R_{b/f} = \sum_{i=1}^{n} \frac{q_i}{[p/(1+R_{b/f})] + 1/K_i} \tag{1}$$

This equation may readily be expressed in terms of $R_{f/b}$ or r (where $R_{f/b}$ = the free to bound activity ratio; r = fraction of total activity bound) by the substitutions:

$$R_{f/b} = \frac{1}{R_{b/f}} \tag{2}$$

$$r = \frac{R_{b/f}}{R_{b/f} + 1} \tag{3}$$

We shall consider the simplest case, where only a single order of reaction site (characterized by a single equilibrium constant) is operative in the system. It then follows, from Eqs. (1)–(3) that:

$$R_{b/f}^2 + R_{b/f}(1 + Kp - Kq) - Kq = 0 \tag{4}$$

$$R_{f/b}^2 + R_{f/b}\left(1 - \frac{p}{q} - \frac{1}{Kq}\right) - \frac{1}{Kq} = 0 \tag{5}$$

$$\left(\frac{r}{1-r}\right)^2 + \left(\frac{r}{1-r}\right)(1 + Kp - Kq) - Kq = 0 \tag{6}$$

Figure 3 shows simple plots of these equations on arithmetic scales.

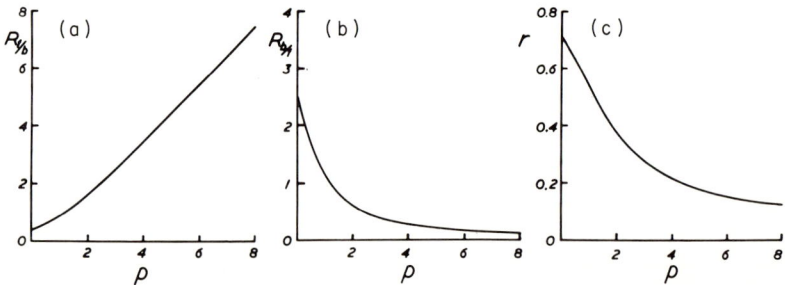

Fig. 3. Standard curves plotted on arithmetic scales in terms of the response metameters: (a) $R_{f/b}$ ("free" to "bound" ratio), (b) $R_{b/f}$ ("bound" to "free" ratio), (c) r (the fraction of total activity "bound"). In each case the following arbitrary values have been ascribed: $q = 1$, $K = 2.5$.

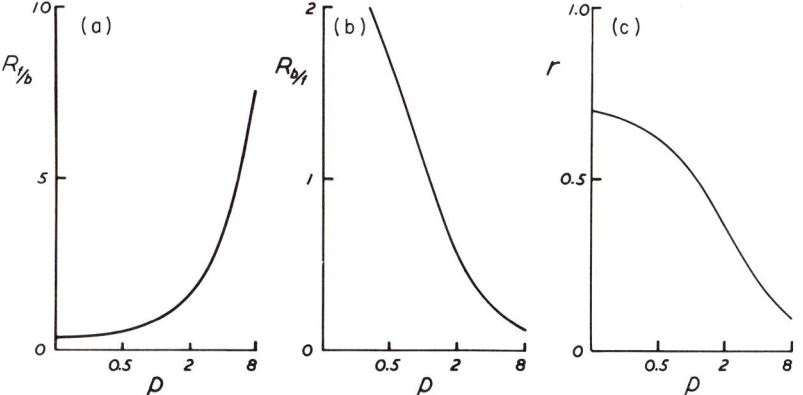

Fig. 4. Standard curves plotted on semilog paper with hormone concentration on a log scale.

Figure 4 shows the same curves plotted on semilog paper, with the concentration of P on a log scale. Figure 5 shows plots of the logit of Y, and Z, against log p where $Y = r/r_0$ (Rodbard et al., 1968; Midgley et al., 1969b)

$$Z = \frac{R_{b/f}}{(R_{b/f})_0} = \frac{R_{b/f}}{Kq}$$

and r_0, $(R_{b/f})_0 = r$, $R_{b/f}$ when $p = 0$.

Finally, Fig. 6 shows a plot, on log paper, of the parameter log $[R_{f/b} - (R_{f/b})_0]$ against log p.

It is evident that, in a single reaction site system, certain methods of presentation yield curves which are effectively straight lines over

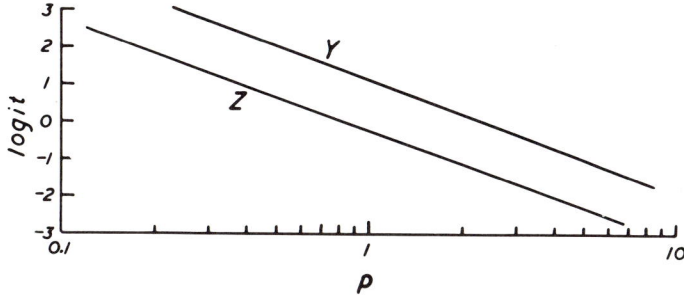

Fig. 5. Standard curves plotted on semilog paper in terms of the response metameters: (a) logit Y ($Y = r/r_0$) (b) logit Z [$Z = R_{b/f}/(R_{b/f})_0$].

much of the range. This is especially true of the logit and log plots shown in Figs. 5 and 6 (which represent algebraically equivalent transforms), but it is also largely true of the simple arithmetic plot of $R_{f/b}$ shown in Fig. 3. Indeed, many presentations, such as of $1/r$, which involve the reciprocal of the bound activity, approach linearity over a large part of the range (Ekins and Samols, 1963).

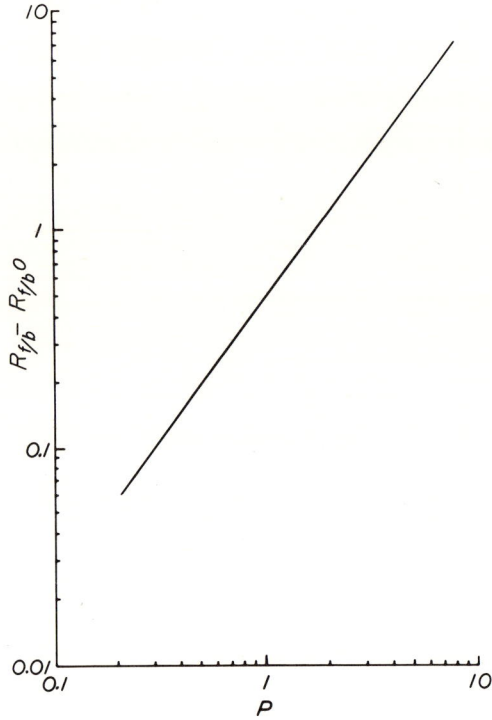

Fig. 6. Response curve plotted on log-log paper. Response metameter: $R_{f/b} - (R_{f/b})_0$.

When more than a single reactive site is operative, response curves are more complex. Figure 7 shows, for a two-site system, a simple $R_{f/b}$ plot. Although in this presentation we shall not explore further the theoretical implications of multiple sites, we should note that, at concentrations of P close to zero, such a mixture behaves as would a single reaction site system with an equivalent site concentration given by:

$$\bar{q} = \frac{[\Sigma K_i q_i]^2}{\Sigma K_i^2 q_i} \tag{7}$$

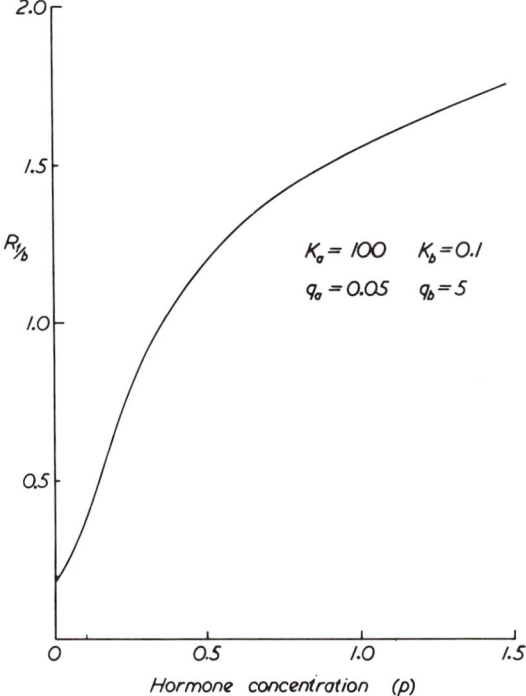

Fig. 7. Typical response curve yielded by two-binding site system.

and an equivalent equilibrium constant of

$$\bar{K} = \frac{\Sigma K_i^2 q_i}{\Sigma K_i q_i} \qquad (8)$$

It is also appropriate, at this stage, to consider the effect in a single-site system of employing tracer (P^*) with an equilibrium constant (K^*) different from that of the inactive hormone. The response equation in terms of $R_{f/b}$ is given by

$$R_{f/b}^2 + R_{f/b}\left(1 - \frac{p^*}{q} - \frac{1}{K^*q}\right) - \frac{1}{K^*q} - \frac{h/q(R_{f/b} + 1)R_{f/b}}{(K^*/K_h)R_{f/b} + 1} = 0 \qquad (9)$$

where K_h is the equilibrium constant of the nonradioactive test compound, and h is the concentration.

The *slope* of the response curve at any point is derived by differentiation of Eqs. (4), (5), or (6) with respect to p. In terms of $R_{f/b}$ the slope is given by

$$\frac{dR_{f/b}}{dp} = \frac{R_{f/b}}{qR_{f/b} + 1/KR_{f/b}} \tag{10}$$

Meanwhile, we must also consider the effect of change in reagent concentrations on the error of the zero response (that is the response, R_0, observed when only radioactive hormone is present in the system). It must be remembered, of course, that the total error in the determination of any point on the response curve is the statistical sum of two independent errors: the counting error (which is a function of the concentration and specific activity of the tracer used, the total counting time, and volume of incubation mixture counted), and the "experimental" error, which reflects the various manipulation errors involved in the technique.

The magnitude and variation of the counting error are theoretically predictable; the "experimental" component is, on the contrary, dependent upon factors (such as the quality of the glassware, the nature of the technique employed to separate "free" and "bound" fractions, the personal skill of the experimenter) which can be assessed only by experimental observation.

For this reason it is difficult, if not impossible, to predict the composition of assay mixtures which will yield maximum sensitivity.† However, provided a relationship between the experimental error and reagent concentrations can (on the basis of preliminary observations) be distinguished, then a logical choice of the optimal reagent mixture can be made—if necessary using empirical computer optimization techniques, although in certain simple situations algebraic solutions are possible.

To illustrate the basic approach, we may consider the simple case in which the "experimental" error is postulated as absent, and only the statistical errors of counting contribute to uncertainty in the magnitude of the response metameter. The distribution of radioactivity following reaction in a saturation assay system is commonly effected either by counting the activities residing in both free and bound fractions, or in one fraction alone. In this presentation two cases will be considered:

---

† This view has been challenged by Rodbard (1970). Recently, Rodbard and his colleagues have met with considerable success in constructing model systems enabling a good estimate to be made of the experimental error incurred in the measurement of the response metameter at any point on the response curve. These interesting developments are not incompatible with the view expressed here, that the prediction of the experimental error relies, at root, on experimental observations.

(i) where bound (B) and free (F) fractions are both counted; (ii) where only the bound fraction is counted, and the total activity in each tube is assumed to be constant.

Case i. Let a total time, T, be employed in counting each assay tube. Let us also assume that the interval T is divided into two parts, t_b and t_f devoted to the counting of bound and free fractions, and that these times are optimally selected so that the relative error in the ratio is minimized. (This is the case when $t_b/t_f = (f/b)^{1/2}$, where b = "bound" count rate, and f = "free" count rate, assuming a negligible background error). Under these circumstances, the standard error in $(R_{f/b})_0$ is given by

$$\frac{\Delta(R_{f/b})_0}{(R_{f/b})_0} = \{1 - [(R_{f/b})_0]^{1/2}\} \left[\frac{(R_{f/b})_0 + 1}{p^*SVT(R_{f/b})_0}\right]^{1/2} \quad (11)$$

where $\Delta(R_{f/b})_0$ is the standard error and S = specific activity of P^*, and V = volume of incubation mixture fractionated and counted. Combining Eqs. (10) and (11), we obtain an expression for Δp, the detection limit:

$$\Delta p (SVT)^{1/2} = \{1 + [(R_{f/b})_0]^{1/2}\} \left[q(R_{f/b})_0 + \frac{1}{K(R_{f/b})_0}\right] \left(\frac{K}{Kq(R_{f/b})_0 - 1}\right) \quad (12)$$

This expression may be partially differentiated with respect to q and p^*, whereby it may be shown that (to reduce Δp to a minimum):

$$\hat{q} = \text{optimal concentration of } Q = 3/K$$

$$\hat{p}^* = \text{optimal concentration of tracer} = 4/K$$

$$(R_{f/b})_0 = 1$$

$$\Delta p_{\min} = \frac{4\sqrt{2}}{(KSVT)^{1/2}}$$

Case ii. A similar approach to that employed above leads to the following expressions: $\hat{p}^* = 9/4K$; $q = 5/4K$; and the detection limit $\Delta p_{\min} = 3\sqrt{3}/(KSVT)^{1/2}$.

Under these conditions $r_0 = 0.33$; i.e., one-third of the tracer is bound.

We note that in this highly artificial situation, in which "experimental" errors are postulated to be absent, a very slight gain in sensitivity stems from counting only a single sequestered fraction. It should also be noted that the optimal composition of assay incubation mixtures is different in the two cases.

When both fractions are counted, the optimal mixture results in equipartition of tracer at the "zero" point, $(R_{f/b})_0 = 1$; in contrast when only the *bound* activity is counted, then in the optimal mixture only one-third of the total radioactivity will be present in this fraction.

Although illustrating the logical approach to assay design, the conclusions derived above are of no practical significance since they depend on the assumption that only counting errors limit sensitivity, an assumption which is, of course, totally unrealistic. We may nevertheless extend the algebraic analysis by postulating an experimental (relative) error (ϵ) in the measurement of the response metameter which may be statistically summed with the counting error to yield the expression of the form:

$$\Delta p = \left(q(R_{f/b})_0 + \frac{1}{(R_{f/b})_0 K}\right) \left\{\frac{(R_{f/b})_0 + 1}{(R_{f/b})_0 p^* SVT}[1 + ((R_{f/b})_0)^{1/2}]^2 + \epsilon^2\right\}^{1/2} \quad (13)$$

Though ϵ will, in general, be a function both of p^* and q, we may simplify the analysis by treating ϵ as a function of $(R_{f/b})_0$ (or r_0) only. By making "reasonable" assumptions regarding the variation of ϵ with the response metameter, we can draw conclusions which, although not necessarily valid in every detail, nevertheless throw considerable light on optimal assay design, and the factors that affect sensitivity. We must, as before, distinguish between the situations in which both free and bound fractions are counted, and those in which only one fraction is used.

Case i. Experimental observation in a number of assays carried out in our own laboratory (such as of protein hormones, T_4, T_3, vitamin B_{12}, using electrophoretic and solid adsorbant methods of separation) have confirmed our intuitive belief that the minimum "experimental" relative error in the free to bound (or bound to free) ratio is observed when the activity is equally distributed† (i.e., $(R_{f/b})_0 = 1$). Since maximal sensitivity when $\epsilon = 0$ is attained when $(R_{f/b})_0 = 1$, we can reasonably suppose that maximum sensitivity will likewise, in the presence of experimental errors, be achieved when reagent concentrations are selected to yield this ratio. By making this assumption and partially differentiating Eq. (13) with respect to p^* and q, the following expressions may be derived:

$$\epsilon^2 STV\left(\hat{q} - \frac{1}{K}\right)^2 + 2\left(\hat{q} - \frac{1}{K}\right) - \frac{4}{K} = 0 \quad (14)$$

† We have observed in certain assays (particularly those in which significant "nonspecific binding" effects occur) that ϵ is a minimum at a value of $(R_{f/b})_0$ which is a little less than 1. Nevertheless the slight invalidity of the assumption made here does not significantly affect the subsequent analysis.

$$\epsilon^2 STV \left(\frac{\hat{p}^*}{2}\right)^2 + \hat{p}^* - \frac{4}{K} = 0 \qquad (15)$$

$$\Delta p_{\min} = \left(\hat{q} + \frac{1}{K}\right)\left(\frac{8}{\hat{p}^* STV} + \epsilon^2\right)^{\frac{1}{2}} \qquad (16)$$

Equations (14) and (15) are plotted in Fig. 8. These curves enable the experimenter, knowing the values of S, T, V, and K relevant to

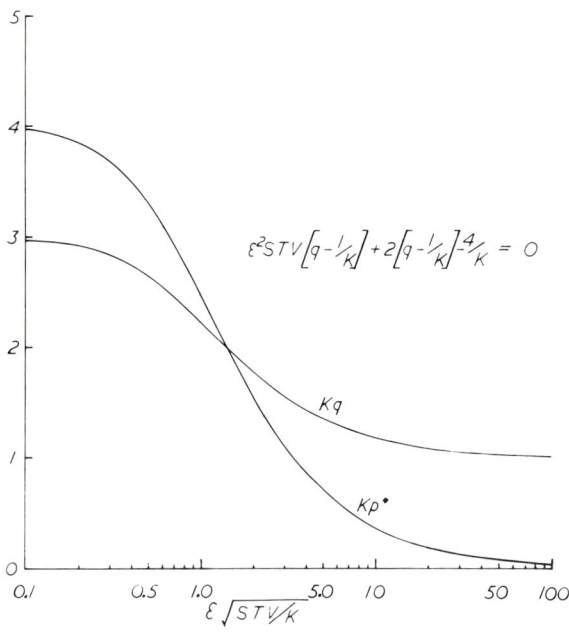

Fig. 8. Curves relating optimal reagent concentrations to the product $\epsilon(SVT/K)^{1/2}$. These curves apply to the case in which both "free" and "bound" fractions are counted, and the minimum experimental error ϵ is incurred for a free:bound activity distribution equal to unity.

his technique, and having ascertained, in previous experiments, the magnitude of ϵ for values of $(R_{f/b})_0$ close to unity, to make a logical choice of optimal reagent concentration yielding maximum sensitivity. The fuller implications of these equations will, however, be delayed until we have considered case ii.

Case ii. A number of assumptions may be made with regard to the relationship between ϵ (note that ϵ here represents the relative error in r) and r (the fraction of radioactivity bound). In a number of assays run in the author's laboratory, the variance in r appears to be approximately proportional to r; in others the standard deviation of r is thus related. (However, neither of these observations holds good for very low values of r.) For the purpose of illustration, we shall consider the latter case, i.e., the standard deviation in r is proportional to r, and hence ϵ is constant.

On the basis of this postulate, we may derive the following equations:

$$\hat{R}^4 - 2\hat{R}^3 - \frac{8\epsilon^2 SVT}{K}\hat{R} - \frac{8\epsilon^2 SVT}{K} = 0 \tag{17}$$

$$\hat{q} = \frac{\hat{R}^2 + 2\hat{R} + 2}{K\hat{R}^3} \tag{18}$$

$$\hat{p}^* = (1 + \hat{R})\left(q - \frac{1}{K\hat{R}}\right) \tag{19}$$

where $\hat{R} = [(1/\hat{r}_0) - 1]$, $\hat{r}_0 = $ optimal fraction bound; whence

$$\Delta p_{\min}(SVTK)^{1/2} = (\hat{R} + 1)\left(K\hat{q} + \frac{1}{\hat{R}^2}\right)\left(\frac{\epsilon^2 SVT}{K} + \frac{\hat{R}}{\hat{R}K\hat{q} - 1}\right)^{1/2} \tag{20}$$

These expressions are plotted in Figs. 9 and 10. Figure 9 shows optimal concentrations of p^* and q as a function of $\epsilon[(SVT)/K]$ together with the resulting optimal fraction of radioactivity appearing in the "bound" moiety. (Because ϵ is not, in fact, constant, particularly at small values of r, these curves are unreliable for large values of $\epsilon[(SVT/K)]^{1/2}$.

Figure 10 exemplifies the representation of Eq. (20) using a value of K of 1 ml/ng which is roughly that observed in an assay system for testosterone (relying on pregnancy serum TBG as the specific binding protein) as set up in the author's laboratory. This set of curves is particularly interesting in that it illustrates the relationship between assay sensitivity and the product STV, (or, assuming that any two of the terms are held constant, between sensitivity and the remaining parameter). Similar curves can be derived from Eq. (16) though, as will be discussed later, they are asymptotic to a different limiting value as STV approaches infinity. The effect of an increase in S, T, or V is to increase the total number of counts accumulated in the radioactive fractions submitted for counting, that is to decrease the magnitude of the counting error. However, as can be observed in Fig. 10, reduction in the "counting" component of the overall error yields decreasing rewards in terms of increased assay sensitivity, the detection limit being progressively determined by the "experimental" errors implicit in the technique.

Equations (16) and (20) clearly enable the experimenter to compute

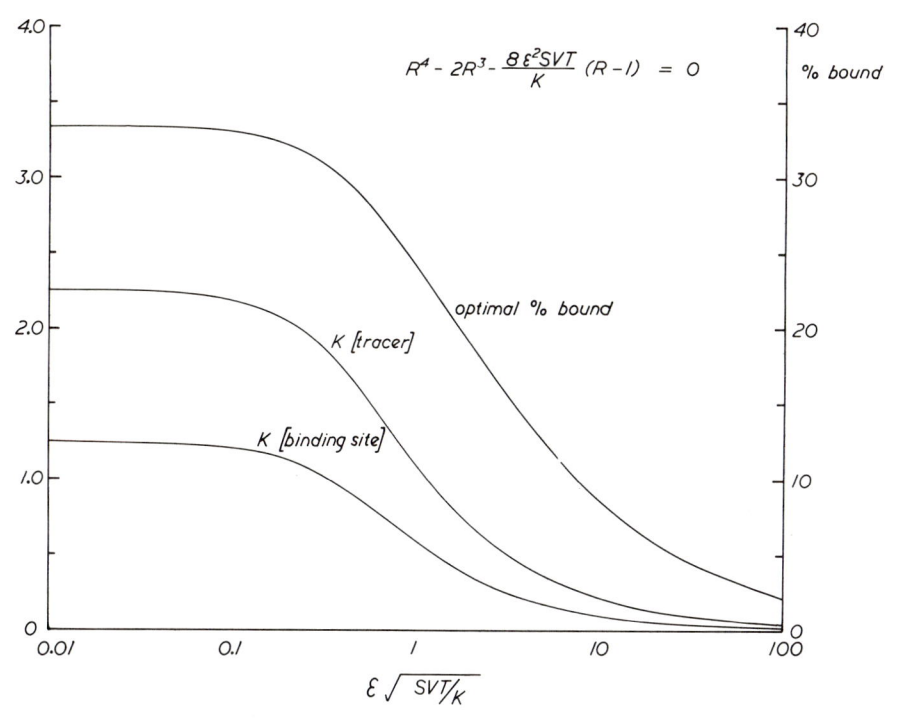

Fig. 9. Curves relating optimal reagent concentrations to the product $\epsilon(SVT/K)^{1/2}$ applicable when only the "bound" activity is counted. They rely on the assumption that ϵ (the relative error in r) is constant for all values of r.

and plot curves as exemplified in Fig. 10 for any assay system provided the relevant value of K is known. Such curves are useful since they not only give guidance relating to the sensitivities likely to be achieved within the assay, but on the likely effect of change in such parameters as tracer specific activity, time of counting of specimens, and so on. It is clear from Fig. 10 that in certain circumstances increase in the specific activity of the tracer used will yield marginal benefit in terms of increased sensitivity. On the other hand, such increase would allow counting times or incubation volumes to be correspondingly decreased without *loss* in sensitivity, benefits which may be of considerable advantage to the experimenter. Likewise the curves can assist in the choice of an optimal counting time for sample radioassay, enabling a balance between the pressures on counter resources and assay sensitivity to be struck. (It should be noted that to preset counting equipment to register large numbers of counts for each sample in circumstances where the resulting counting errors are very small in relation to the "experimental"

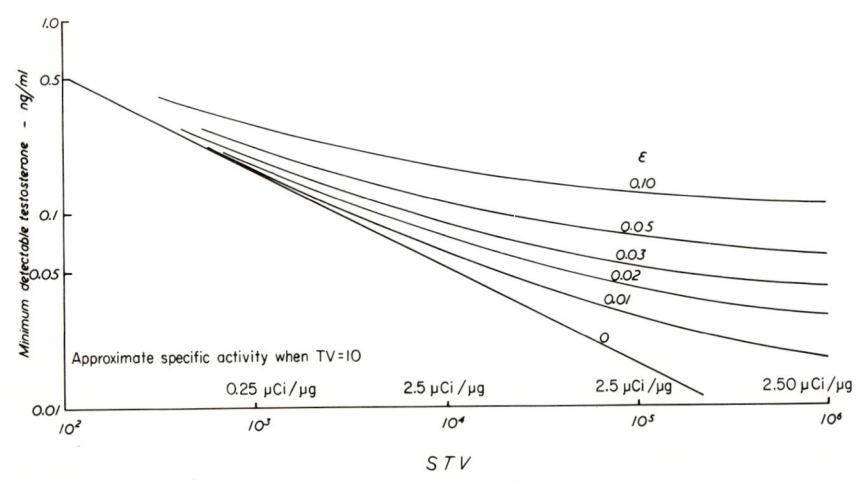

Fig. 10. The detection limit (i.e., "sensitivity") of a testosterone assay as a function of the product STV. The curves are based on an assumed K value of 1 ml/ng testosterone.

error may represent a gross misuse of the equipment. In many circumstances the choice of counting time to yield 1000 or 2000 counts per sample may yield sensitivities very close to the limiting values determined by other factors.)

The curves shown in Fig. 10 are asymptotic to the value ϵ/K; reference to Eq. 16 indicates that under the conditions postulated in case i, Δp_{min} approaches 2 ϵ/K as the product STV approaches infinity. It must be emphasized that in case i, ϵ represents the relative error in the ratio $R_{f/b}$, in case ii, ϵ refers to the relative error in the fraction of radioactivity bound (r_0). These will not normally be numerically identical. Moreover, the assumption on which the former value rests are unlikely to hold true as STV approaches infinity (and $\hat{r}_0$ approaches zero); hence the expression 2 ϵ/K is probably more realistic in indicating the maximum sensitivity attainable in a saturation assay system. As this expression implies, the higher the equilibrium constant of the fundamental reaction, the lower the detection limit (i.e., the higher the sensitivity) achievable.

D. *Sensitivity in "Competitive" Assays (i.e., Tracer Differing Chemically from the Test Compound)*

In many saturation assay systems, the specificity of the fundamental binding reaction is such as to permit the use of labeled compounds differing chemically (and hence in reaction energy) from the test compound P. The effects of such a choice on assay sensitivity are subtle and essentially unpredictable since they depend on the magnitude of experimental errors, and their variation as a function of the response metameter.

Some insight into the problem can be gained from simple algebraic analysis as described by Ekins *et al.* (1968). By taking Eq. (9) as a starting point, and applying the same approach as outlined in previous sections of this chapter, it may be shown that, in the absence of experimental errors, a slight increase in sensitivity results from the use of competitor displaying an equilibrium constant either higher *or lower* than that of the unlabeled test compound. This somewhat unexpected result reflects two contradictory effects. On the one hand, labeled material of lower equilibrium constant is more readily displaceable; on the other, if the labeled material reacts with higher energy, then smaller amounts of reagents are required to achieve an optimal distribution of radioactivity, with a consequent increase in sensitivity. However, such sensitivity increase is achieved only by the choice of particular optimum reagent concentrations which suffer from the disadvantage that they are likely to yield activity distributions associated with especially elevated experimental errors when these are present. For this reason the net effect may be a fall in sensitivity. Nevertheless, it can be shown that, in the conditions under which many assay systems are actually set up in practice (i.e., with approximate equidistributions of radioactivity in bound and free fractions in the absence of competing unlabeled compounds), best sensitivity is probably achieved using labeled material displaying a slightly higher equilibrium constant than that of the competing unlabeled compound (see Fig. 11).

In summary, it is difficult, on simple theoretical grounds, to predict the effect on sensitivity resulting from the use of a labeled competitor compound differing from the test material. Computer methods are, in principle at least, applicable to this problem providing sufficient information is available regarding the magnitude and variation of experimental errors in the assay system and that the equilibrium constants of both active and inactive compounds are known. However, it is unlikely that the advantage to be gained from such detailed analysis would ever be justified by startling gains in assay sensitivity.

E. Assay Precision

The theoretical approach to the optimization of assay precision with respect to *any* selected hormone concentration essentially represents a generalization of the particular problem posed by the attainment of optimal sensitivity. Unfortunately the equations that emerge from the analysis are more complex, and the assumptions that must be made

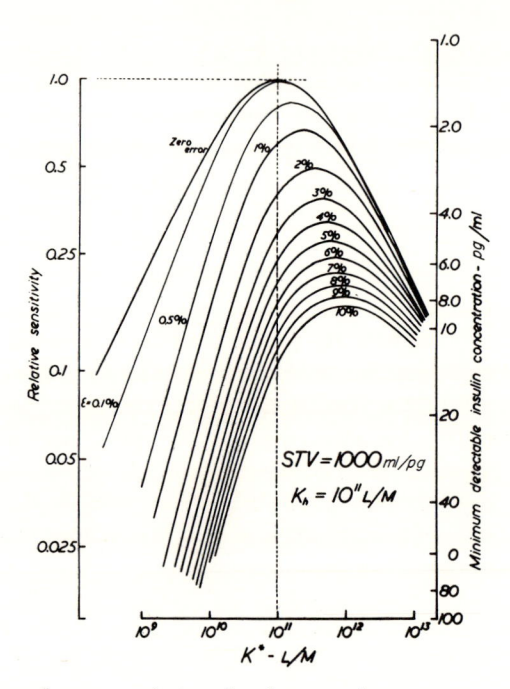

Fig. 11. Computed curves relating the detection limit in an assay for insulin to the equilibrium constant (K^*) of the labeled hormone in the system. The equilibrium constant of the unlabeled insulin is assumed to be 10^{11} L/M. Maximum sensitivity is observed (for usual experimental errors) when the labeled hormone is the more reactive.

with regard to the variation of "experimental errors" less dependable. In consequence, relatively simple algebraic solutions are neither achievable, nor, if they were, would they be reliable. It is therefore perhaps wiser to restrict the analysis simply to the presentation of the general equations which govern assay precision. The fundamental equations are as follows:

$$q = \frac{1}{K^*R} + \frac{p^*}{R+1} + \frac{h}{K_rR+1} \tag{21}$$

$$(\Delta R)^2 = R(R+1)(1+\sqrt{R})^2/(p^*SVT) + R^2(\epsilon)^2 \tag{22}$$

or

$$(\Delta R)^2 = (R+1)^2 \left(\frac{R+1}{p^*SVT} + \epsilon_b^2\right) \tag{23}$$

$$\Delta h = \Delta R((K_rR+1)(1/(K^*R^2) + p^*/(R+1)^2) + K_rh/(K_rR+1) \tag{24}$$

where R has been used for $(R_{f/b})_h$ = the free to bound ratio in the presence of unlabeled compound h; ΔR = total standard error in the determination of R; h = concentration of unlabeled hormone to be measured; $K_r = K^*/K_h$; $\epsilon = f(R)$ = "experimental" component of the standard error in R; $\epsilon_b = f(r)$ = "experimental" component of the standard error in r. [Note that, though these equations are phrased in terms of R (i.e., $R_{f/b})_h$, they are equally applicable to the choice of the optimal reagent mixture and isotopic distribution if the chosen response metameter is $R_{b/f}$ or r [$=1/(R+1)$]. In the latter case, Eq. (23) is applicable as an expression of the total error in the measurement of the response, assuming that only the bound fraction is counted.

These equations may be solved by standard computer methods to yield values of p^* and q such that Δh, the standard error in h, is minimized. Additionally, the computer may be programmed to yield estimates of the precision of measurement of all other concentrations of the test compound between specified limits embracing the initial selected value. In this way, the experimenter may be reassured that all likely

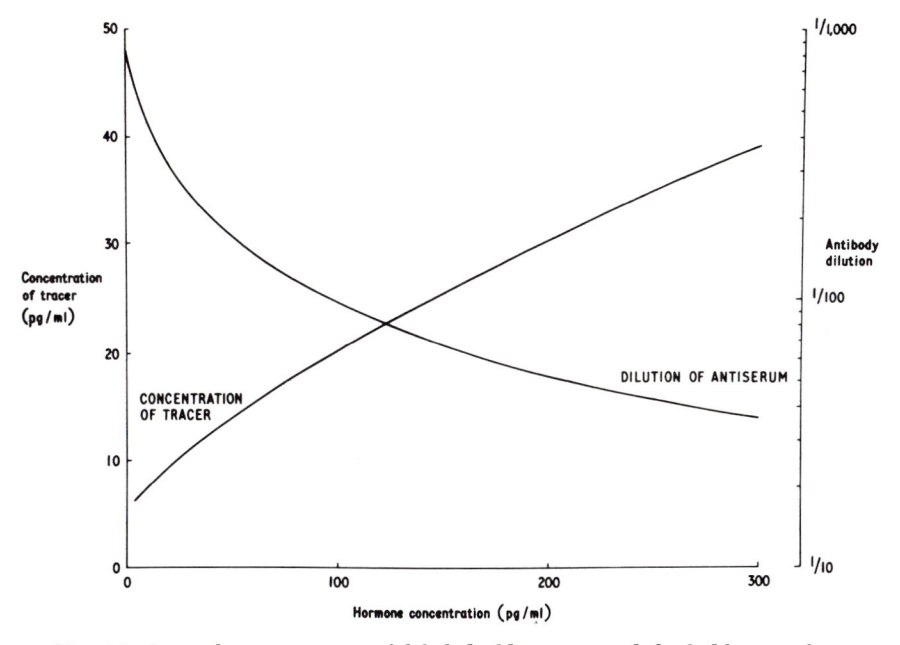

Fig. 12. Optimal concentration of labeled aldosterone and final dilution of antialdosterone antiserum as a function of "target" hormone concentration. These values have been computed assuming an equilibrium constant for both labeled and unlabeled hormones of 0.094 ml/pg; specific activity $(S) = 153$ cmp/pg; incubation volume $(V) = 0.3$ ml; counting time $(T) = 20$ min. ϵ was taken as 4% (0.04) over the working range of response. [Note: the computations illustrated here are based on an assay system in which the "free" radioactivity only is counted. Equations relevant to this situation have been presented by Ekins et al. (1971).]

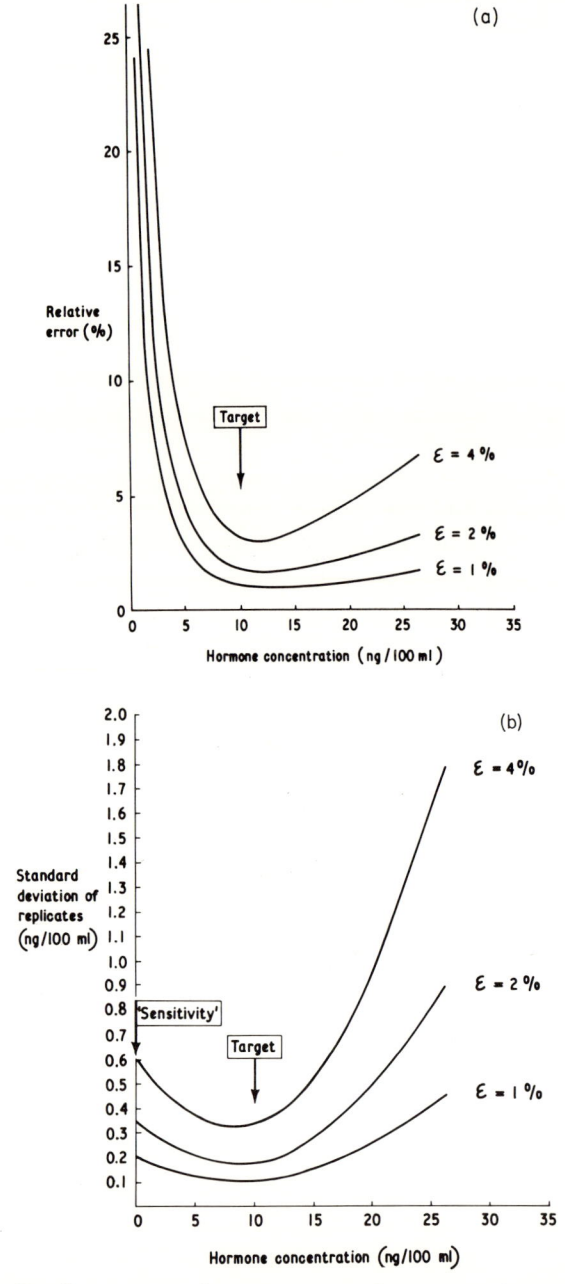

Fig. 13. Predicted precision of measurement of a range of serum aldosterone hormone concentration in an assay optimized with respect to a "target" concentration of 10 ng/100 ml. (a) Refers to the relative, or percentage, error of measurement. (b) Indicates the absolute error. A recovery of 50% is assumed in the extract from a starting volume of 1 ml of serum. Incubation volume 0.3 ml. Other parameters as indicated in Fig. 12.

concentrations within a desired range will be measured with acceptable precision (or whether, as sometimes occurs, he must set up a second assay using different reagent concentrations to satisfactorily encompass all anticipated values). Figures 12 and 13 show results plotted from a typical computer optimization study relating to a radioimmunoassay for aldosterone (Ekins et al., 1971). Figure 12 shows the optimal concentration of labeled aldosterone and dilution of antibody as a function of the "target" hormone concentration. Figure 13 indicates the anticipated precision of measurement of other hormone concentrations assuming the assay has been optimized with respect to a serum aldosterone concentration of 10 ng/100 ml.

It must be emphasized that the above equations assume a single "order" of binding sites reacting with uniform energy, albeit differently vis-a-vis labeled and unlabeled compounds. A more general set of equations can, in principle, be derived applicable to the multiple binding site situation.

F. Assay Specificity

The "response" equations derived earlier in this chapter can also be used to shed light on some of the problems of assay specificity. It should be noted that nonspecific effects can arise at two stages of the assay: at the primary reaction stage between P and Q, and subsequently at the separation stage when free hormone is sequestered from bound.

Effects on the reaction between P and Q may take one of two principal forms: (a) competition of a compound (other than P) for the reaction sites on Q; (b) an effect on the energy of reaction between P and Q.

Case a. In considering the first of these two possibilities, we must immediately distinguish the situations in which (i) only a single reaction site is effectively involved in reaction with P; (ii) two or more sites are so involved.

Case i. We may suppose that a competitor (N) reacts with equilibrium constant K_n while P reacts with constant K_p. We may now consider two assay systems, in one of which labeled P is present together with a range of concentrations of unlabeled P, while in the other concentrations of unlabeled N are substituted for P. Under these circumstances we shall observe response curves given by:

$$R_{f/b}^2 + R_{f/b}\left(1 - \frac{p^*}{q} - \frac{1}{K^*_p q}\right) - \frac{1}{K^*_p q} - \frac{h_p/q(R_{f/b}+1)R_{f/b}}{(K^*_p/K_p)R_{f/b}+1} = 0 \quad (25)$$

$$R_{f/b}^2 + R_{f/b}\left(1 - \frac{p^*}{q} - \frac{1}{K^*_p q}\right) - \frac{1}{K^*_p q} - \frac{h_n/q(R_{f/b}+1)R_{f/b}}{(K^*_p/K_n)R_{f/b}+1} = 0 \quad (26)$$

Combining these two equations we see that, for any given value of the response $R_{f/b}$:

$$h_n/h_p = \frac{(K^*_p/K_n)R_{f/b} + 1}{(K^*_p/K_p)R_{f/b} + 1} \tag{27}$$

or

$$h_n/h_p = \frac{(K^*_p/K_n)R_{f/b} + 1}{R_{f/b} + 1} \tag{28}$$

assuming that $K^*_p = K_p$.

Equation (28) implies that when $R_{f/b}$ is small (i.e., when $R_{f/b} \ll K_n/K_p$), h_n/h_p approaches unity, and the two response curves are essentially identical. Conversely when $R_{f/b} > K_n/K_p$ the relative "potency" of the two compounds tends toward the value K_p/K_n.[†]

These conclusions imply that, in certain circumstances, two hormones both of which react with an identical binding site will yield response curves which, when plotted in terms of log concentration, are almost (though not exactly) parallel. In such situations parallelism of response curves, often taken as necessary though not conclusive evidence of identity between standard and unknown hormones, clearly serves as an unreliable criterion of such identity. On the other hand, there are circumstances in which, though only a single binding site is implicated, the response curves will clearly be far from parallel.

These predictions are well exemplified by assay systems for thyroxine (T_4) and triiodothyronine (T_3) represented in Figs. 14 and 15. In Fig. 14 the response curves yielded by T_4 and T_3 in a system relying on thyroxine-binding globulin (TBG) as specific reagent and using radioactive T_4 to quantitate the response are plotted. Assay conditions have been selected so that all values of $R_{b/f}$ fall below unity (i.e., $R^2_{f/b} > 1$). Since K_{T_3}/K_{T_4} is of the order of 0.25, $R_{f/b}$ is $> K_{T_3}/K_{T_4}$ at all points of the response curves, and the relative potencies are of the order of the ratio of the equilibrium constants.

In Fig. 15 the response curves yielded by the two compounds in a system relying on TBG and labeled T_3 are shown. In this example, reagent concentrations have likewise been chosen so that all values of $R_{f/b}$ are of the order of unity or greater. However, K_{T_4}/K_{T_3} is now in the region of 4, and for values of $R_{f/b}$ significantly less than this, we may anticipate, as in fact is well demonstrated in this study, that T_4 will react with a potency (on a molar basis) of the order of that of T_3. We see, in addition, increasing potency manifested by T_4 vis-a-vis T_3 as $R_{b/f}$ falls (i.e., as $R_{f/b}$ increases).

[†] These theoretical observations have recently been expanded upon by Rodbard and Lewald (1970).

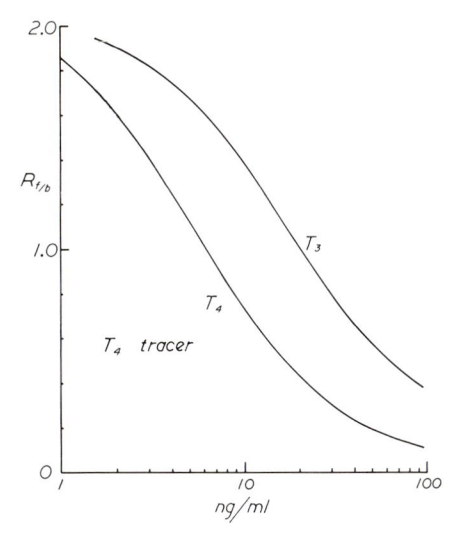

Fig. 14. Response curves yielded by thyroxine (T_4) and triiodothyronine (T_3) in a system relying on the distribution of labeled T_4.

These observations demonstrate that the potency ratios of cross-reacting hormones in saturation assay systems will vary significantly depending upon the conditions under which they are tested. They emphasize that a strongly reacting compound may demonstrate quite a low potency in certain circumstances, and conversely, that a weakly reacting compound may show relatively high potency in others. The possible complexity of this situation is underlined when we consider, as an example, the effects of T_4 as a contaminant in T_3 extracts in an assay for the

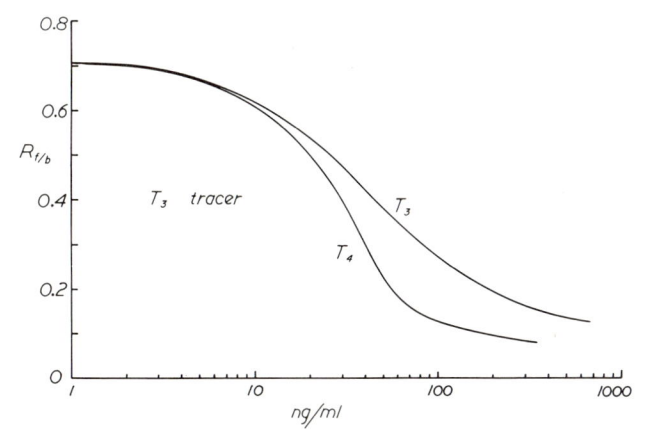

Fig. 15. Response curves yielded by T_4 and T_3 using labeled T_3.

latter compound. If the T_3 concentration in the extract is low, then the contaminating T_4 may react relatively weakly and the increment due to the latter compound in the T_3 measurement (in absolute terms) may be small. Conversely if the T_3 concentration is high, and the free to bound ratio is elevated in consequence, then the T_4 present will show a much more marked effect.

Case ii. When a multiplicity of binding sites is associated with the specific reagent (as will probably be the case if the latter comprises a dilution of antiserum), the situation is clearly more complex. A simple illustration of the possibilities is provided by a system comprising two orders, or species, of binding site, one of which reacts with both compounds (P and N), the other which is reactive with P only. Assuming labeled P is used in the system, it is clear that the addition of excess amounts of the competitor N will not result in a diminution of the binding of the labeled compound with those sites reactive only with P. Response curves *cannot*, under these circumstances, be parallel over the entire range of hormone concentrations, whatever the range of values of the response metameter encountered.

More complex mixtures clearly offer a wide range of possibilities; however, it is evident that the probability of distinguishing between two cross-reacting hormones (using the criterion of parallelism of dilution curves) is greatly increased when a number of different species of binding site are present in the system.

Case b. Nonspecific effects on the energy of reaction between P and Q are more difficult to quantify. We may postulate, for example, that the presence of certain ions [which display marked effects in radioimmunoassay systems (e.g., Girard and Greenwood, 1968)] results in a diminution in the reaction energy which is proportional to the ionic concentration in the incubation mixture. In these circumstances it is not unlikely that the dilution curve yielded by the "nonspecific solute" will be approximately parallel to that yielded by the standard hormone. Girard and Greenwood have indeed observed near-parallelism between the response curves yielded by standard growth hormone preparation and, in contrast, by dilutions of urine, an observation which they have attributed largely to the effect of "nonspecific" reactants in urine.

G. "Linearization" of Assay Response Curves

Many of the statistical treatments developed for bioassay methods are not immediately applicable to saturation assay. This is largely because saturation assay data are frequently much more precise than those encountered in bioassay and assumptions (such as of linearity of the response curve and of homoscedasticity of the variance of the response metameter) upon which statistical analysis of bioassay results frequently rely are demonstrably untenable in the case of the saturation methods. Nevertheless attempts have recently been made (see Bliss, 1970; Rodbard *et al.*, 1968) to rectify this situation by employing transforms which have the effect of linearizing assay response curves, thereby rendering them more amenable to accepted statistical treatment. Perhaps the most promising approach reported at the present time is that of Rodbard and his colleagues (1969), who, by plotting the logit of the parameter Y (i.e., $\log_e Y/1 - Y$ where $Y = r/r_0$) against the log hormone concentration obtain curves which are essentially linear over a large part of the concentration range. Similar results have been obtained in the author's laboratory by plotting the parameter $\log_e [R_{f/b} - (R_{f/b})_0]$ against log hormone concentration (see Fig. 6). Midgley and co-workers (1969b) have reported excellent straight-line fits to assay data by adopting the logit transform.

These results must nevertheless be treated with caution. The exact shape of the response curve in a saturation system is dependent upon several factors, including the number and relative significance of the different "orders" of binding site which are operative, identity, or otherwise, of the labeled or unlabeled hormones, presence of radioactive impurities in the labeled preparation. Empirical transforms which successfully linearize data in one system may therefore be totally inapplicable to another.

As an example, Fig. 16 illustrates results from a saturation assay for vitamin B_{12} (Ekins and Sgherzi, 1965) plotted in logit form. This assay method performs, in the author's hands, with a remarkable stability; response curves are almost exactly reproducible from day to day, and points on the curve are routinely determined with overall precision of the order of 1–2%. The typical set of data plotted in Fig. 16 demonstrate that the logit plot is not linear but sigmoid for this system, and that errors of up to 10% in estimates of B_{12} concentration could stem from assuming a linearity which in practice is not normally displayed.

III. Some Practical Aspects of Saturation Assay Procedures

It is not possible, in a presentation of restricted length, to discuss in detail the experimental problems encountered in saturation assay procedures. Nevertheless, insofar as the theoretical treatment outlined in this chapter points to certain practical conclusions, it is apposite that

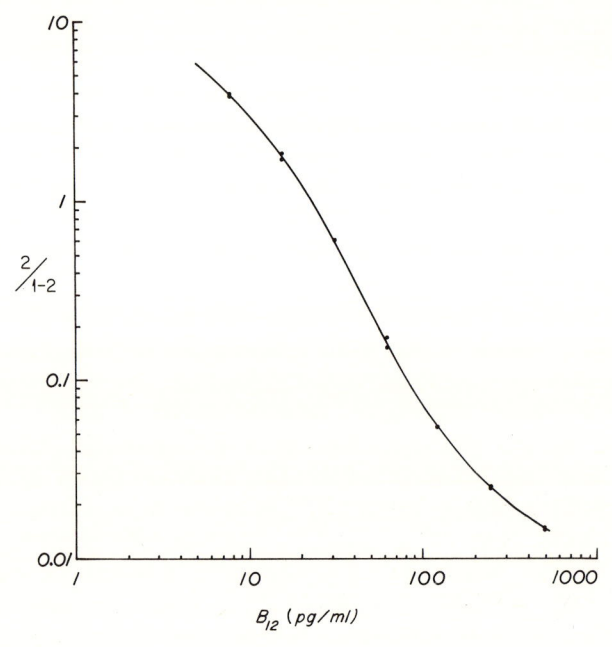

Fig. 16. Response curve observed in a saturation assay for vitamin B_{12}. The response metameter is log $2/(1-2)$ [where $2 = R_{b/f}/(R_{b/f})_0$], i.e., logit 2. The sigmoid shape is almost invariably observed in this assay system.

these should be briefly considered. Reference to Fig. 1 reveals that the general method may be subdivided into the following steps:

1. Extraction (if necessary) of P.
2. Reaction with specific reagent Q.
3. Separation of reacted and unreacted moieties.
4. Measurement of the distribution of P between reacted and unreacted fractions.

We may consider briefly each of these steps in turn.

Step 1. Extraction. Extraction of the compound under test from its biological milieu may be necessary if (a) the endogenous compound is bound to binding protein or other similar material; (b) cross-reacting compounds are present at a concentration sufficient to affect the final estimate of P; (c) compounds are present which affect the equilibrium constant of the reaction between P and Q; (d) compounds are present which affect the efficiency of the separation of "free" and "bound" fractions; (e) there exist components which significantly degrade the test compound either during storage or during the assay incubation period;

(f) the initial concentration of P is below the detection limit of the assay system.

Clearly any extraction and purification steps involved must be sufficiently rigorous to overcome disturbing effects arising from any or each of these sources. Moreover, it is essential that these steps must in themselves not contribute chemical contaminants in the final extract which can influence the assay, either by reacting with Q, or affecting the equilibrium or "affinity" constant of the reaction, or the characteristics of the separation method.

Many extraction methods in practice fall far short of these requirements. It is a common observation that many chromatographic techniques (applied, for example to the isolation of the steroid hormones) contribute important differences between standards and unknowns, as is reflected by the reported observation of significant "blank" values (i.e., apparent measurements of P when none is known to be present in the system) in many saturation assays for these compounds.

Assay "blanks" may be positive or negative; i.e., the effect of contaminants in the extract may be such as to decrease or increase the extent to which the labeled compound apparently reacts with the specific reagent. (One possible explanation for the latter is competition by contaminants for adsorbant sites on materials, such as activated charcoal, Florisil, Fuller's earth, which are frequently used to separate reacted and unreacted moieties.)

It is important to recognize that a "blank" value observed in a saturation assay procedure cannot be regarded as might a small additional weight on a balance pan which can subsequently be subtracted from all other observations. Whether a contaminant competes with P for reaction sites on Q, or otherwise affects the reaction between P and Q, or whether, in contrast, it influences only the separation method, the quantitative effects will normally be dependent upon the relative concentrations of the other reactants in the system. Only in the unlikely event of the contaminant competing with reaction sites on Q with an equilibrium constant identical to that of P will it exert a constant effect (expressed as a positive or negative increment in the apparent concentration of P) in the assay system. The practical implication of this conclusion is that a necessary step in the validation of any assay procedure involving extraction is that the response curve observed in "blank" extracts (i.e., the curve resulting from addition of varying standard amounts of hormone to blank extracts) should be superimposable onto the normal buffer response curve over the entire range of hormone concentrations. Any departure of the two curves will almost certainly manifest itself as a variable "blank" correction at different hormone concentrations.

An estimate of the recovery of P through the extraction procedure is usually effected by the addition of labeled P to the original biological mixture, followed by the measurement of recovered activity in the final incubation mixture. For such measurements to be valid, it is essential that the tracer material should exactly parallel the unlabeled compound through each of the steps, and this usually implies that it must be identical to the unlabeled compound and radiochemically pure. Two distinct consequences stem from the use of radiochemically *impure* tracer. The first is that the estimate of recovery will be in error. The second arises only in those procedures where the same labeled material is used to reveal the distribution P between reacted and unreacted moieties. In these circumstances, radioactive material which has passed through the extraction step may be of a different degree of purity from that which is added directly to standards, and distribution ratios observed in "unknowns" will not legitimately be referable to the standard response curve.

A similar problem may arise if the labeled compound is *chemically* impure. If unlabeled contaminants are present in the preparation which are capable of reacting with, or affecting the reactivity of, Q, the possibility exists that purified "unknowns" may be significantly different from the "standards" in which such contaminants remain. One method of distinguishing this possibility is by estimating the apparent specific activity of the labeled compound before and after successive purification steps, using the assay system itself to effect this (see Ekins and Sgherzi, 1965).

Step 2. Reaction with Specific Reagent Q. As discussed earlier in this chapter, the prime characteristics required of the specific reagent Q are a high reaction energy and specificity with a respect to P. Such characteristics are notably displayed by certain serum- and tissue-binding proteins, antibodies, and enzymes. In general it is unnecessary for the specific reagent to be employed in pure form. However, it may be so diluted by other proteins or other similar reagents which themselves react with P that both the effective equilibrium constant displayed by the mixture, or its specificity, may be severely reduced. In such circumstances it may be advantageous to isolate the specific protein, antibody, or enzyme from other less specific, or less "energetic," reactants, though fragility of the purified material may in practice vitiate attempts to do this.

Several methods may be employed to estimate the "effective" equilibrium constant of the specific reagent. One of the most common is the plotting of assay data in the form of a "Scatchard" plot (Scatchard, 1949) relating the ratio $R_{b/f}$ to the calculated total concentration of "bound" hormone in the system. The slope of the resulting straight line yields an estimate of the equilibrium constant governing the reaction. In most systems, however, a curvilinear plot is obtained, an observation which is customarily interpreted as indicating the presence of multiple binding sites each characterized by a different equilibrium constant. It should be noted that a difference in the equilibrium constants displayed by labeled and unlabeled hormone molecules present in the system can likewise give rise to nonlinearity of the Scatchard plot, as also can inefficiency of the method adopted to sequester free and bound fractions. In short, the observed equilibrium constant cannot be regarded as possessing any absolute significance but should be treated merely as a useful parameter describing the kinetic behavior of the reaction under the conditions of the assay. Nevertheless, it constitutes a useful measurement since the observed equilibrium constant at zero hormone concentration (the tangent to the Scatchard curve at this point) can legitimately be used as a guide in calculating optimal reagent concentrations to yield maximum sensitivity as described earlier.

If labeled hormone is introduced in the assay system immediately before reaction with Q (i.e., in those circumstances in which prior extraction of the endogenous hormone is not necessary, or in which a recovery figure through the extraction step is assumed), then the criteria the labeled hormone must fulfill are, in principle, less rigorous than if it is also used to monitor recovery. Unreactive radioactive contaminants, provided they behave identically in all incubation tubes, may alter either the precision of measurement of radioactivity distributions, or the slope of the response curve, or both, and hence contribute to the lowering of the precision of the final estimate. However, provided the amounts of contaminant are constant and small, their existence is not usually of great importance. Likewise the presence of unlabeled chemically reactive contaminants is of little significance except insofar as they may greatly reduce the "effective" specific activity of the labeled hormone in the system, and thus significantly reduce assay sensitivity.

The specific activity of the tracer employed need not, indeed, be known with great precision provided that, as is customary, exactly identical amounts of tracer are added to each assay tube; its value must be known only within the relatively broad limits which enable a roughly optimal concentration of tracer to be used.

Finally, as we have seen, it is not essential that the labeled hormone be identical to the unlabeled hormone under test, provided that it reacts with identical sites on Q and its distribution is affected by, and hence a measure of, the concentration of P in the system. Nevertheless, it is usually preferable to employ a labeled material which reacts slightly more avidly for highest sensitivity. On the other hand, sensitivity may in practice be restricted by the specific activity of available labeled hormones and a reduction in the reaction energy of the labeled material be more than offset by the gains resulting from an increase in specific activity. It is presumably with such considerations in mind that Midgley and his collaborators (1969b) have employed an ^{131}I-labeled steroid protein conjugate as the labeled competitor in systems for the assay of nonconjugated estrogenic steroids relying on specific antibodies directed against the haptenic determinant.† However, as emphasized earlier, the necessity for higher specific activity labeled competitors (a requirement perhaps overemphasized in the past) depends upon a number of factors, and the advantages of Midgley's approach may lie more in the ease with which radioiodine may be counted than in any associated dramatic increase in assay sensitivity.

Step 3. Separation of Free (Unreacted) and Bound Moieties. It is not intended or possible to review here the many separation techniques currently employed in saturation assay methods. Ideally, the separation method must totally separate the two fractions instantaneously; simultaneously, association and dissociation reactions between the reactants should be halted. In addition, the efficiency of the separation should be totally unaffected by incubation mixture constituents.

Few, if any, separation methods meet all these demands. Failure to meet the first two may result in a significant loss of assay precision and sensitivity, particularly in those cases (exemplified by certain steroid/protein interactions) where the rate of dissociation with the bound complex is high. Failure to meet the third may lead to a loss of specificity unless extreme care is taken to ensure identity in composition of all incubation mixtures. Thus differences in protein concentration are well known to show marked effects upon the characteristics of adsorbants such as charcoal, and a large discrepancy in the protein content of standards and unknowns will, in the circumstances, lead to erroneous results.

It should be noted that the effective equilibrium constant displayed by the reacting system may be a function of the separation method employed, and there is little doubt that both sensitivity and precision in general can thereby be affected. Observations in our own laboratory, for example (Lejeune-Lenain, 1970), suggest that the effective equilibrium constant displayed by *some* (if not all) antibodies is reduced in

---

† Steiner *et al.* (1969) have similarly employed an iodine-labeled tyrosine-cyclic AMP (as labeled competitor in his radioimmunoassay for this nucleotide). The advantages of this approach have been discussed by Brown *et al.* (1971).

systems relying on prior adsorption of antibody to plastic surfaces as described by Catt and his colleagues (Catt *et al.*, 1970), and this technique, although more convenient than many separation methods, may consequently lead to lower assay sensitivity.

Step 4. Measurement of the Distribution of Labeled Hormone between Reacted and Unreacted Moieties. Perhaps the most important conclusion emerging from the analysis relating to the counting of the separated fractions is that the total number of counts accumulated for each sample is secondary in importance to the counting time. In short, an experimenter incurring experimental errors of 5% and meticulously counting samples to 10,000 counts may greatly improve sensitivity (while maintaining the same overall counting time) by using a lower concentration of labeled hormone, such that perhaps no more than 1000 counts are accumulated for each sample.

This proposition (which, as emphasized earlier, is essentially relevant to the optimization of the assay with respect to a single hormone concentration) breaks down when the range of concentrations likely to be encountered is very wide. The precision of measurement at extremities of the range may then be greatly reduced in consequence of the low count rates observed in certain of the fractions. In practice, therefore, counter settings must be judiciously selected so that the samples showing low count rates are counted for longer times than the time T used in calculating optimal reagent concentrations.

IV. Conclusions

The fundamental purpose of this presentation has been the exemplification of the basic principles underlying saturation assay techniques. In a survey of restricted length, it is clearly impossible to consider the many variants of the basic principles which are currently employed. Clearly the equations governing "radioenzymatic" assays would be different in detail from those presented here, as will also those relevant to "disequilibrium" assays (those, for example, in which labeled and unlabeled hormones are added at different times). For this reason at least, some of the theoretical material presented here is not immediately relevant, in detail, to practical assay procedures. Nevertheless, it is sufficient that the importance of a clear understanding of the concepts of sensitivity and precision, and of the broad factors which influence their maximization, should have been adequately demonstrated by the particular situations that have been discussed.

References

Avivi, P., Simpson, S. A., Tait, J. F., and Whitehead, J. K. (1954). *Radioisotope Conf. Proc. Int. Conf., 2nd, Oxford 1954* 1, 313.
Berson, S. A., and Yalow, R. S. (1968). *J. Clin. Invest.* 47, 2725.
Bliss, C. I. (1970). In "Statistics in Endocrinology" (J. W. McArthur and T. Colton, eds.), p. 431. MIT Press, Cambridge, Massachusetts.
Borth, R. (1957). *Vitam. Horm.* 15, 259.
Brodie, A. H., and Tait, J. F. (1969). In "Methods in Hormone Research" (R. I. Dorfman, ed.), 2nd Ed., Vol. 1, p. 323. Academic Press, New York.
Brown, B. L., Ekins, R. P., and Tampion, W. (1970). *Biochem. J.* 120, 8 p.
Brown, B. L., Ekins, R. P., and Albano, J. D. M. (1971). *Recent Advan. Cyclic Nucleotide Res.* In press.
Catt, K. J., Tregear, G. W., Burger, H. G., and Skermer, C. (1970). *Clin. Chim. Acta* 27, 267.
Ekins, R. P. (1960). *Clin. Chim. Acta* 5, 453.
Ekins, R. P. (1968). In "Protein and Polypeptide Hormones" (M. Margoulies, ed.), Int. Congr. Ser. No. 161, p. 612. Excerpta Med. Found., Amsterdam.
Ekins, R. P., and Samols, E. (1963). *Lancet* ii, 114.
Ekins, R. P., and Sgherzi, A. M. (1965). In "Radiochemicals Methods of Analysis," Vol. II, p. 239. IAEA, Vienna.
Ekins, R. P., Newman, G. B., and O'Riordan, J. L. H. (1968). In "Radioisotopes in Medicine: *In Vitro* Studies" (R. I. Hayes, F. A. Goswitz, and B. E. P. Murphy, eds.), p. 59. USAEC, Oak Ridge, Tennessee.
Ekins, R. P., Newman, G. B., Piyasena, R., Banks, P., and Slater, J. D. H. (1971). *Proc. Int. Symp. Interact. Ster. Macromol.* In press.
Finney, D. J. (1964). "Statistical Method in Biological Assay." Griffin, London.
Gaddum, J. H. (1933). *Spec. Rept. Med. Res. Council London, No. 183.*
Girard, J., and Greenwood, F. C. (1968). In "Protein and Polypeptide Hormones" (M. Margoulies, ed.), Int. Congr. Ser. No. 161, p. 332. Excerpta Med. Found., Amsterdam.
Jones, R. C. (1959). *Proc. IRE* 47, 1495.
Kaiser, H., and Specker, H. (1956). *Fresenius' Z. Anal. Chem.* 149, 46.
Keston, A. S., Udenfriend, S., and Cannan, R. K. (1946). *J. Amer. Chem. Soc.* 68, 1390.
Lejeune-Lenain, C. H. D. (1970). Unpublished observations.
Macurdy, L. B., Alber, H. K., Benedetti-Pichler, A. A., Carmichael, H., Corwin, A. H., Fowler, R. H., Huffman, E. W. D., Kirk, P. L., and Lashof, T. W. (1954). *Anal. Chem.* 26, 1199.
Midgley, A. R., Niswender, G. D., and Ram, J. S. (1969a). *Steroids* 13, 731.
Midgley, A. R., Niswender, G. D., and Rebar, R. W. (1969b). In "Immunoassay of Gonadotrophins" (E. Diczfalusy, ed.), p. 163. Stockholm.
Miles, L. E. M., and Hales, C. N. (1968). In "Protein and Polypeptide Hormones" (M. Margoulies, ed.), Int. Congr. Ser. No. 161, p. 61. Excerpta Med. Found., Amsterdam.
Morrison, G. H., and Skogerboe, R. K. (1965). In "Trace Analysis: Physical Methods" (G. H. Morrison, ed.), p. 1. Wiley (Interscience), New York.
Peterson, R. E. (1959). *Recent Progr. Horm. Res.* 15, 231.

Rodbard, D., Rayford, P. L., Cooper, J. A., and Ross, G. T. (1968). *J. Clin. Endocrinol. Metab.* **28**, 1412.

Rodbard, D., Bridson, W., and Rayford, P. L. (1969). *J. Lab. Clin. Med.* **74**, 770.

Rodbard, D. (1970). *Acta Endocrin. Suppl. 147*, 30.

Rodbard, D. and Lewald, J. E. (1970). *Acta Endocrin. Suppl. 147*, 79.

Scatchard, G. (1949). *Ann. N.Y. Acad. Sci.* **51**, 660.

Steiner, A. L., Kipnis, D. M., Utiger, R. D., and Parker, C. (1969). *Proc. Nat. Acad. Sci. U.S.* **64**, 367.

Whitehead, J. K., and Beale, D. (1959). *Clin. Chim. Acta* **4**, 710.

Wilson, A. L. (1961). *Analyst* **86**, 72.

Yalow, R. S., and Berson, S. A. (1960). *J. Clin. Invest.* **39**, 1157.

Yalow, R. S., and Berson, S. A. (1968a). In "Radioisotopes in Medicine: *In Vitro* Studies" (R. L. Hayes, F. A. Goswitz, and B. E. P. Murphy, eds.), p. 7. USAEC, Oak Ridge, Tennessee.

Yalow, R. S., and Berson, S. A. (1968b). In "Protein and Polypeptide Hormones" (M. Margoulies, ed.), Int. Congr. Ser. No. 161, p. 71. Excerpta Med. Found., Amsterdam.

Yalow, R. S., and Berson, S. A. (1970a). In "Statistics in Endocrinology" (J. W. McArthur and T. Colton, eds.), p. 327. MIT Press, Cambridge, Massachusetts.

Yalow, R. S., and Berson, S. A. (1970b). In "*In Vitro* Procedures with Radioisotopes in Clinical Medicine and Research" (E. H. Belcher and T. Nagai, eds.), p. 455. IAEA, Vienna.

STEROID HORMONES AND THE DIFFERENTIATION OF THE CENTRAL NERVOUS SYSTEM

Béla Flerkó

DEPARTMENT OF ANATOMY
UNIVERSITY MEDICAL SCHOOL
PÉCS, HUNGARY

I. General Introduction	42
II. The Androgen-Sterilized Rat	42
A. The Polyfollicular Ovary Syndrome (POS) Induced by Perinatal Administration of Androgen	42
B. Effect of Age and Dosage	43
C. Pituitary Content of Ovulating Hormone in Rats with POS	45
III. The Possible Site of Action of Androgen	48
A. A Dual Hypothalamic Mechanism Controlling Gonadotropin Secretion	48
B. Factors Responsible for the Development of POS in Rats with Electrolyte Lesions or a Frontal Cut in the Anterior Hypothalamus	54
C. Data Suggesting That Hypothalamic LH and FSH Mechanisms Are Deranged in the Androgen-Sterilized Rat	56
IV. The Possible Mechanism of Action of Androgen	62
A. Characteristic Pattern of Uptake and Retention of Tritiated Estradiol by Certain Hypothalamic Areas	62
B. Effect of Neonatal Androgen Treatment in Reducing the Estradiol Binding Capacity of Neural and Nonneural Target Tissues	63

V. Effects of Neonatal Treatment with Steroid Hormones Other
    Than Androgen on Subsequent Fertility 67
    A. The POS Induced by Neonatal Estrogen Administration . 67
    B. Anestrous State Induced by Neonatal Estrogen Treatment . 68
    C. Other Steroid Hormones Inducing Sterility in the Rat When
        Administered Neonatally 68
    D. The Possible Mechanism of Action 69
VI. Protection Against Steroid-Induced Sterility 70
VII. Summary and Conclusions 74
    References 75

I. General Introduction

It is not the purpose of this review to cover the whole field indicated by the title. Rather, this contribution will summarize what the author considers to be pertinent studies that have led him to a concept of how steroid hormones might influence the differentiation of certain brain structures instrumental in the control of gonadotropin secretion. These studies were carried out mainly on androgen-sterilized rats. Modifications in reproductive function after exposure to steroid hormones during the neonatal period were recently summarized by Barraclough (1967), and this excellent review is particularly helpful in that pertinent studies carried out before 1967 can be treated very briefly in this chapter.

II. The Androgen-Sterilized Rat

A. *The Polyfollicular Ovary Syndrome (POS) Induced by Perinatal Administration of Androgen*

It has long been known that the ovary transplanted to any region of the male rat, except the spleen, does not develop a corpus luteum. Pfeiffer (1936) was the first to observe that ovaries grafted to adult intact female rats or to adult male rats which had been castrated at birth showed normal follicular development and formation of corpora lutea. However, when testes were implanted into newborn females, the ovaries of these animals, when they became adults, contained only growing follicles and interstitial tissue without a corpus luteum (the so-called polyfollicular ovary), and persistent vaginal cornification ensued after puberty.

It turned out later on that the condition of polyfollicular ovary associated with persistent vaginal cornification and permanent sterility, termed the polyfollicular ovary syndrome, could be induced by administration of testosterone given repeatedly from birth or 6 days of age to either 5-6 or 25 weeks of age (Shay et al., 1939; Bradbury, 1941).

To evaluate more carefully the effect and duration of effect of a hormone administered at a given time in development, Barraclough and Leathem (1954) and Barraclough (1955) using the mouse, and Barraclough (1961) using the rat, studied the effect of a single injection of testosterone given in the first 20 days of life. As a consequence of these studies, Barraclough (1961) assumed that there is a "critical period" in the development of the female mouse and rat during the first 10 days of life when injection of a single 1.25-mg dose of testosterone will induce subsequent anovulatory sterility associated with the POS.

B. Effect of Age and Dosage

Androgen treatment at 10 days of age had a less drastic effect, as the ovaries of only 4 of 10 rats lacked corpora lutea at 100 days of age. In mice treated at 10 days of age, ovulation was delayed approximately 10 days, but at 60 days of age 85% of the ovaries contained corpora lutea as compared with 90% of the littermate controls. All ovaries of rats or mice treated with androgen at 20 days of age were normal at autopsy (Barraclough, 1967).

While 99.8% of the rats treated with a single injection of 1.25 mg of testosterone propionate (TP) at 5 days of age, were sterile, as little as 10, 5, or 1 μg, administered on day 5, produced sterility in 70.6, 44.0, and 30.0%, respectively, of the treated rats (Barraclough, 1961; Gorski and Barraclough, 1963).

Later, it became clear that a delineation of the "critical period" is complicated by several variables as Swanson and van der Werff ten Bosch (1964b) pointed out. They showed that the full "early androgen" syndrome may not exist at the time of puberty but may develop after an initial period of normal female ovarian activity (Swanson and van der Werff ten Bosch, 1964a,b). Second, the relation between the time of androgen administration and the effect on reproductive function is greatly influenced by variations in the dose of androgen administered. In other words, as maturation of the brain-pituitary-gonadal axis proceeds with age (from 1 to 10 days of age), "masculinization" may still be produced, provided that the dosage of administered androgen is increased. Similar observations were reported also by Gorski (1968) and Kurcz et al. (1969; Kurcz and Gerhardt, 1968).

The effects of androgen administered prior to birth on subsequent fertility have also been studied. After a single dose of 2.5 mg of TP into pregnant rats, Swanson and van der Werff ten Bosch (1964b) did not observe any alteration in the cyclic pattern of gonadotropin secretion of the female offspring. They interpreted their finding to mean that androgen given to the mother animal did not pass, presumably, the placental barrier in such a measure that it could get into the fetuses in an effective amount. Obviously, the amount of androgen injected into pregnant rats was insufficient, since Swanson and van der Werff ten Bosch (1965) gave an account of successful treatment in their next paper. A single dose of 10–25 mg of TP given to pregnant rats, or injection of 20–100 μg TP into the fetuses, did convert the female (cyclic) hormonal pattern into a male (acyclic) pattern. Flerkó *et al.* (1967) also observed the masculinizing effect of TP injected either directly into fetuses or into pregnant rats.

1. TP Injection into Fetuses

Nineteen females were anesthetized on day 19 of pregnancy, and the uterus was exposed. All fetuses were injected with 0.5 mg of TP. Thirteen out of the 19 aborted shortly after operation. The remaining 6 pregnant animals spontaneously delivered a total of 15 females which were reared by the mothers. All these female offspring had abnormal masculinized external genitalia, from which vaginal smears could not be taken. They were killed at the age of 100 days. The ovaries contained no corpora lutea, but growing and cystically dilated follicles and interstitial tissue were found.

2. A Single Dose of TP to Mothers

A single dose of 5.0 mg of TP was injected intramuscularly into 5 rats on day 19 of pregnancy. These animals delivered a total of 15 females 2 or 3 days later and breast-fed the offspring successfully. After the opening of the vaginal orifice, daily smears of the female young were recorded. They had irregular vaginal cycles with estrus predominating. Their ovaries were cyclic in character and contained corpora lutea at the age of 100 days, when the animals were killed.

3. Repeated Doses of TP to Mothers

Six pregnant rats, in three subgroups, received testosterone injections from day 19 of pregnancy until birth in the following doses: daily 2 × 0.5, 1.0, or 2.0 mg of TP, respectively. With these doses, three effects were noted: (a) intrauterine death, (b) delayed parturition, in 5 pregnant animals out of 6, and (c) failure to lactate. In consequence of the latter only 9 female offspring survived, and only two of these were born at term. In the daily vaginal smears they had persistent vaginal cornification irrespective of the amount of androgen their mothers received. At the age of 100 days, when killed, their ovaries were polyfollicular and contained no copora lutea.

These results, in accordance with those of Swanson and van der Werff ten Bosch (1965) show clearly that androgen sterilization can be induced before birth by administration of sufficiently large doses of testosterone either directly in the rat fetus or to the pregnant animal.

C. *Pituitary Content of Ovulating Hormone* in Rats with POS*

The POS induced by a single injection of testosterone given to newborn rats is similar to that induced by constant illumination (Browman, 1937; Hemmingsen and Krarup, 1937; Fiske, 1939, 1941; Dempsey and Searles, 1943), by anterior hypothalamic lesions (Hillarp, 1949; Greer, 1953; Alloiteau, 1954; Flerkó, 1954), or by neural isolation of the preoptic–anterior hypothalamic area from the rest of the hypothalamus (Halász and Pupp, 1965; Halász and Gorski, 1967; Tima and Flerkó, 1967). Since it was reasonable to assume that the absence of corpora lutea in this syndrome might reflect a deficiency in the secretion of LH, the pituitary and plasma LH content was investigated in various forms of the POS.

Barraclough (1963) has proposed that the constant levels of estrogen secreted by the ovaries of androgen-sterilized or brain-lesioned rats might prevent normal storage of LH in the pituitary gland. Thus, even though this gland might be activated by neural stimuli, LH would not be present in sufficient quantity to cause ovulation and luteinization. This proposition was supported by the observations of Gorski and Barraclough (1962a) showing that hypophyses of androgen-sterilized rats contain approximately one-third of the LH of the glands of normal rats in proestrus, and also that progesterone permits LH to be stored in sufficient concentration to cause ovulation when released by hypothalamic activation (Barraclough and Gorski, 1961). Also in anterior hypothalamus-lesioned rats, Taleisnik and McCann (1961), using the ovarian ascorbic acid depletion test of Parlow (1958), found that pituitary LH content was diminished to 33% of normal.

This is in disagreement with the findings of Segal and Johnson (1959) on the pituitary LH content of androgen-sterilized rats, and with those of van der Werff ten Bosch *et al.* (1962) on the LH content of pituitaries of rats with POS following anterior hypothalamic lesion. Segal and Johnson's (1959) assays on the LH content of the 60-day-old androgen-steril-

---

* For the sake of simplicity, luteinizing hormone (LH) is considered to be the ovulation-inducing hormone. Whether follicle-stimulating hormone (FSH) is a part of the hormone causing rupture of the follicle is not clear as yet. For detailed discussion of this question, the reader is referred to the review by Everett (1969).

ized rat pituitary (Weaver-Finch method) indicated that the concentration of LH was high, and comparable to that of the male rat. Using the ventral prostate assay, in rats having normal cycles, van der Werff ten Bosch et al. (1962) found the highest content of LH in the pituitary and serum during late diestrus. In further experiments, the pituitary LH content of rats with POS from an anterior hypothalamic lesion was high as compared with late diestrus, but serum LH was barely detectable. They believe, therefore, that the production of LH may not be inhibited in pituitaries of rats with POS, but that LH is not released from the pituitary gland in the normal way.

Bradshaw and Critchlow (1966), using the Parlow (1958) test, found that pituitaries of rats with POS produced by constant illumination or by neonatal androgen administration had lower LH levels than those of controls. However, after an anterior hypothalamic lesion, the pituitaries of persistent-estrus rats contained more LH than those of intact rats on the day of estrus.

There is an apparent discrepancy between the findings of the different authors concerning the LH content of the hypophysis of rats with POS. The relatively high or low LH contents, found in pituitaries of permanently estrous rats, supports alternative explanations for the absence of ovulation and/or luteinization in these rats. We (Tima and Flerkó, 1967, 1968) decided, therefore, to clarify the problem of whether or not the pituitaries of rats with POS contained sufficient LH to elicit ovulation.

Four groups of animals were studied. In group I, electrolytic lesions were produced in the anterior hypothalamus, just above the optic chiasma, with the aid of a Horsley-Clarke instrument. In group II, the preoptic-anterior hypothalamic area was isolated neurally from the rest of the hypothalamus with the aid of the Halász knife (Halász and Pupp, 1965). The half-dome-shaped cut extended from the base of the brain up to the paraventricular nuclei. It was situated just behind the optic chiasma, and laterally reached the lateral border of the ventromedial nuclei. This type of neural isolation will be referred to later as the "frontal cut" (Tima and Flerkó, 1967). In a third group, androgen-sterilization was performed by giving a single injection of 1.25 mg of testosterone phenylpropionate (TPP) at the age of 2 days. In group IV, the rats, at the age of 45 days, were kept under constant illumination (175 lux) for different periods (2.5–8 months: Tima and Flerkó, 1968). Vaginal smears were recorded daily for different periods (1.5–8 months), and animals without persistent cornification were discarded. From the four groups, 51 rats with constant vaginal cornification were investigated at different intervals (1.5–8 months) after operation. Forty-eight hours before killing, the left (so-called control) ovary and the pituitary gland were removed. A gonadotropin extract was made from the pituitary gland and injected intraperitoneally into the same animal within 2 hours after hypophysectomy. Fallopian tubes were examined for the presence of tubal ova 48 hours after injection of the pituitary extract. Animals were then killed by bleeding, and the remaining (test) ovary was removed and examined for the presence of fresh corpora lutea. Results are summarized in Table I.

Table I

Number and Percentage of Persistent-Estrus Rats Showing Ovulation and Corpus Luteum Formation after Administration of Autologous Pituitary Extract[a]

Group No.	Experimental procedure	Ovulation No. of rats	Percent	Luteinization, fresh corpora lutea No. of rats	Percent
I	Anterior hypothalamic lesion	8/14	57.1	14/14	100.0
II	Frontal cut in the anterior hypothalamus	10/15	66.6	14/15	93.3
III	Androgen sterilization	8/12	66.6	11/12	91.7
IV	Constant illumination	7/10	70.0	7/10	70.0

[a] From Tima and Flerkó (1967, 1968), by permission.

Results presented in Table I show unequivocally that pituitaries of the sterile rats with POS contain a sufficient amount of LH to elicit ovulation. This finding indicates that the pituitaries of these rats synthesize LH but they are unable to release an ovulatory dose of the hormone. Furthermore, it was suggested by these findings that a mechanism essentially similar to that operating in the rats with a hypothalamic lesion is responsible for inducing sterility associated with POS also in the androgen- or light-sterilized rat.

Serum FSH levels were similar in controls and in female rats androgenized with 1.0 mg of TP (Cheng and Li, 1965). Pituitary FSH and hypothalamic FSH-releasing factor content were found to be slightly reduced or normal in rats given 1.25 mg of TP on day 4 of life (Carraro et al., 1966).

According to Kurcz *et al.* (1967), the hypophyses of androgenized female rats contain significantly less prolactin than those of the control animals.

III. The Possible Site of Action of Androgen

A. *A Dual Hypothalamic Mechanism Controlling Gonadotropin Secretion*

Originally, it was proposed by Pfeiffer (1936) that the mechanism by which androgen of testicular origin produced the POS was by "masculinization" of the anterior pituitary, which resulted in a permanent imbalance in gonadotropin secretion. This interpretation was reasonable at that time since very little was known of the central nervous control of anterior pituitary function.

The mechanism enabling the female anterior pituitary to release gonadotropins cyclically is apparently absent in the male. The experiments of Harris and Jacobsohn (1952) as well as of Martinez and Bittner (1956) made it clear that this mechanism cannot be hypophysial, but must be situated in the central nervous system. The observations of Segal and Johnson (1959) pointed in the same direction. These authors observed that pituitaries of anovulatory female rats with POS induced by androgen treatment during the first week after birth were capable of producing cyclic reproductive functions when transplanted in contiguity with the hypothalamus of intact females. Having thus demonstrated that the functional capacity of the hypophysis itself was unaltered, it was reasonable to assume that it was the hypothalamic mechanism which was influenced by androgen either when given neonatally or when acting in the male animal before or after birth.

On the basis of suggestive experiments, Yazaki (1959, 1960) was the first to conclude that the noncyclicity of the hypothalamohypophysial function in the adult male rat is established only around the third day after birth, and the presence of testes in the first few days of postnatal life determines the male specificity of the hypothalamus. The same conclusion was reached also by Harris and Levine (1962) as well as Gorski and Wagner (1965). All these experiments suggest that the hypothalamus of the newborn rat of either sex has the inherent ability to maintain cyclic release of gonadotropins. It is only in the first few postnatal days that normal male rats under the influence of testicular androgens, or female rats that are given testosterone, lose the ability to release gonadotropins in a cyclic manner and, thereby, to cause ovulation. It seems probable that the same conditioning by androgen occurs also in the human, but the hypothalamic structures instrumental in determining the cyclic pattern of gonadotropin secretion and ovulation may be organized at an earlier stage, so that the male or female pattern of gonadotropin release might be established earlier in fetal life.

Current concepts invoke a dual mechanism controlling gonadotropin secretion (Barraclough and Gorski, 1961; Flerkó, 1962; Halász, 1969).

1. Tonic Mechanism of Gonadotropin Secretion

The first of these, termed a tonic mechanism by Barraclough and Gorski (1961), stimulates follicular growth and estrogen secretion without ovulation or formation of corpora lutea. Tuberoinfundibular neurons (Szentágothai, 1962, 1964) in the "hypophysiotropic area" (Halász et al., 1962) producing FSH- and LH-releasing factors (FRF and LRF) are responsible for this mechanism.

The half-moon-shaped area of the hypothalamus (Fig. 1), which maintained the normal cytological characteristics and hormone function of anterior pituitary grafts transplanted into it, was termed by Halász et al. (1962) "hypophysiotropic area" (HTA). In order to explore the functional capacity of the HTA, Halász and Pupp (1965) developed a stereotaxic technique to interrupt the neural connections of the HTA without altering its contact with the pituitary gland. With respect to the gonadotropic hormones (GTH), the findings following the neural isolation of HTA were as follows. In male rats, gonadotropin secretion was fairly well maintained after interruption of all neural connections of the HTA (Halász and Pupp, 1965; Halász et al., 1967). Testicular weight and histology were nearly normal; only a slight decrease in seminal vesicle weight was observed. Voloschin et al. (1968) published similar findings recently. There was no gonadal atrophy in female rats, but FSH and LH secretion appeared to be seriously altered (Halász and Pupp, 1965; Halász and Gorski, 1967). Such animals were not able to ovulate; their ovaries were polyfollicular without corpus luteum. The vaginal smears indicated permanent cornification.

Thus, interruption of the neural connections of the HTA interferes with pituitary gonadotropic function in the female, but not in the male. This difference might be related to the fact that FSH and LH secretion is tonic in the male and cyclic in the female, and the HTA is responsible only for tonic secretion of anterior pituitary hormones (for details, see Halász, 1968, 1969). As shown by Fig. 1, the tonic mechanism acts directly on the anterior pituitary cells by the releasing and inhibiting factors carried by the portal circulation to the anterior lobe.

A considerable body of evidence supports the assumption that the nerve cells contributing to the tonic mechanism, i.e., the cells of the

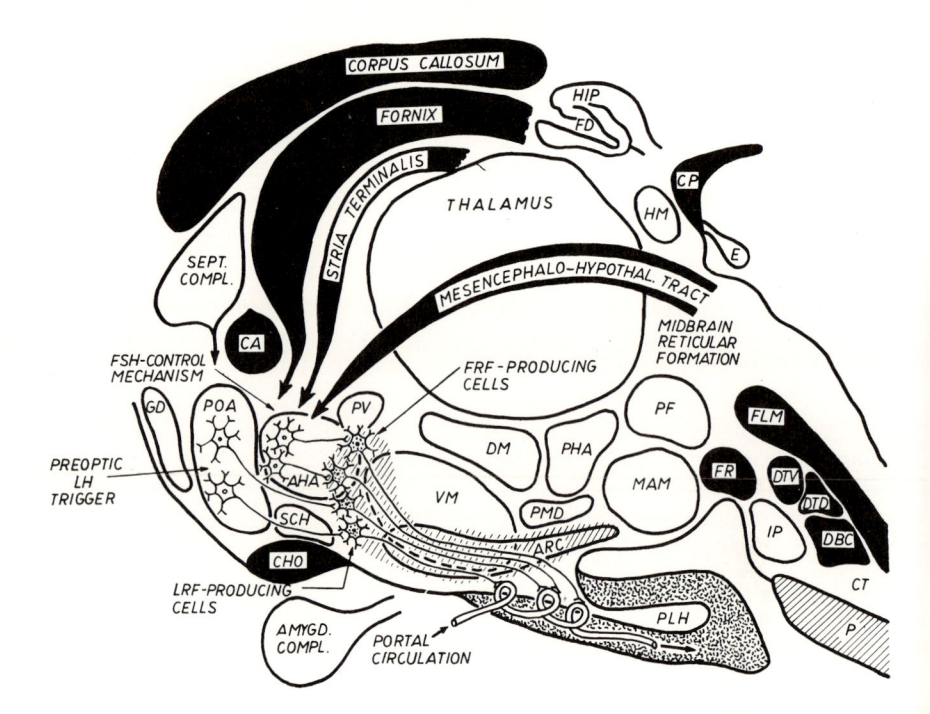

Fig. 1. Schematic representation of the hypothalamic and limbic control mechanisms for FSH and LH secretion. Arrows show the direction of the blood flow in the hypothalamohypophysial portal system, the special capillary loops of which penetrate the median eminence. The FSH- and LH-releasing factors that produce neurons of the "tonic mechanism" are indicated by the neural units with dotted cell bodies. They are situated in the hypophysiotropic area (hatched), and their nerve endings terminate on the capillary loops of the portal system. Perikarya of the neurons belonging to the hypothalamic "cyclic mechanism" (preoptic LH trigger + FSH control mechanism) are represented by clear cell bodies located in the preoptic and anterior hypothalamic area, respectively. Abbreviations used: AHA, anterior hypothalamic area; AMYGD. COMPL., amygdaloid complex; ARC, arcuate nucleus; CA, anterior commissure; CHO, optic chiasma; CP, posterior commissure; CT, nucleus centralis tegmenti; DBC, decussatio brachiorum conjunctivorum; DM, dorsomedial nucleus; DTD, decussatio tegmenti dorsalis; DTV, decussatio tegmenti ventralis; E, pineal gland; FD, fascia dentata; FLM, fasciculus longitudinalis medialis; FR, fasciculus retroflexus; GD, gyrus diagonalis; HIP, hippocampus; HM, medial habenular nucleus; IP, interpeduncular nucleus; MAM, mamillary nucleus; P, pons; PF, nucleus parafascicularis thalami; PHA, posterior hypothalamic area; PLH, posterior lobe of the hypophysis; PMD, dorsal premamillary nucleus; POA, preoptic area; PV, paraventricular nucleus; SCH, suprachiasmatic nucleus; SEPT. COMPL., septal complex; VM, ventromedial nucleus. From Flerkó (1970a), by permission from Academic Press, New York.

HTA which produce FRF, LRF and PIF (prolactin inhibiting factor), are influenced by the sexual steroids in the sense of a neurohormonal (negative or positive) feedback (Lisk, 1960, 1962, 1963; Davidson and Sawyer, 1961a,b; Flerkó and Bárdos, 1961b; Arai, 1962, 1963; Desclin *et al.*, 1962; Ifft, 1962; McCann, 1962; Kanematsu and Sawyer, 1963a,b, 1964; Kobayashi *et al.*, 1963; Hilliard *et al.*, 1964; Ramirez *et al.*, 1964; David *et al.*, 1965; Davidson and Smith, 1967; Kobayashi *et al.*, 1966; Meites *et al.*, 1967; Palka *et al.*, 1966; Piacsek and Meites, 1966; Pasteels, 1970). Further support for this assumption comes from the finding that a considerable number of neurons in the HTA, especially in the arcuate nucleus, accumulate estradiol (Stumpf, 1968), and the medial hypothalamus shows a pattern of uptake and retention of tritiated estradiol which is similar to the pattern found in the uterus, vagina, and anterior pituitary, i.e., in the peripheral estrogen-reactive tissues (Flerkó *et al.*, 1969, 1971).

2. CYCLIC MECHANISM OF GONADOTROPIN SECRETION

The second or higher level of the neural control of gonadotropin secretion modulates (i.e., enhances or inhibits) the activity of the FRF- and LRF-producing neurons according to the changes in the external and internal environment. This level includes brain structures outside of the HTA and may be termed a "cyclic mechanism" being indispensable in the maintenance of the cyclic release of FSH and LH. Hypothalamic parts of the cyclic mechanism* are the preoptic-anterior hypothalamic LH-trigger and FSH-control mechanism.

a. Preoptic LH Trigger. Critchlow (1958) was the first to localize the center for the neural mechanism that triggers the burst of LH secretion responsible for ovulation in the preoptic area of the rat. Stimulation involving electrolysis with electrodes of ferrous alloys combined with hypothalamic deafferentation has been used by Everett (1964, 1965), Everett and Radford (1961), and Tejasen and Everett (1967) in mapping the localization of the LH-releasing neural structures approaching the HTA from the rostral side of the brain. On the basis of these investigations, it was postulated that a diffuse system of LH-releasing neurons originates throughout the septal complex, converges, as it enters the medial preoptic area and anterior hypothalamus, and rapidly assumes a restricted basal location as it reaches the HTA. Recent investigations of Köves and Halász (1970) indicate that the neurogenic stimulus, caus-

---

* For detailed description of extrahypothalamic parts of the cyclic mechanism, the reader is referred to the review by Flerkó (1970a).

ing the release of LRF in amounts necessary for ovulation, comes from the preoptic area itself. The findings, however, that in their experiments ovulation was subnormal and the rats had irregular cycles, indicate that neural structures outside the preoptic area are also involved in the control of an entirely normal, cyclic ovulatory output of LRF and LH.

The preoptic LH trigger or LH control mechanism does not act directly on the anterior lobe, but exerts its influence via the HTA. It has been shown that only the HTA exhibits LRF activity (McCann, 1962; Mess et al., 1967) and is capable of maintaining gonadotropic function of the pituitary graft (Halász et al., 1965; Flament-Durand, 1965). The neurons of the HTA have their nerve endings in the surface zone of the median eminence (Réthelyi and Halász, 1970). Further support for the aforementioned assumption has been recently furnished by Terasawa and Sawyer (1969). These authors have found that during the critical period of proestrus in rats with spontaneous ovulation blocked by pentobarbital, electrochemical stimulation in the medial preoptic area always caused an elevation in integrated multiple unit activity in the median eminence–arcuate nuclear region. The rise in activity started immediately, reached a peak around 9 minutes, and lasted about 30 minutes. Interestingly enough, changes were observed only in those cases in which electrochemical stimulation in the preoptic region was effective in releasing an ovulating amount of LH. No elevation in multiunit activity of the arcuate region appeared in rats that failed to ovulate in response to the preoptic stimulus.

A positive estrogen-progesterone feedback has also been shown to play a role in ovulatory LH release (Everett and Sawyer, 1949; Sawyer et al., 1949; Critchlow and Sawyer, 1955; Ralph and Fraps, 1960; Barraclough et al., 1964; Döcke and Dörner, 1965). Thus, it can be assumed with considerable certainity that the preoptic LH trigger (Fig. 1) responds under proper environmental and hormonal circumstances (which are fulfilled on the day of proestrus) by stimulation of the HTA cells producing LRF that, in turn, elicits the sudden and intensive discharge of LH which is necessary for ovulation.

b. *Anterior Hypothalamic FSH-Control Mechanism.* The HTA requires afferent impulses reaching it from the oral border of the anterior hypothalamic area, not only for the ovulatory LH surge, but also for the complete control of FSH secretion.

It was found a decade ago that electrolytic lesions in the oral part of the anterior hypothalamic area (AHA) prevented compensatory ovarian hypertrophy following the removal of one ovary (D'Angelo and Kravatz, 1960; Flerkó and Bárdos, 1961a). Similarly, Halász and Gorski (1967) reported that no compensatory ovarian hypertrophy occurred in rats bearing a frontal cut which separated the AHA from the HTA. These results indicate that the neural structures responsible for the occurrence of enhanced FSH release after hemispaying are located outside the HTA. Such an assumption is consistent with the view that estrogen-sensitive neurons occur in the preoptic anterior hypothalamic area and are involved in the negative feedback action of estrogen on FSH release (Flerkó and Szentágothai, 1957).

Another aspect of this negative neurohormonal feedback, i.e., that rats with anterior hypothalamic lesions showed less inhibition of FSH secretion following treatment with physiological amounts of estrogen than did nonlesioned animals, has been shown more than ten years ago (Flerkó, 1956, 1957a,b; Flerkó and Bárdos, 1960). On the basis of these and similar findings (Donovan and van der Werff ten Bosch, 1956a,b, 1959a,b; Bogdanove and Schoen, 1959; Hohlweg and Daume, 1959; Kreici and Critchlow, 1959; Littlejohn and de Groot, 1963; Fendler and Endröczi, 1965–1966; Köves and Halász, 1969), the existence of an FSH control mechanism (Fig. 1) was assumed in the oral part of the anterior hypothalamic area through which estrogen exerts its feedback influence on FSH secretion.

The postulate that estrogen-sensitive neurons are present in the preoptic–anterior hypothalamic area is supported by the findings that individual neurons in this part of the brain accumulate estrogen (Michael, 1962; Attramadal, 1964; Stumpf, 1968), and the anterior hypothalamus, including the preoptic area, takes up and retains estradiol in the same way as the peripheral estrogen-reactive tissues (Kato and Villee, 1967a; Flerkó et al., 1969, 1971).

It may be assumed with considerable certainty that the sensitivity or responsiveness to estrogen of the neurons contributing to the cyclic mechanism is not identical with that of the neurons of the tonic mechanism. Ovarian compensatory hypertrophy was blocked in animals with a frontal cut behind the anterior hypothalamus, but this deafferentation did not interfere with the pituitary response to castration (Köves and Halász, 1969). Similar observations have been reported in animals with complete deafferentiation of the HTA; ovarian compensatory hypertrophy did not occur in these rats, but at the same time pituitary LH content increased and castration cells developed in the anterior pituitary after bilateral gonadectomy (Halász and Gorski, 1967). These findings suggest that the neurons of the preoptic—anterior hypothalamic cyclic mechanism are more sensitive to the changes in blood estrogen levels than are the elements of the HTA-pituitary complex, i.e., neurons of the hypothalamic tonic mechanism and the estrogen-sensitive cells of the anterior pituitary.

B. Factors Responsible for the Development of POS in Rats with Electrolytic Lesions or a Frontal Cut in the Anterior Hypothalamus

Data summarized in Section III, A indicate that the HTA controls the tonic discharge of FSH and LH, which maintains follicular development and estrogen secretion. For ovulation to occur however, the participation of the preoptic LH trigger is also required. It appears, therefore, that electrolytic lesions or a frontal cut in the anterior hypothalamus may inhibit both ovulation and luteinization by the same mechanism, i.e., by separating the preoptic trigger from the HTA. Furthermore, this assumption seems to be in fair agreement with the findings presented in Table I, i.e., that pituitaries of sterile rats with POS contain sufficient LH to elicit ovulation, but they are unable to release an ovulatory dose of LH in the absence of the preoptic trigger. Although the above interpretation appears to be correct so far as ovulation is concerned, the following data suggest that the absence of luteinization and development of the POS cannot be attributed solely to the separation of the preoptic LH trigger from the HTA.

1. In the majority of our rats with anterior hypothalamic lesions the complete absence of luteinization, indicated by persistent vaginal cornification, sets in about 2–3 weeks after the operation. As a rule, the lesions are followed by a "transition period" of prolonged estrous phases interrupted by short diestrous intervals, usually associated with the formation of new corpora lutea (Flerkó and Bárdos, 1959).

2. Greer (1953) found that rats with POS from anterior hypothalamic lesions, when injected with 0.5 mg progesterone daily, resumed normal cyclic activity, and this continued after cessation of progesterone administration in approximately half the animals. Everett (1943) observed the same effect in a strain of rats with persistent vaginal cornification. During the period of regular cycles evoked by progesterone administration, corpora lutea were also seen to develop. The termination of constant vaginal cornification by progesterone—even with smaller daily doses than those used by Greer (1953)—was confirmed also by Alloiteau (1954) and by van Dyke et al. (1957). However, these authors failed to find copora lutea under these circumstances.

3. In rats with POS following anterior hypothalamic lesions, massive luteinization can be induced simply by abruptly lowering the estrogen level in the blood (Flerkó and Bárdos, 1961b; Desclin et al., 1962). It is hardly conceivable that either progesterone treatment or lowering the estrogen level in the blood could induce resumption of luteinization in rats deprived of the preoptic LH trigger, if the latter were essential for the LH release necessary for luteinization without ovulation.

4. It is beyond question that a permanent estrogen action exists in rats with POS. Besides the permanent vaginal cornification, this is evidenced by the presence of cystically dilated endometrial glands as well as by the pituitary hypertrophy and cytological picture, the latter being characteristic of the adenohypophysis of rats under prolonged estrogen treatment (Flerkó and Bárdos, 1960). It is well known, however, that continuous estrogen action, even within physiological limits, inhibits FSH output in the intact rat (Hertz and Meyer, 1937; Byrnes and Meyer, 1951; Flerkó, 1957b). The explanation of Hillarp (1949) for POS fails to answer the question why the constant action of estrogen should not inhibit the continuous secretion of FSH that is so clearly indicated by the permanent follicular development and estrogen action.

In the light of the aforementioned data, the following hypothesis attempts to explain the mechanism by which electrolytic lesions or a frontal cut in the anterior hypothalamus may elicit the POS. These operative interferences partly destroy, and partly separate, the preoptic–anterior hypothalamic LH trigger and FSH control mechanism from the HTA. These animals do not ovulate because of the absence of the neural impulses indispensable for the ovulatory output of gonadotropins. On the other hand, in the absence of a neurohormonal feedback, which in the intact animal operates via the preoptic–anterior hypothalamic FSH and LH control mechanism, a moderate but continuous degree of gonadotropin release is maintained by the spontaneous activity of the FRF- and LRF-producing neurons in the HTA. This moderate but continuous output of GTH—similar to the situation existing in spayed rats with intrasplenic ovarian grafts (Lipschütz, 1946; Flerkó and Illei, 1957)—stimulates permanently follicular growth, estrogen secretion and, at irregular intervals, also the formation of copora lutea. This is indicated by the fact that even properly localized lesions or a frontal cut in the anterior hypothalamus do not evoke constant vaginal cornification and absence of luteinization immediately after the operation. As mentioned in item 1 above, in most lesioned rats the "transition period" lasts 2–3 weeks, and complete absence of luteinization, indicated by the permanent vaginal cornification, sets in only after this period.

Apparently, less LH, in synergism with FSH, is required for maintaining follicular growth and estrogen secretion than for the formation of corpora lutea. A certain inhibition of LH release is reflected, therefore, in the shift from the "transition period" to the steady state of permanent vaginal cornification and absence of luteinization. This inhibition may be brought about and maintained by the continuous estrogen action on the LRF-producing neurons of the HTA. Experimental results have shown that implantation of crystalline estradiol into the HTA induced gonadal atrophy in rats and rabbits (Lisk, 1960; Davidson and Sawyer, 1961a; Kanematsu and Sawyer, 1963b), and that postovariectomy elevation of plasma LH was prevented by estrogen implants into the same region (Kanematsu and Sawyer, 1964).

When, however, in rats with POS the negative estrogen feedback on the HTA was greatly reduced or eliminated by partial ovariectomy, or by removing both ovaries and reimplanting one of these into the spleen, the tonic mechanism of the HTA was once more able to stimulate the pituitary to release LH in sufficient amounts for luteinization to occur (Flerkó and Bárdos, 1961b; Desclin et al., 1962). Probably, progesterone also elicited its effect, mentioned in item 2 above, by counteracting the continuous negative estrogen feedback which blocked the activity of the LRF-producing neurons in the HTA.

These observations suggest that in rats with anterior hypothalamic lesions, the decisive factors in inducing sterility associated with POS might be the simultaneous disconnection of the FSH and LH control mechanism from the HTA. In the absence of this "higher" neural control, the tonic mechanism in the HTA still maintains the tonic release of gonadotropins. However, the continuous negative estrogen feedback on the HTA reduces gonadotropin release to such an extent that it is no longer sufficient to elicit formation of corpora lutea.

C. Data Suggesting That Hypothalamic LH and FSH Mechanisms Are Deranged in the Androgen-Sterilized Rat

The POS induced by a single injection of androgen given to newborn rats is similar to that elicited by electrolytic lesions or a frontal cut in the anterior hypothalamus. The pituitaries of both androgen-sterilized rats and rats with anterior hypothalamic lesions contain an amount of LH which is sufficient for ovulation (see Section II, C), and formation of corpora lutea in the polyfollicular ovaries of androgen-sterilized rats could be induced by lowering the estrogen level in the blood (Kovács, 1966) to a level similar to that in rats with POS from anterior hypothalamic lesions (see Section III, B, item 1). The identity of the two types of experimental anovulatory syndrome suggested that identical brain structures might suffer damage in both cases.

1. Neonatal Androgen Effect on the Preoptic LH Trigger

Barraclough and Gorski (1961) have shown that high doses of androgen produced a refractory hypothalamus which could be activated only after progesterone priming plus electrical stimulation of the HTA (arcuate-ventromedial complex). Low doses of androgen (10 μg) produced the same anovulatory POS, but the rats did not require progesterone priming in order to respond to electrical stimulation of the HTA with the release of LH. Furthermore, when the rats treated with 10 μg of androgen were primed with progesterone, ovulation could be induced by stimulation of the preoptic area, a phenomenon never observed in the animals sterilized with 1.25 mg of androgen. These observations indicate that the degree of hypothalamic alteration produced by androgen treatment is dosage dependent (Gorski and Barraclough, 1963; Barraclough, 1966). The high dosage of androgen affects the arcuate–ventromedial nuclear region of the HTA as well as the preoptic area, whereas the lower dosage alters only preoptic thresholds. The latter circumstance may represent the normal "physiological" state in male rats where cyclic regulatory processes are not necessary and only the tonic control is required (Barraclough, 1967).

2. Neonatal Androgen Effect on the Anterior Hypothalamic FSH Control Mechanism

From the findings summarized in the preceding section, it follows that the neonatal androgen effect alters neuronal responsiveness in the preoptic LH trigger. On the basis of the concept described in Section III, B, it seems likely that not only the preoptic LH trigger but, simultaneously, the anterior hypothalamic FSH control mechanism might also be affected by neonatal androgen action. Furthermore, if the hypothesis of Yazaki (1959, 1960) and Harris and Levine (1962), mentioned in the introductory part of Section III, A, and that of Barraclough (1967) is correct, it would be expected that male rats castrated immediately after birth might have an intact anterior hypothalamic FSH control mechanism which is apparently absent in the intact adult male rat. Results shown in Table II appear to support this assumption.

The experiment (Petrusz and Flerkó, 1965) was carried out on 30 male rats divided into two groups. In group I, the testes were removed at the age of 2 days. When the animals reached 120–125 gm body weight at the age of 60 days, one ovary was grafted into the dorsal neck muscles and estradiol (0.1 μg/day) was injected intramuscularly for a period of 1 month from the day of ovarian implantation. Group II animals were the same as those in group I except that testes were removed simultaneously with ovarian implantation and the commencement of estradiol treatment at the age of 60 days.

The grafted ovaries were taken from females 9–13 days old and weighed 5 ± 0.2 mg at the time of transplantation. As shown in Table II, the higher FSH output in rats of group II is reflected by the higher weight of ovarian graft in this group as compared to group I. This finding suggests that, in the neonatal male rat, testicular androgen re-

Table II

Mean Weight of Endocrine Organs of Male Rats Castrated at the Age of 2 Days (Group I) or 2 Months (Group II), Bearing Ovarian Grafts and Treated with 0.1 μg of Estradiol per Day for 1 Month[a]

Group	No. of rats	Castration	Ovarian transplantation and beginning of estradiol treatment	Mean body weight at the end of experiment	Pituitary	Thyroid	Adrenals	Ovarian graft
I	15	Day 2 after birth	Day 60 after birth	150 ± 5.6	14 ± 3.2	11 ± 3.1	56 ± 3.9	31 ± 3.5[b]
II	15	Day 60 after birth	Day 60 after birth	158 ± 5.6	13 ± 0.9	12 ± 0.5	53 ± 2.6	48 ± 3.7[b]

Average weight of endocrine organs (mg)

[a] From Petrusz and Flerkó (1965), by permission from the editor of *Acta Biol. (Budapest)*.
[b] $p < 0.02$.

duces the responsiveness to estradiol of the anterior hypothalamic neurons contributing to the FSH control mechanism which is indispensable to the negative neurohormonal feedback, by which physiological amounts of estrogen inhibit the release of FSH (Section III, A, 2, b). In rats castrated only after puberty, these neurons have become functionally inactive because of the "desensitizing" action of testicular androgen during the critical period of development. Therefore, physiological amounts of exogenous estradiol do not inhibit the FSH output in these rats to the same measure as in animals castrated immediately after birth. In the latter animal, the responsiveness of the neurons contributing to the FSH control mechanism remained intact, owing to the absence of testicular androgen during the critical period of the first few days after birth.

Simultaneously with our publication, Harris and Levine (1965) reported that the responsiveness to estrogen of the uterus was reduced in the androgen-sterilized rat. Later, van Rees and Gans (1966), Petrusz and Flerkó (1968) and Takewaki (1968) observed that responsiveness to estradiol of the so-called estrogen-responsive tissues (i.e., uterus, anterior pituitary, and vagina) was diminished in rats injected with TP a few days after birth. It appears, therefore, that neural and nonneural target tissues of estrogen are similarly affected by the early postnatal androgen action.

In androgen-sterilized persistent-estrus rats, Gorski and Barraclough (1962b), Swanson and van der Werff ten Bosch (1964a) as well as Schapiro (1965) failed to observe any change in the degree of ovarian compensatory hypertrophy (COH) following unilateral ovariectomy. This led these authors to conclude that it is not necessary to postulate any imbalance in FSH secretion, to explain the development of POS, at least in the androgen-sterilized animals. In our opinion, however, from experiments comparing the degree of COH of rats with and without neonatal androgenization, no conclusion can be drawn as to whether or not the negative estrogen-FSH feedback was disturbed by the neonatal androgen treatment. In this regard, the comparison between the degree of inhibition by estrogen of the COH in androgenized and nonandrogenized rats might furnish some evidence. Therefore, in the experiment of Petrusz and Nagy (1967), the inhibition of the COH by estradiol was used as a measure of the estrogen responsiveness of the anterior hypothalamic neurons.

The degree of the COH after treatment with different doses of estradiol is diagrammatically shown in Fig. 2. In group I, the left ovaries of forty, 70-day-old rats were removed and then the animals were distributed into four subgroups. Ten hemispayed rats served as untreated

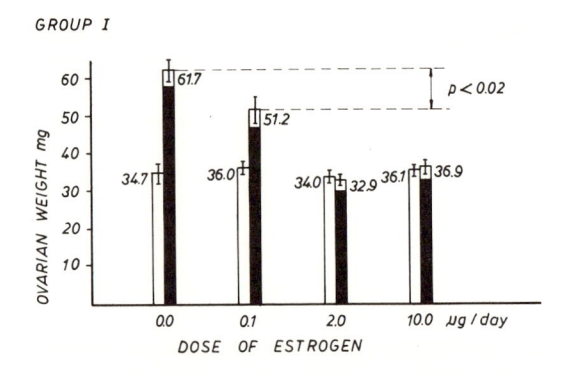

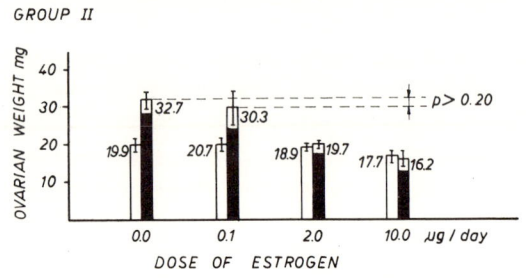

Fig. 2. Diagrammatic representation of compensatory ovarian hypertrophy and its inhibition by exogenous estrogen in adult hemispayed rats. Group I without, group II with, pretreatment with 1.0 mg of testosterone. Mean weights of the excised ovaries are represented by open columns, those of the remaining ones by black columns. The first double columns represent the data from rats without estrogen administration, the following ones indicate the data from rats treated with 0.1, 2.0, and 10.0 μg/day estradiol, respectively. Average weights in milligrams are given above the columns. From Petrusz and Nagy (1967), by permission from the editor of *Acta Biol. (Budapest)*.

controls, the remaining ones, in three subgroups of 10 animals, received daily injection of estradiol propionate (0.1, 2.0, and 10.0 μg, respectively, dissolved in 0.1 ml of oil) for the next 30 days.

In group II, 48 females were pretreated with 1.0 mg of testosterone phenylpropionate (TPP) dissolved in 0.05 ml of oil at the age of 2 days. After the opening of the vaginal orifice, vaginal smears were recorded daily, and they revealed persistent cornification in all animals at least for a period of 1 month before the left ovaries were removed at the age of 70 days. The animals were then divided into four subgroups. Twelve hemispayed rats remained without estrogen treatment, and served as controls for the androgenized group. The remaining ones, in three subgroups of 13, 10, and 13 animals, respectively, received the same treatment for the next 30 days as the animals in the three estrogen-treated subgroups of group I. All the rats in both groups were killed on day 30 of estrogen treatment, at the age of 100 days.

Unilateral ovariectomy without administration of estrogen resulted in COH of considerable degree, while administration of a daily estrogen dose of 2.0 or 10.0 μg abolished this effect completely in both groups. Treatment daily with 0.1 μg of estradiol gave, however, dichotomic results in the two groups. This dose of estradiol inhibited significantly the COH in group I—ovarian weight, 51.2 mg vs. 61.7 mg ($p < 0.02$)—while in the androgenized animals of group II it resulted only in a slight, nonsignificant inhibition (ovarian weight, 30.3 mg *vs.* 32.7 mg, $p > 0.20$). The results of the subgroups given 0.1 μg of estradiol daily support the assumption that inactivity (or at least, inadequate function) of preoptic–anterior hypothalamic neurons instrumental in the neurohormonal feedback action of estrogens plays an important role in the disturbance of gonadotropin secretion following neonatal androgen treatment. Various explanations for this inactivity or inadequate function could be advanced; the most simple, however, being the assumption of a reduction of the responsiveness to estradiol of the preoptic–anterior hypothalamic neurons contributing to the FSH and LH control mechanism.

Furthermore, in accordance with the findings of Barraclough and Gorski (1961), mentioned in Section III, C, 1, the results of the experiment of Petrusz and Nagy (1967) suggest that perinatal androgen treatment affects the different hypothalamic estrogen target tissues to different degrees. Sterilization with 1.0 mg of TPP rendered the anterior hypothalamic FSH control mechanism unresponsive to estrogen since physiological doses (0.1 μg/day) of estradiol, acting through the anterior hypothalamic FSH control mechanism, were not able to inhibit COH. The HTA or the anterior pituitary or both, however, retained at least a part of their estrogen responsiveness, since larger (unphysiological) doses of estradiol (2.0 and 10.0 μg/day), probably acting at the HTA and/or pituitary level, were capable of inhibiting FSH secretion also in androgen-sterilized rats.

Similar observations were reported by Kurcz *et al.* (1969; Kurcz and Gerhardt, 1968) which led these authors also to the assumption that neonatal androgen action might have a double effect on the hypothalamic mechanisms controlling gonadotropin secretion. Besides desensitizing the preoptic–anterior hypothalamic cyclic mechanism, neonatal androgen—when given in adequate doses at the appropriate time—might also damage the HTA neurons that the capacity of these neurons to produce the releasing factors might be reduced as compared to intact animals.

IV. The Possible Mechanism of Action of Androgen

Results mentioned in Section III, C, 2 indicate that neonatal androgen action, if not too powerful, "desensitizes" the estrogen-responsive neurons contributing to the preoptic–anterior hypothalamic cyclic mechanism, leaving intact the FRF- and LRF-producing elements of the tonic mechanism. In other words, the neonatal androgen action "switches off" the cyclic mechanism while the tonic mechanism maintains male type (acyclic) gonadotropin release.

At this point, the question arose: What is the mechanism whereby perinatal androgen action reduces the sensitivity or responsiveness to estrogen of hypothalamic neurons instrumental in neurohormonal estrogen feedback and, hence, in the maintenance of cyclic release of GTH?

A. *Characteristic Pattern of Uptake and Retention of Tritiated Estradiol by Certain Hypothalamic Areas*

Michael (1962) and Attramadal (1964) were the first to observe that estrogens were taken up selectively by certain hypothalamic areas. Later, Kato and Villee (1967a,b) showed that the anterior hypothalamus takes up and retains estradiol, converting very little to other products. According to the findings of these authors, the pattern of incorporation of estradiol into the anterior hypothalamus is similar to that of the uterus and vagina described by Jensen and Jacobson (1962), Stone et al. (1963), Stone (1963, 1964), and Martin (1964). Similar observations were reported by Eisenfeld and Axelrod (1967) as well as by McGuire and Lisk (1968) and Woolley et al. (1968).

On the basis of their observations, Kato and Villee (1967a) suggested that the anterior hypothalamus is a direct target tissue of estradiol and that the specific trapping mechanism in the target tissue, which retains the estradiol in an unconverted form, may serve to initiate a sequence of reactions by which estradiol exerts its feedback control on gonadotropin secretion. Our findings (Flerkó et al., 1969, 1971) agree with those of Kato and Villee (1967a), except for the fact that in our experiment not only the anterior, but also the middle, hypothalamus took up and retained significantly more radioactive estradiol than the posterior hypothalamus and the parietal cortex, used as control brain tissue in these experiments. This finding of ours is in accordance with our earlier assumption that the preoptic–anterior hypothalamic area (Flerkó, 1956, 1957a,b; Flerkó and Szentágothai, 1957) as well as the medial-basal part of the middle hypothalamus (Flerkó, 1962) contains estrogen-responsive neurons [for details see Section III, A and Flerkó (1966, 1967, 1968)].

B. Effect of Neonatal Androgen Treatment in Reducing the Estradiol Binding Capacity of Neural and Nonneural Target Tissues

Jensen et al. (1967) and King (1967) suggested that uptake and retention of estradiol occurs at receptor sites that are specific for estrogens. The specificity of action of estradiol on the estrogen-responsive tissues has been explained by the ability of these tissues to take up and retain estradiol in an unconverted form. A preliminary experiment of ours (Flerkó and Mess, 1968) revealed that the estradiol-binding capacity of pituitaries and uteri of androgen-sterilized rats was significantly reduced as compared to intact controls. This raised the possibility that early postnatal androgen action might interfere with the development of the estrogen-receptor proteins and in this way, interferes with estradiol uptake or retention by the estrogen-responsive tissues. Since the findings mentioned in the Section IV, A indicate that the anterior and middle hypothalamus are direct target tissues for estradiol, one might postulate that the early postnatal androgen action might damage the specific trapping mechanism in the estrogen-responsive hypothalamic neurons. If so, estradiol-binding capacity of the hypothalamic areas containing estrogen-responsive neurons should be reduced in the androgen-sterilized rat.

In order to study this hypothesis, the radioactivity present in the anterior, middle, and posterior hypothalamus, in the anterior pituitary and uterus was measured by liquid scintillation counting 2 hours after intravenous injection of 50 μCi of tritiated estradiol into control and androgen-sterilized rats spayed 9 days before the injection of the labeled estradiol. For control brain tissue, the cortical region was excised from the parietal lobe of the brain. Three androgen-sterilized and three control rats were taken from each litter, and a total of 18 androgen-sterilized and 18 control animals was investigated in 6 experiments. Tissue samples from three androgen-sterilized and three control rats, respectively, were jointly homogenized, extracted with ether and measured in a liquid scintillation counter (Flerkó et al., 1969; Flerkó, 1970b). The radioactivity of the different parts of the brain, the anterior pituitary, and the uterus is shown in Table III.

In the control group, the anterior pituitary and the uterus accumulated 9–10 times more tritiated estradiol than the anterior and middle hypothalamus. This difference may possibly indicate the relative concentration of cells in the anterior and middle hypothalamus and peripheral target tissues which can accumulate estradiol. The radioactivity in the anterior and middle hypothalamus was significantly higher ($p < 0.01$) than in the parietal cortex, a part of the brain which probably does

Table III
Radioactivity[a] Following Injection of 50 μCi Tritiated Estradiol into Spayed Rats with and without Early Postnatal Administration of Androgen
(Pooled Results from 3 Animals)[b]

Expt. No.	Anterior hypo-thalamus	Middle hypo-thalamus	Posterior hypo-thalamus	Cerebral cortex	Anterior pituitary	Uterus
			Controls			
1	16.0	10.1	4.9	3.9	150.6	72.3
2	16.1	14.1	4.1	5.0	248.4	123.5
3	19.0	11.5	0.0	1.9	197.8	146.7
4	17.6	8.1	6.6	5.3	169.2	134.9
5	17.0	12.9	4.3	1.3	209.2	180.6
6	11.8	9.8	9.2	5.3	51.6	240.8
Mean:	16.2[c]	11.0[c]	4.8[f]	3.7[e]	171.1[d]	149.8[c]
			Androgen-sterilized rats			
1	10.2	6.0	7.1	4.9	136.3	65.6
2	11.9	10.3	3.1	0.1	120.6	60.6
3	10.0	7.1	4.1	2.7	146.7	92.1
4	8.5	6.8	2.7	2.1	115.4	92.5
5	15.2	8.8	2.9	1.8	197.3	120.4
6	8.0	7.6	7.3	5.3	25.8	133.3
Mean:	10.6[c]	7.7[c]	4.5[f]	2.8[e]	123.6[d]	94.0[c]

[a] Expressed as counts per minute per milligram of wet tissue.
[b] From Flerkó et al. (1969), by permission from S. Karger AG, Basel.
[c] $p < 0.01$.
[d] $p < 0.05$.
[e] $p > 0.30$.
[f] $p > 0.50$.

not contain estrogen-responsive neurons. The radioactivity in the posterior hypothalamus did not differ significantly ($p > 0.70$) from that in the parietal cortex. On the other hand, the estradiol-binding capacity of the anterior and middle hypothalamus and of the nonneural target tissues was significantly reduced in androgen-sterilized rats (for statistical analysis see Table III). No change occurred in the posterior hypothalamus and parietal cortex of the same animals.

Similar findings have been reported by McGuire and Lisk (1969), Tuohimaa et al. (1969), and Vértes and King (1969). Green et al. (1969) also found that 30 min after an injection of tritiated estradiol, certain hypothalamic parts of the brain and pituitaries of spayed rats retained more radioactivity than did similar tissues in castrated males or spayed neonatally androgenized females. In the first experiment of Green et *al.* (1969), however, the males and neonatally androgenized females were heavier than the control female rats. To estimate the role of body weight in the uptake of estradiol, a second experiment was conducted using male and female rats of equal group body weight but of different age, the males being approximately 3 weeks younger than the females. Both sets of animals were, however, sexually mature. In this second experiment, Green *et al.* (1969) did not find any difference between sexes in the binding of estradiol by any tissue, and concluded that the effect observed by us might reflect weight differences rather than a blockage of estrogen-receptor sites by neonatal androgenization, as we had suggested. We repeated, therefore, our original experiment using control and androgen-sterilized females of approximately equal group body weight since control and androgenized rats used in our earlier experiments (Flerkó and Mess, 1968; Flerkó *et al.*, 1969; Flerkó, 1970b) were of equal age but differed in body weights. Results of this experiment are shown in Table IV.

In agreement with our previous findings, the radioactivity in the anterior and middle hypothalamus was significantly higher in the control group than in the parietal cortex ($p < 0.01$), used as control brain tissue. The radioactivity of the posterior hypothalamus did not differ significantly from that of the parietal cortex ($p > 0.20$). Furthermore, similarly to our previous findings on control and androgenized rats of equal age but different body weight, the estradiol-binding capacity of the neural (anterior and middle hypothalamus) and of the nonneural (uterus) target tissues was significantly reduced in androgen-sterilized rats as compared to controls of approximately equal body weight (for statistical analysis see Table IV). The only difference between the results of these experiments and those of the previous ones was that the difference between control and androgenized pituitary samples failed to reach statistical significance. This, in agreement with the finding of Green *et al.* (1969), suggests that weight differences rather than age differences between control and androgenized rats have to be eliminated in similar experiments.

Nevertheless, the finding that androgen-sterilized rats had significantly lower anterior and middle hypothalamic radioactivity levels than controls of approximately equal weight supports our hypothesis that perinatal androgen action might interfere with normal development of estrogen-receptor proteins and, hence, with normal uptake or retention of estradiol by the hypothalamic estrogen-responsive neurons. In this way, these neurons might become desensitized and functionally inactive in mediating positive and negative estrogen feedback on the anterior pituitary cells producing gonadotropic hormones. These results, taken together

Table IV
Radioactivity[a] Following Injection of 50 μCi of Tritiated Estradiol into Spayed Controls and into Rats Injected with 1.25 mg of Testosterone Propionate 2 Days after Birth (Group I) and with 0.6 mg/Day of Testosterone Propionate for the First 10 Days of Life (Group II) (Pooled Samples from 3 Animals)[a]

Expt. No.[c]	Anterior hypo-thalamus	Middle hypo-thalamus	Posterior hypo-thalamus	Cerebral cortex	Anterior pituitary	Uterus
\multicolumn{7}{c}{Controls ($\bar{X}$ = 179.3 gm)}
1	13.2	7.9	4.5	3.0	162.1	97.8
2	19.8	13.9	8.7	4.8	257.6	197.1
3	13.4	12.4	4.7	2.7	142.9	131.8
4	9.5	6.2	3.2	2.0	113.4	71.2
5	16.2	14.5	10.9	3.7	337.0	202.9
Mean (1–5)	14.4	10.9	6.4	3.2	202.6	140.1
6	15.3	11.1	6.3	3.6	229.2	235.5
7	13.2	10.8	7.8	10.5	175.8	243.6
8	17.0	11.6	9.3	5.2	209.7	245.9
Mean (6–8)	15.1	11.1	7.8	6.2	204.9	241.6
Mean (1–8)	14.7[d]	11.0[e]	6.9[f]	4.4[h]	203.4[g]	178.2[e]
\multicolumn{7}{c}{Group I ($\bar{X}$ = 185.8 gm)}
1	8.8	6.2	3.5	3.6	147.3	105.5
2	10.9	10.4	8.3	4.1	102.0	100.7
3	7.6	4.4	3.3	1.2	124.3	121.3
4	7.2	5.7	3.7	2.0	104.9	57.2
5	13.0	10.3	7.1	5.3	234.5	128.4
Mean (1–5)	9.5	7.4	5.1	3.4	142.2	102.6
6	10.5	10.2	4.5	5.1	198.0	198.3
7	12.9	7.5	5.7	9.3	151.8	175.5
8	8.6	7.8	5.0	4.3	166.9	145.8
Mean (6–8)	10.3	8.5	5.0	6.2	172.2	173.1
Mean (1–8)	9.9[d]	7.8[e]	5.1[f]	4.3[h]	153.7[g]	129.0[e]
\multicolumn{7}{c}{Group II ($\bar{X}$ = 195.7 gm)}
1	8.3	5.1	4.2	1.6	98.8	89.8
2	12.1	9.0	4.5	3.3	134.9	92.8
3	7.8	5.6	—	1.2	109.6	102.4
4	5.8	5.2	5.5	1.8	73.5	71.2
5	—	—	—	—	—	—
Mean (1–5)	8.5	6.2	4.7	1.9	104.2	89.0
6	10.8	9.3	8.4	4.8	196.8	163.5
7	11.1	7.2	3.9	4.8	140.1	171.6
8	12.3	10.3	8.8	7.3	194.3	198.8
Mean (6–8)	11.4	8.9	7.0	5.6	177.0	177.9
Mean (1–8)	9.7	7.3	5.8	3.5	135.4	127.1

[a] Expressed as counts per minute per milligram of wet tissue.
[b] From Flerkó et al. (1971), by permission from the editor of Acta Biol. (Budapest).
[c] The experiments were carried out in two series, Nos. 1–5 and 6–8, with different tritiated estradiol preparation; experiment 5 contains only controls and rats of group I.
[d] $p < 0.01$.
[e] $p < 0.05$.
[f] $p > 0.10$.
[g] $p > 0.20$.
[h] $p > 0.50$.

with the findings mentioned in Section III, C, furnish evidence that the reduction of estradiol binding and the consequent loss of neurohormonal feedback, induced by perinatal androgen action, might account for the noncyclic pattern of gonadotropin secretion and for the presence of anovulatory sterility in the androgen-sterilized female and probably also in the male rat.

It is well established that the relationship between the time of androgen administration and the effect on the brain (–pituitary–ovarian axis) is greatly influenced by the dose of androgen (see Section II, B). We have compared, therefore, the effect of continuous administration of larger amounts of TPP (0.6 mg/day for the first 10 days of life) on the estradiol-binding capacity of neural and nonneural target tissues with that experienced following a single injection of 1.25 mg of TPP 2 days after birth. As can be seen from Table IV (Groups I and II), radioactivity of tissue samples from female rats treated with daily doses of 0.6 mg TPP during the first 10 days of life were not significantly different from those of animals treated with a single dose of 1.25 mg TPP 2 days after birth ($p > 0.50$). This indicates that the latter had a maximal reducing effect on the estradiol binding capacity of the neural and nonneural target tissues.

V. Effects of Neonatal Treatment with Steroid Hormones Other Than Androgen on Subsequent Fertility

A. The POS Induced by Neonatal Estrogen Administration

Turner (1941) treated newborn female rats with 100–200 IU of estrogen at days 1–10 of age, and he observed 10 months later that the ovaries of these rats contained many follicles in various stages of growth and atresia but no corpora lutea. Following Turner's observation, several authors (Hale, 1944; Takasugi, 1952a; Kikuyama, 1963a) reported that the POS can be induced by repeated injections of estrogen during the first few days of life.

Gorski (1963a) has studied the frequency of occurrence of the POS when various amounts of estradiol benzoate were administered as a single injection to the 5-day-old rat. He has found that 5 μg of estradiol benzoate is the minimal dose capable of inducing POS in more than 60% of the rats injected. The single injection of 100 μg of estradiol benzoate induces the POS in 93.4% of animals. When adult, these rats exhibit anovulatory vaginal cycles in which the stage of vaginal cornification predominates. They mate, but not in correlation with the vaginal cycle.

Ovulation is not induced by mating or by progesterone injections, and only infrequently following electrical stimulation of the hypothalamus.

Ladosky (1967) has confirmed the previous data of Hale (1944) in showing that a single small dose of stilbestrol can also elicit the POS if given during the first few days of life.

B. Anestrous State Induced by Neonatal Estrogen Treatment

The effects of early postanatal estrogen administration on the brain–pituitary–ovarian axis also differ according to the dose of estrogen and the length of the administration period. Whereas daily injections of small doses for a short period (e.g., for 5–7 days) result in the POS, prolonged treatment of rats with large doses for the first 30 days of life produces persistent anestrus. The ovaries of these anestrous rats contain small follicles, but neither maturing ones nor corpora lutea (Takasugi, 1952b, 1956). In contrast to the rats with POS, in the persistent anestrous rats, the hypothalamus is no longer capable of eliciting an increase in the secretion of gonadotropins after ovariectomy. This is evidenced by the fact that neither follicular growth nor luteinization takes place in ovaries autografted into the spleen (Takasugi, 1953a), the low pituitary GTH potency is not raised by ovariectomy in contrast to the GTH potency of the estrogen- or androgen-induced persistent-estrus rat (Noumura, 1958), and that ovariectomy is not followed by the occurrence of typical castration cells in the anterior pituitary (Arai, 1964, 1965). Furthermore, in persistent-anestrus rats both the content of LH in the anterior pituitary and that of LH-releasing factor in the hypothalamus are decidedly lower than in intact female rats (Arai, 1963).

Although the corpora lutea formed after treatment with gonadotropins do not become functional spontaneously in the persistent-anestrus rat, administration of reserpine or transplantation of the hypophysis under the kidney capsule elicits the secretion of luteotropic hormone (LTH). Assays of the LTH content of the pituitaries demonstrated that such content was significantly lower in persistent-anestrus rats than in persistent-estrus or normal rats (Kikuyama, 1963b; Takewaki, 1964).

C. Other Steroid Hormones Inducing Sterility in the Rat When Administered Neonatally

Selye and Friedman (1940) and later Takasugi (1953b) have found that after 50 mg and 62 μg/day, respectively, of deoxycorticosterone acetate administered over a 40-day period and for the first 20 days, respectively, starting from birth, corpora lutea were not formed in the rat ovary and persistent vaginal cornification ensued after puberty.

Turner (1941) has reported persistent estrus after perinatal treatment with progesterone, and Takasugi (1953b) observed that 83 μg of progesterone per day for 20 days or 8 mg of cholesterol per day for 50 days from birth produced the POS.

Gorski (1963b) has also studied the effects of a variety of different steroids on the development of brain mechanisms controlling GTH secretion. He observed that the following compounds, administered as a single injection at 5 days of age, failed to alter the normal reproductive pattern: 0.05 ml peanut oil, 1 mg androstenedione, 1.25 mg norethandrolone, 6.25 mg hydroxyprogesterone caproate, 1.25 mg cortisone acetate, 2.5 mg hydrocortisone, 5 mg cholesterol, and 1 mg of conjugated estrogens. In contrast, Jacobsohn (1964) has reported that various anabolic steroids injected into newborn rats will induce sterility. Apparently most steroid hormones, if given in sufficiently high doses for prolonged periods immediately after birth are capable of inducing sterility associated with POS or with permanent anestrus.

D. The Possible Mechanism of Action

No studies characterizing the mechanism of action of the above steroids have been performed except for estrogens. Nevertheless, the fact that any substance bearing the cyclopentane ring may have POS-inducing action, suggests that all steroid hormones might act in a similar way during the perinatal period, i.e., they reduce the responsiveness to estrogen of these structures by diminishing the estradiol binding of the hypothalamic estrogen-responsive neurons.

Concerning the estrogens, there are some experimental data supporting the above assumption. Taksugi and Kimura (1967) as well as Mori (1967, 1969) have shown that both the uterus and vagina were less sensitive to exogenous estrogen in neonatally estrogenized adult mice than in normal mice. Increase in uterine weight following estrogen treatment when adult was less marked in spayed rats which received estrogen neonatally than in controls without neonatal estrogen treatment (Hayashi, 1968). In ovarian grafts in estrogenized, spayed rats with POS, given daily injections of 32 or 128 μg of estrone, corpora lutea were absent or highly degenerate, while ovarian grafts in ovariectomized control rats similarly treated with estrone exhibited many well developed corpora lutea (Hayashi, 1969). This may indicate that the secretion of LTH stimulated by injections of estrogen was smaller in amount in spayed, estrogenized rats than in spayed "normal" rats. Greater increase in weight of the anterior hypophysis in ovariectomized "normal" rats than in spayed, estrogenized rats following estrogen administration (Hayashi, 1967) seems to lend support to this assumption. Furthermore, similarly to the androgen sterilized rat (Section IV, *B*), the estradiol-binding capacity of the anterior and middle hypothalamus as well as that of the anterior pituitary was significantly reduced also in estrogen-sterilized rats (McGuire and Lisk, 1969).

VI. Protection Against Steroid-Induced Sterility

The use of various drugs to counteract the sterility-inducing action of androgen and estrogen, proved to be a fruitful approach to the study of the mechanism of action of steroid sterilization.

Kikuyama (1961) has shown that if reserpine was administered concurrently with TP or estradiol to infantile rats, the effects of the steroids inducing the POS were attenuated or nullified and in the ovaries of the treated rats both follicles and copora lutea developed after the animals attained sexual maturity. In a control experiment, administration of the vehicle of reserpine together with androgen or estrogen did not interfere at all with the induction of the POS by the steroid. In Kawashima's (1964) experiment, male rats were injected with reserpine for the first 10 days of life and castrated on day 11 after birth. The animals were given subcutaneous ovarian grafts when they reached 30 days of age and were killed 50 days later. Histological studies revealed that the ovarian grafts in these animals invariably contained both follicles and corpora lutea. In a control series of experiments, rats were orchidectomized at 10 days of age with no preceding treatment with reserpine and given subcutaneous ovarian grafts at 30 days of age. The grafts recovered 50 days later exhibited follicles of varying sizes but no corpora lutea.

From these experiments, it seems evident that reserpine nullified, or at least attenuated, the effects of estrone or testosterone on the brain–pituitary–ovarian axis. However, reserpine failed to interfere with the precocious vaginal opening which occurs in steroid-sterilized rats (Takewaki, 1962). It is evident, therefore, that reserpine cannot antagonize the effect of the steroids on the accessory organs.

Chlorpromazine, given concurrently with estrone to newborn female rats, also nullified the effect of perinatal estrogen administration, the estrous cycles and ovarian function of the animals remaining almost undisturbed (Kikuyama, 1962). Takasugi (1965) has shown that, if injected together with progesterone, chlorpromazine nullifies the luteinization-inducing effect of the steroid in the persistent-estrus rat. Gorski and Barraclough (1962a) suggested that in androgen-sterilized rats, progesterone acts on the anterior pituitary to increase the storage of

LH. However, the possibility cannot be excluded that progesterone influences LH release in rats with POS indirectly, i.e., through the central nervous system (CNS), since chlorpromazine is capable of nullifying the effect of progesterone in stimulating LH release in persistent-estrus rats.

As mentioned in Section V, the POS can be elicited also by the perinatal administration of ovarian steroids. However, relatively large doses of ovarian hormones—well above the physiological range—are required for this effect. The minimal dose of 5 μg estradiol benzoate given to rats at 5 days of age (Gorski, 1963a) or 83 μg of progesterone per day administered for the first 20 days of life (Takasugi, 1953b) results in permanent sterility. Interestingly, very small amounts of ovarian

Table V
Number and Percentage of Luteinized Ovarian Grafts in Adult Male Rats Castrated 10 Days after Birth after Pretreatment with Ovarian Hormones[a]

Group	Treatment at the age of 1–10 days	No. of rats	Rats with luteinized ovarian graft No.	Percent
I	No treatment	12	0	0
II	Daily 0.1 μg estradiol benzoate (EB)	13	6	46.1
	Daily 0.1 μg EB + 0.5 μg progesterone	13	8	61.5
	Daily 0.1 μg EB + 2.5 μg progesterone	12	9	75.0

[a] From Flerkó et al. (1967), by permission from the editor of Acta Biol. (Budapest).

steroids, e.g., 0.1 μg of estradiol alone or with 0.5 to 2.5 μg of progesterone per day given during 10 days to newborn male rats, prevented the masculinizing effect of testicular androgen on the hypothalamus (Flerkó et al., 1967). The results of this investigation are summarized in Table V.

In this experiment, 50 newborn male rats were distributed into two groups. In Group I, the testes of 12 rats were removed 10 days after birth. At the age of 70 days, one ovary and a piece of vagina were transplanted into the dorsal neck muscles of the castrated rats. In group II, 38 newborn rats, prior to undergoing the same operation as the animals in group I, received a daily treatment of ovarian hormones in three subgroups (see doses in Table V). None of the ovarian grafts in group I had corpora lutea; they contained only growing follicles and interstitial tissue. The noncyclic pattern of GTH secretion in this group was clearly shown also by the histological picture of the vaginal tissue transplanted close to the ovarian grafts. The epithelium of the vaginal grafts was filled with concentric layers of cornified cells. In contrast, the majority of the ovarian grafts in group II contained corpora lutea. In these cases also, the histological picture of the vaginal grafts gave evidence of the cyclic pattern of gonadotropin secretion. The lumen of the grafts was filled with detached cell layers in which cornified layers alternated with layers of nucleated epithelial cells in association with a great number of leukocytes. The percentage of the luteinized ovaries in the three different subgroups increased with the daily doses of ovarian steroids administered before castration (see Table V).

The mechanism of this effect is unknown. Possibly a countereffect of the ovarian steroids might antagonize the masculinizing action of the testicular androgens. The other possibility involves the negative feedback action of ovarian hormones, which might inhibit the GTH secretion and, in turn, the androgen production in the treated males. The findings of Cagnoni et al. (1965), Kincl and Maqueo (1965), and Arai and Gorski (1968a) do not support the second assumption, and give preference to the former one. Their data suggest that progesterone can protect the hypothalamic-hypophysial–gonadal axis against the action of early postnatal androgen administration. This may explain why androgen, when given in insufficiently large doses to pregnant rats, cannot change the pattern of gonadotropin secretion of the offspring, while masculinizing the external and internal genitalia, as was the case in the experiments of Swanson and van der Werff ten Bosch (1964b) and Kincl and Maqueo (1965).

Apparently the hormonal environment of the pregnant animal can protect the sex steroid-responsive hypothalamic structures, at least to a certain extent, against the densitizing effect of androgen action. This may account for the fact that masculinization of the hypothalamo–pituitary axis occurs also in the genetically male rat only after birth, i.e., when the male offspring is no longer under the influence of the maternal hormonal environment. When, however, the concentration of androgen rises above a certain level in the fetus, maternal estrogen and progesterone can no longer protect the hypothalamic structures of the fetus against the densensitizing action of androgen. Evidence for this has been mentioned in Section II, B. It may be concluded from the above findings that the critical period, during which testicular, or exogenously administered androgen can imprint the masculine pattern of control on the hypothalamic regulation of gonadotropin secretion, depends on the hormonal environment existing in the fetus and in the mother. The other decisive factor in this respect is the developmental stage of the sex steroid-responsive hypothalamic neurons.

Among the agents that can protect the developing hypothalamus from androgen or estrogen, Arai and Gorski (1968a) found that barbiturates, e.g., pentobarbital and phenobarbital, are most effective in blocking androgen sterilization. According to their observations, 10 μg of reserpine, 500 μg of chlorpromazine, 2500 μg of progesterone, 1000 μg of deoxycorticosterone acetate, or 1500 μg of pregnanedione, given simultaneously with 30 μg of TP to the 5-day-old female rat, reduced markedly the incidence of sterility during the immediate postpubertal period. This protection was found to be incomplete, however, as the incidence of sterility approached control levels by 90 days of age. In contrast, pentobarbital or phenobarbital affords the 5-day-old female marked protection against the effect of androgen and only 5% of the androgen–barbiturate injected females were found to be anovulatory at 90 days of age. The protective effect of pentobarbital was eliminated by simultaneous injection of Metrazol, a stimulant of the CNS. Since depression of neural activity is a common feature after injection of the above agents, among other possibilities, Arai and Gorski (1968a) assumed that their CNS-depressing capacity might underlie their protective action.

In order to determine the length of time neural elements must be exposed to androgen to induce sterility, Arai and Gorski (1968b) injected pentobarbital and phenobarbital simultaneously with 30 μg of TP or at 3, 6, 9, 12, or 24 hours after TP injection. Results of this experiment suggest that androgen can exert its inductive action on the developing brain during a very short period of 12 hours or less. They are also consistent with the hypothesis that androgen action can be divided into two phases. A brief phase (approximately 3 hours in length) of androgen uptake by neurons is followed by a more prolonged phase (approximately another 9 hours) of intraneuronal biochemical action.

The simultaneous injection of cyproterone acetate (CA), an antiandrogen, also protects the female rat against the hypothalamic masculinizing action of TP (Wollman and Hamilton, 1967; Arai and Gorski, 1968c). When CA was administered 6 or more hours after androgen injection, however, its effectiveness was markedly reduced in the experiment of Arai and Gorski (1968c). They concluded that a CA-labile component of the process of hypothalamic masculinization, which lasts for less than 6 hours, may consist of the uptake of androgen by hypothalamic neurons.

The results of the experiment of Kobayashi and Gorski (1970) are also consistent with the view that androgen exerts its sterility-inducing action on the developing brain for a short time after its injection. Actinomycin D or puromycin administered at various intervals before or after injecting TP prevented its action. However, almost all rats injected with either actinomycin D or puromycin 12 hours after TP administration possessed ovaries without corpora lutea at both 45 and 90 days of age, suggesting that androgen modifies hypothalamic mechanisms within this short period. Actinomycin D and puromycin have been shown to inhibit DNA-dependent RNA and protein synthesis, respectively (Hurwitz et al., 1962). Therefore, the observation of Kobayashi and Gorski (1970) that antibiotics administered at various intervals before or after TP administration can prevent its action, implicate these intracellular biochemical processes in the differentiation of the developing hypothalamus. These biochemical processes might be disturbed by the perinatal steroid action leading to diminished estradiol binding, and hence to reduced responsiveness to estradiol in the hypothalamic estrogen-responsive neurons.

VII. Summary and Conclusions

Most steroid hormones, if given in sufficiently high doses for prolonged periods immediately after birth, are capable of inducing sterility associated with the polyfollicular ovary syndrome (POS) or with permanent anestrus. Injection of a single dose of 10–1250 μg of testosterone propionate or of 5–100 μg of estradiol benzoate will induce anovulatory sterility associated with POS, a phenomenon termed androgen, or estrogen, sterilization.

Pituitaries of androgen-sterilized rats are capable of maintaining cyclic reproductive functions when transplanted in contiguity with the hypothalamus of intact females. This indicates that neonatal androgen administration induces sterility by altering hypothalamic mechanisms controlling the cyclic release of gonadotropic hormones (GTH).

Current concepts invoke a dual mechanism for the neural control of the secretion of GTH.

The first, termed the tonic mechanism, stimulates a tonic, basal discharge of follicle-stimulating and luteinizing hormone (FSH and LH). Tuberoinfundibular neurons in the hypophysiotropic area (HTA) of the hypothalamus, which produce the FSH- and LH-releasing factors (FRF and LRF), are responsible for this mechanism.

The second mechanism modulates the activity of the FRF- and LRF-producing neurons. This involves brain structures outside the HTA, and may be termed a cyclic mechanism, being indispensable for the maintenance of the cyclic release of FRF-FSH and LRF-LH, respectively. Hypothalamic parts of the cyclic mechanism are the preoptic LH trigger and the anterior hypothalamic FSH control mechanism. A number of experimental data indicate that the neurons contributing to the hypothalamic FSH and LH control mechanisms are instrumental in the neurohormonal steroid feedback controlling cyclic gonadotropin release.

The POS induced by neonatal androgenization is similar to that evoked by electrolytic lesions or a frontal cut in the anterior hypothalamus. This is true even to the extent that pituitaries of both androgen-sterilized and hypothalamus-lesioned rats contain an amount of GTH sufficient for ovulation. However, the pituitaries of these rats are unable to release an ovulatory dose of GTH in the absence of the necessary hypothalamic mechanisms. The identity of the two types of POS suggested that damage to identical brain structures may occur in both types of the syndrome. While electrolytic lesions or a frontal cut in the anterior hypothalamus destroy or separate the anterior hypothalamic FSH control mechanism and the preoptic LH trigger from the tonic mechanism of the HTA, responsiveness to estradiol of the neurons contributing to the preoptic anterior hypothalamic FSH and LH control mechanism is considerably reduced in androgen- and estrogen-sterilized rats as well as in the male rats.

When trying to clarify the way in which neonatal androgen or estrogen action results in reduced responsiveness and, hence, in diminished functional capacity of the hypothalamic estrogen-responsive neurons, the estradiol binding capacity of the neural (anterior and middle hypothalamic) and of the nonneural target tissues was found to be reduced significantly in the androgen- and estrogen-sterilized rat. These and other findings suggest that neonatal androgen or estrogen action might interfere with the normal development of the estrogen-receptor proteins and, in this way, reduce the responsiveness to estradiol of the neural and nonneural target tissues. Thus, the absence of the specific trapping mechanism of the estrogen-responsive hypothalamic neurons may account for the loss of the neurohormonal estrogen feedback and hence, for the loss of cyclic gonadotropin release and ovulation in the androgen- and estrogen-sterilized rat.

References

Alloiteau, J. J. (1954). *C. R. Soc. Biol.* **148**, 223.
Arai, Y. (1962). *Dobutsugaku Zasshi* **71**, 333.
Arai, Y. (1963). *Proc. Jap. Acad.* **39**, 605.
Arai, Y. (1964). *J. Fac. Sci. Univ. Tokyo, Sect. 4* **10**, 369.
Arai, Y. (1965). *Proc. Jap. Acad.* **41**, 163.
Arai, Y., and Gorski, R. A. (1968a). *Endocrinology* **82**, 1005.
Arai, Y., and Gorski, R. A. (1968b). *Endocrinology* **82**, 1010.
Arai, Y., and Gorski, R. A. (1968c). *Proc. Soc. Exp. Biol. Med.* **127**, 590.

Attramadal, A. (1964). *Proc. Int. Congr. Endocrinol., 2nd, London.* Excerpta Med. Found. Intern. Congr. Ser. **83**, Part I, 612–616.
Barraclough, C. A. (1955). *Amer. J. Anat.* **97**, 493.
Barraclough, C. A. (1961). *Endocrinology* **68**, 62.
Barraclough, C. A. (1963). *Advan. Neuroendocrinol., Proc. Symp., Miami, 1961,* pp. 224–233.
Barraclough, C. A. (1966). *Endocrinology* **78**, 1053.
Barraclough, C. A. (1967). *In* "Neuroendocrinology" (L. Martini and W. F. Ganong, eds.),Vol. 2, pp. 61–99. Academic Press, New York.
Barraclough, C. A., and Gorski, R. A. (1961). *Endocrinology* **68**, 68.
Barraclough, C. A., and Leathem, J. H. (1954). *Proc. Soc. Exp. Biol. Med.* **85**, 673.
Barraclough, C. A., Yrarrazaval, S., and Hatton, R. (1964). *Endocrinology* **75**, 838.
Bogdanove, E. M., and Schoen, H. C. (1959). *Proc. Soc. Exp. Biol. Med.* **100**, 664.
Bradbury, J. T. (1941). *Endocrinology* **28**, 101.
Bradshaw, M., and Critchlow, B. V. (1966). *Endocrinology* **78**, 1007.
Browman, L. G. (1937). *J. Exp. Zool.* **75**, 375.
Byrnes, W. W., and Meyer, R. K. (1951). *Endocrinology* **49**, 449.
Cagnoni, M., Fantini, F., Morace, G., and Ghetti, A. (1965). *J. Endocrinol.* **33**, 527.
Carraro, A., Caviezel, F., Fochi, M., and Martini, L. (1966). *Atti Accad. Med. Lomb.* **21**, 1.
Cheng, S., and Li, M. (1965). *Sheng Li Hsueh Pao* **28**, 140.
Critchlow, B. V. (1958). *Amer. J. Physiol.* **195**, 171.
Critchlow, B. V., and Saywer, C. H. (1955). *Fed. Proc. Fed. Amer. Soc. Exp. Biol.* **14**, 32.
D'Angelo, S. A., and Kravatz, A. S. (1960). *Proc. Soc. Exp. Biol. Med.* **104**, 130.
David, M. A., Fraschini, F., and Martini, L. (1965). *C. R. Acad. Sci.* **261**, 2249.
Davidson, J. M., and Sawyer, C. H. (1961a). *Acta Endocrinol. (Copenhagen)* **37**, 385.
Davidson, J. M., and Sawyer, C. H. (1961b). *Proc. Soc. Exp. Biol. Med.* **107**, 4.
Davidson, J. M., and Smith, E. R. (1967). *Proc. Int. Congr. Horm. Steroids, 2nd, Milan, 1966,* pp. 805–813.
Dempsey, E. W., and Searles, H. F. (1943). *Endocrinology* **32**, 119.
Desclin, L., Flament-Durand, J., and Gepts, W. (1962). *Endocrinology* **70**, 429.
Döcke, F., and Dörner, G. (1965). *J. Endocrinol.* **33**, 491.
Donovan, B. T., and van der Werff ten Bosch, J. J. (1956a). *J. Physiol. (London)* **132**, 57.
Donovan, B. T., and van der Werff ten Bosch, J. J. (1956b). *Nature (London)* **178**, 745.
Donovan, B. T., and van der Werff ten Bosch, J. J. (1959a). *J. Physiol. (London)* **147**, 78.
Donovan, B. T., and van der Werff ten Bosch, J. J. (1959b). *J. Physiol. (London)* **147**, 93.
Eisenfeld, A. J., and Axelrod, J. (1967). *Biochem. Pharmacol.* **16**, 1781.
Everett, J. W. (1943). *Endocrinology* **32**, 285.
Everett, J. W. (1964). *In* "Major Problems in Neuroendocrinology" (E. Bajusz and G. Jasmin, eds.), pp. 346–366. Karger, Basel.

Everett, J. W. (1965). *Endocrinology* **76**, 1195.
Everett, J. W. (1969). *Annu. Rev. Physiol.* **31**, 383.
Everett, J. W., and Radford, H. M. (1961). *Proc. Soc. Exp. Biol. Med.* **108**, 604.
Everett, J. W., and Sawyer, C. H. (1949). *Endocrinology* **45**, 581.
Fendler, K., and Endröczi, E. (1965–1966). *Neuroendocrinology* **1**, 129.
Fiske, V. M. (1939). *Proc. Soc. Exp. Biol. Med.* **40**, 189.
Fiske, V. M. (1941). *Endocrinology* **29**, 187.
Flament-Durand, J. (1965). *Endocrinology* **77**, 446.
Flerkó, B. (1954). *Acta Morphol.* **4**, 475.
Flerkó, B. (1956). *Acta Physiol.* **9**, Suppl. 17.
Flerkó, B. (1957a). *Endokrinologie* **34**, 202.
Flerkó, B. (1957b). *Arch. Anat. Microsc. Morphol. Exp.* **46**, 159.
Flerkó, B. (1962). *In* "Hypothalamic Control of the Anterior Pituitary" (J Szentágothai, B. Flerkó, B. Mess, and B. Halász, eds.), 1st Ed. pp. 192–264. Akadémiai Kiadó, Budapest.
Flerkó, B. (1966). *In* "Neuroendocrinology" (L. Martini and W. F. Ganong, eds.), Vol. 1, pp. 613–668. Academic Press, New York.
Flerkó, B. (1967). *In* "Symposium on Reproduction" (K. Lissák, ed.), pp. 11–37. Akadémiai Kiadó, Budapest.
Flerkó, B. (1968). *In* "Hypothalamic Control of the Anterior Pituitary" (J. Szentágothai, B. Flerkó, B. Mess, and B. Halász, eds.), 3rd Rev. Ed., pp. 249–342. Akadémiai Kiadó, Budapest.
Flerkó, B. (1970a). *In* "The Hypothalamus" (L. Martini, M. Motta, and F. Fraschini, eds.), pp. 351–363. Academic Press, New York.
Flerkó, B. (1970b). *La fisiopatologia dell"ovulazione, Milano, 1968, Torino,* pp. 27–44, Atti Convegni Farmitalia No. 51. Minerva Med., Torino.
Flerkó, B., and Bárdos, V. (1959). *Acta Neuroveg.* **20**, 248.
Flerkó, B., and Bárdos, V. (1960). *Acta Endocrinol. (Copenhagen)* **35**, 375.
Flerkó, B., and Bárdos, V. (1961a). *Acta Endocrinol. (Copenhagen)* **36**, 180.
Flerkó, B., and Bárdos, V. (1961b). *Acta Endocrinol. (Copenhagen)*, **37**, 418.
Flerkó, B., and Illei, G. (1957). *Acta Morphol.* **7**, 377.
Flerkó, B., and Mess, B. (1968). *Acta Physiol.* **33**, 111.
Flerkó, B., and Szentágothai, J. (1957). *Acta Endocrinol. (Copenhagen)* **26**, 121.
Flerkó, B., Petrusz, P., and Tima, L. (1967). *Acta Biol. (Budapest)* **18**, 27.
Flerkó, B., Mess, B., and Illei-Donhoffer, A. (1969). *Neuroendocrinology* **4**, 164.
Flerkó, B., Illei-Donhoffer, A., and Mess, B. (1971). *Acta Biol. (Budapest)* **22**, 125.
Gorski, R. A. (1963a). *Amer. J. Physiol.* **205**, 842.
Gorski, R. A. (1963b). *Anat. Rec.* **145**, 234.
Gorski, R. A. (1968). *Endocrinology* **82**, 1001.
Gorski, R. A., and Barraclough, C. A. (1962a). *Acta Endocrinol. (Copenhagen)* **39**, 13.
Gorski, R. A., and Barraclough, C. A. (1962b). *Proc. Soc. Exp. Biol. Med.* **110**, 298.
Gorski, R. A., and Barraclough, C. A. (1963). *Endocrinology* **73**, 210.
Gorski, R. A., and Wagner, J. W. (1965). *Endocrinology* **76**, 226.
Green, R., Luttge, W. G., and Whalen, R. E. (1969). *Endocrinology* **85**, 373.
Greer, M. A. (1953). *Endocrinology* **53**, 380.
Halász, B. (1968). *In* "Hypothalamic Control of the Anterior Pituitary" (J. Szentágothai, B. Flerkó, B. Mess, and B. Halász, eds.), 3rd Rev. Ed., pp. 110–149. Akadémiai Kiadó, Budapest.

Halász, B. (1969). In "Frontiers in Neuroendocrinology, 1969" (W. F.Ganong and L. Martini, eds.), pp. 307–342. Academic Press, New York.
Halász, B., and Gorski, R. A. (1967). *Endocrinology* 80, 608.
Halász, B., and Pupp, L. (1965). *Endocrinology* 77, 553.
Halász, B., Pupp, L., and Uhlarik, S. (1962). *J. Endocrinol.* 25, 147.
Halász, B., Pupp, L., Uhlarik, S., and Tima, L. (1965). *Endocrinology* 77, 343.
Halász, B., Florsheim, W. H., Corcorran, N. L., and Gorski, R. A. (1967). *Endocrinology* 80, 1075.
Hale, H. B. (1944). *Endocrinology* 35, 499.
Harris, G. W., and Jacobsohn, D. (1952). *Proc. Roy. Soc. Ser. B* 139, 263.
Harris, G. W., and Levine, S. (1962). *J. Physiol. (London)* 163, 42P.
Harris, G. W., and Levine, S. (1965). *J. Physiol. (London)* 181, 379.
Hayashi, S. (1967). *J. Fac. Sci. Univ. Tokyo, Sect. 4* 11, 227.
Hayashi, S. (1968). *Endocrinol. Jap.* 15, 229.
Hayashi, S. (1969). *Annot. Zool. Jap.* 42, 13.
Hemmingsen, A. M., and Krarup, N. B. (1937). *Kgl. Dan. Vidensk. Selsk., Biol. Medd.* 13, 1.
Hertz, R., and Meyer, R. K. (1937). *Endocrinology* 21, 756.
Hillarp, N. Å. (1949). *Acta Endocrinol. (Copenhagen)* 2, 11.
Hilliard, J., Hayward, J. N., and Sawyer, C. H. (1964). *Proc. Int. Congr. Endocrinol., 2nd, London.* Excerpta Med. Found. Int. Congr. Ser. 83, Part II, 1275–1276.
Hohlweg, W., and Daume, E. (1959). *Endokrinologie* 38, 46.
Hurwitz, J., Furth, J. J., Malamy, M., and Alexander, M. (1962). *Proc. Nat. Acad. Sci. U.S.* 48, 1222.
Ifft, J. D. (1962). *Anat. Rec.* 142, 1.
Jacobsohn, D. (1964). *Acta Endocrinol. (Copenhagen)* 45, 402.
Jensen, E. V., and Jacobson, H. I. (1962). *Recent Progr. Horm. Res.* 18, 387.
Jensen, E. V., Desombre, E. R., Hurst, D. J., Kawashima, T., and Jungblut, P. W. (1967). *Arch. Anat. Microsc. Morphol. Exp.* 56, Suppl. Nos. 3/4, 547.
Kanematsu, S., and Sawyer, C. H. (1963a). *Endocrinology* 73, 687.
Kanematsu, S., and Sawyer, C. H. (1963b). *Amer. J. Physiol.* 205, 1073.
Kanematsu, S., and Sawyer, C. H. (1964). *Endocrinology* 75, 579.
Kato, J., and Villee, C. A. (1967a). *Endocrinology* 80, 567.
Kato, J., and Villee, C. A. (1967b). *Endocrinology* 80, 1133.
Kawashima, S. (1964). *Annot. Zool. Jap.* 37, 79.
Kikuyama, S. (1961). *Annot. Zool. Jap.* 34, 111.
Kikuyama, S. (1962). *Annot. Zool. Jap.* 35, 6.
Kikuyama, S. (1963a). *Annot. Zool. Jap.* 36, 145.
Kikuyama, S. (1963b). *J. Fac. Sci. Univ. Tokyo, Sect. 4* 10, 231.
Kincl, F. A., and Maqueo, M. (1965). *Endocrinology* 77, 859.
King, R. J. B. (1967). *Arch. Anat. Microsc. Morphol. Exp.* 56, Suppl. Nos. 3/4, 570.
Kobayashi, F., and Gorski, R. A. (1970). *Endocrinology* 86, 285.
Kobayashi, T., Kobayashi, T., Kigawa, T., Mizuno, M., and Amenomori, Y. (1963). *Endocrinol. Jap.* 10, 16.
Kobayashi, T., Kobayashi, T., Kato, J., and Minaguchi, H. (1966). In "Steroid Dynamics" (G. Pincus, J. Tait, and T. Nakao, eds.), pp. 303–337. Academic Press, New York.
Köves, K., and Halász, B. (1969). *Neuroendocrinology* 4, 1.

Köves, K., and Halász, B. (1970). *Neuroendocrinology* **6**, 180.
Kovács, K. (1966). *Acta Anat.* **63**, 167.
Kreici, M. E., and Critchlow, B. V. (1959). *Anat. Rec.* **33**, 300.
Kurcz, M., and Gerhardt, V. J. (1968). *Endocrinol. Exp.* **2**, 29.
Kurcz, M., Kovács, K., Tiboldi, T., and Orosz, A. (1967). *Acta Endocrinol. (Copenhagen)* **54**, 663.
Kurcz, M., Maderspach, K., and Horn, G. (1969). *Acta Biol. (Budapest)* **20**, 303.
Ladosky, W. (1967). *Endokrinologie* **52**, 259.
Lipschütz, A. (1946). *Nature (London)* **157**, 551.
Lisk, R. D. (1960). *J. Exp. Zool.* **145**, 197.
Lisk, R. D. (1962). *Acta Endocrinol. (Copenhagen)* **41**, 195.
Lisk, R. D. (1963). *Anat. Rec.* **146**, 281.
Littlejohn, M., and De Groot, J. (1963). *Fed. Proc. Fed. Amer. Soc. Exp. Biol.* **22**, 571.
McCann, S. M. (1962). *Amer. J. Physiol.* **202**, 395.
McGuire, J., and Lisk, R. D. (1968). *Fed. Proc. Fed. Amer. Soc. Exp. Biol.* **27**, 270.
McGuire, J., and Lisk, R. D. (1969). *Nature (London)* **221**, 1068.
Martin, L. (1964). *J. Endocrinol.* **30**, 337.
Martinez, C., and Bittner, J. J. (1956). *Proc. Soc. Exp. Biol. Med.* **91**, 506.
Meites, J., Piacsek, B. E., and Mittler, J. C. (1967). *Proc. Int. Congr. Horm. Steroids, 2nd, Milan, 1966,* pp. 958–965.
Mess, B., Fraschini, F., Motta, M., and Martini, L. (1967). *Proc. Int. Congr. Horm. Steroids, 2nd, Milan, 1966,* pp. 1004–1013.
Michael, R. P. (1962). *Science* **136**, 322.
Mori, T. (1967). *Annot. Zool. Jap.* **40**, 82.
Mori, T. (1969). *Proc. Jap. Acad.* **45**, 931.
Noumura, T. (1958). *J. Fac. Sci. Univ. Tokyo, Sect. 4* **8**, 317.
Palka, Y. S., Ramirez, V. D., and Sawyer, C. H. (1966). *Endocrinology* **78**, 487.
Parlow, A. F. (1958). *Fed. Proc. Fed. Amer. Soc. Exp. Biol.* **17**, 402.
Pasteels, J. L. (1970). *In* "The Hypothalamus" (L. Martini, M. Motta, and F. Fraschini, eds.), pp. 385–399. Academic Press, New York.
Petrusz, P., and Flerkó, B. (1965). *Acta Biol. (Budapest)* **16**, 169.
Petrusz, P., and Flerkó, B. (1968). *Acta Biol. (Budapest)* **19**, 159.
Petrusz, P., and Nagy, É. (1967). *Acta Biol. (Budapest)* **18**, 21.
Pfeiffer, C. A. (1936). *Amer. J. Anat.* **58**, 195.
Piacsek, B. E., and Meites, J. (1966). *Endocrinology* **79**, 432.
Ralph, C. L., and Fraps, R. M. (1960). *Endocrinology* **66**, 269.
Ramirez, V. D., Abrams, R. M., and McCann, S. M. (1964). *Endocrinology* **75**, 243.
Réthelyi, M., and Halász, B. (1970). *Exp. Brain Res. (Berlin)* **11**, 145.
Sawyer, C. H., Everett, J. W., and Markee, J. E. (1949). *Endocrinology* **44**, 218.
Schapiro, S. (1965). *Endocrinology* **77**, 585.
Segal, S. J., and Johnson, D. C. (1959). *Arch. Anat. Microsc. Morphol. Exp.* **48**, 261.
Selye, H., and Friedman, S. M. (1940). *Endocrinology* **27**, 857.
Shay, H., Gershon-Cohen, J., Paschkis, K. E., and Fels, S. S. (1939). *Endocrinology* **25**, 933.
Stone, G. M. (1963). *J. Endocrinol.* **27**, 281.
Stone, G. M. (1964). *Acta Endocrinol. (Copenhagen)* **47**, 433.

Stone, G. M., Baggett, B., and Donnelly, R. B. (1963). *J. Endocrinol.* **27**, 271.
Stumpf, W. E. (1968). *Science* **162**, 1001.
Swanson, H. E., and van der Werff ten Bosch, J. J. (1964a). *Acta Endocrinol. (Copenhagen)* **45**, 1.
Swanson, H. E., and van der Werff ten Bosch, J. J. (1964b). *Acta Endocrinol. (Copenhagen)* **47**, 37.
Swanson, H. E., and van der Werff ten Bosch, J. J. (1965). *Acta Endocrinol. (Copenhagen)* **50**, 379.
Szentágothai, J. (1962). *In* "Hypothalamic Control of the Anterior Pituitary" (J. Szentágothai, B. Flerkó, B. Mess, and B. Halász, eds.), 1st Ed., pp. 19–105. Akadémiai Kiadó, Budapest.
Szentágothai, J. (1964). *Progr. Brain Res.* **5**, 135.
Takasugi, N. (1952a). *Annot. Zool. Jap.* **25**, 120.
Takasugi, N. (1952b). *Annot. Zool. Jap.* **25**, 337.
Takasugi, N. (1953a). *Annot. Zool. Jap.* **26**, 91.
Takasugi, N. (1953b). *Annot. Zool. Jap.* **26**, 52.
Takasugi, N. (1956). *J. Fac. Sci. Univ. Tokyo, Sect. 4* **7**, 625.
Takasugi, N. (1965). *Annot. Zool. Jap.* **38**, 20.
Takasugi, N., and Kimura, T. (1967). *Gumma Symp. Endocrinol. (Proc.)* **4**, 185.
Takewaki, K. (1962). *Gen. Comp. Endocrinol. Suppl.* **1**, 309.
Takewaki, K. (1964). *Endocrinol. Jap.* **11**, 1.
Takewaki, K. (1968). *Sci. Rep. Tokyo Woman's Christian Coll.* 1/6, 31.
Taleisnik, S., and McCann, S. M. (1961). *Endocrinology* **68**, 263.
Tejasen, T., and Everett, J. W. (1967). *Endocrinology* **81**, 1387.
Terasawa, W., and Sawyer, C. H. (1969). *Endocrinology* **85**, 143.
Tima, L., and Flerkó, B. (1967). *Endocrinol. Exp.* **1**, 193.
Tima, L., and Flerkó, B. (1968). *Arch. Anat. Histol. Embryol.* **51**, 699.
Tuohimaa, P., Johansson, R., and Niemi, M. (1969). *Scand. J. Clin. Lab. Invest. Suppl.* **23**, 42.
Turner, C. D. (1941). *Amer. J. Physiol.* **133**, 471.
van der Werff ten Bosch, J. J., van Rees, G. P., and Wolthuis, O. L. (1962). *Acta Endocrinol. (Copenhagen)* **40**, 103.
van Dyke, D. C., Simpson, M. E., Lepkovsky, S., Koneff, A. A., and Brobeck, J. R. (1957). *Proc. Soc. Exp. Biol. Med.* **95**, 1.
van Rees, G. P., and Gans, R. (1966). *Acta Endocrinol. (Copenhagen)* **52**, 471.
Vértes, M., and King, R. J. B. (1969). *J. Endocrinol.* **45**, xxii.
Voloschin, L., Joseph, S. A., and Knigge, K. M. (1968). *Neuroendocrinology* **3**, 141.
Wollman, A. L., and Hamilton, J. B. (1967). *Endocrinology* **81**, 350.
Woolley, D., Holinka, C., and Timiras, P. (1968). *Fed. Proc. Fed. Amer. Soc. Exp. Biol.* **27**, 270.
Yazaki, I. (1959). *Jap. J. Zool.* **12**, 267.
Yazaki, I. (1960). *Annot. Zool. Jap.* **33**, 217.

RECENT TRENDS IN THE PHYSIOLOGY OF THE POSTERIOR PITUITARY

T. Chard

DEPARTMENT OF CHEMICAL PATHOLOGY
ST. BARTHOLOMEW'S HOSPITAL MEDICAL COLLEGE
LONDON, ENGLAND

I. Introduction	82
II. Neurosecretion	83
A. The Synthesis of Oxytocin and Vasopressin in the Hypothalamus	83
B. The Release of Oxytocin and Vasopressin from the Posterior Pituitary	85
III. Neurophysin	86
A. The Properties of Neurophysin	87
B. Neurophysin as a Precursor of Oxytocin and Vasopressin	88
C. Circulating Neurophysin	89
IV. Vasopressin	93
A. The Control of Vasopressin Release	93
B. Vasopressin as a Corticotropin-Releasing Factor (CRF)	95
C. The Release of Vasopressin by the Human Fetal Pituitary during Parturition	97
V. Oxytocin	98
A. The Measurement of Circulating Oxytocin	98
B. Oxytocin and Lactation	100
C. Oxytocin as a Releasing Factor	101
D. Oxytocin and Sperm Transport	103
E. Oxytocin and Salt and Water Metabolism	104

F. Other Functions of Oxytocin 107
G. Oxytocin and Parturition in Animals 107
H. Oxytocin and Parturition in the Human 107
I. Oxytocin Release by the Human Fetus 111
VI. The Natriuretic Hormone 114
VII. Summary and Conclusions 114
References 115

I. Introduction

The posterior pituitary was among the first organs clearly recognized as having endocrine function (Oliver and Schäfer, 1895). Its extracts were shown to cause vasoconstriction and a rise in blood pressure, and it was thought that it might play a role in the control of the circulation in conjunction with the adrenal gland (Howell, 1898). Subsequently, its oxytocic (Dale, 1906; Blair-Bell, 1909), galactokinetic (Ott and Scott, 1910), and antidiuretic effects (von Konschegg and Schuster, 1915) were demonstrated. The existence of two major principles, pressor and oxytocic, was shown by Dudley (1919) and confirmed by Kamm and his colleagues (1928). These principles were shown to be associated, in the posterior pituitary, with a larger peptide molecule, the van Dyke protein (van Dyke et al., 1942). Analysis and synthesis of oxytocin followed some years later (du Vigneaud, 1956). In the meantime, it was shown that the active peptides were synthesized in the hypothalamus, and that the posterior pituitary itself served only to store and release them (Bargmann and Scharrer, 1951).

It is arguable whether any advance, comparable in importance with these, has been made in the decade 1960–1970. Rather, the developments have consisted of exploitation of the processes and materials described above. These developments fall into two groups: chemical and morphological analysis of the process of neurosecretion; and detailed studies on the control and control pathways of the release of the hormone. Many of these studies have been made possible by another important advance, less easily recognized than the above, namely, a great improvement in the methods for the assay of the hormones in biological fluids. It is common to find that work on plasma levels of oxytocin and vasopressin, reported up till 1960 or even later, are now dismissed with the comment that the possibility of interference by nonspecific factors was not sufficiently recognized. Often these comments are well justified. More recently, close attention has been given to both the specificity and the sensitivity of assays for oxytocin and vasopressin. As a result, current work using hormone assays is more reliable than that performed a decade ago, though many pitfalls remain.

The availability of specific and sensitive assays has also led to advances in the study of the physiological functions of the peptides. There have been few developments in this field since the earliest investigations. Thus, following the work of Dale (1906) and Blair-Bell (1909) on the uterotonic effects of oxytocin, it has been assumed that the posterior pituitary plays a role in normal parturition. Similarly, a role in lactation has been accepted since the description of its galactokinetic effects (Ott and Scott, 1910). Vasopressin, after a false start when only its pressor activities had been recognized, soon achieved its rightful place as the antidiuretic hormone (von Konschegg and Schuster, 1915). Subsequent work has not altered the original views on these functions, although a number of additional roles have been suggested. No function has yet been attributed to neurophysin, other than as a carrier for the octapeptides in the hypothalamic–neurohypophyseal tract.

The purpose of the present chapter is to review some aspects of posterior pituitary function which have been the subject of recent advances and to speculate where these advances may lead within the next few years. In some cases, these speculations are based on flimsy evidence, often from the study of a few plasma or urine samples. Nevertheless, they cannot be dismissed in the light of existing evidence, and should be capable of verification or dismissal by the application of current techniques.

II. Neurosecretion

The concept that oxytocin and vasopressin are synthesized in hypothalamic nuclei and transported to the posterior pituitary in association with a larger peptide, neurophysin, is now so familiar that it requires no further comment. Two aspects of neurosecretion will be discussed here: the process by which the peptides are synthesized in the hypothalamus, and the process by which they are released into the circulation in response to stimuli.

A. *The Synthesis of Vasopressin and Oxytocin in the Hypothalamus*

The studies by Sachs and his group on the hypothalamic synthesis of vasopressin and oxytocin (Sachs, 1967) are a major contribution to endocrinology. The basic experimental system is simple, synthesis of the peptides being followed by the incorporation of ^{35}S-labeled cysteine. The system has been applied to both *in vivo* studies, when the labeled material is infused into the third ventricle, and to *in vitro* studies, when the label is added to the culture medium. Since the hypothalamus and pituitary contain large quantities of ill-defined peptides (Winnick *et al.*, 1955), the hormones, including those carrying the ^{35}S-label, must be purified. This is achieved either by a battery of chromatographic fractionations, or by the use of neurophysin coupled to an insoluble support, which behaves similarly to an immunoadsorbent (Portanova and Sachs, 1967).

These studies have yielded valuable information. First, they have confirmed that vasopressin is synthesized in the hypothalamus. Second, they have shown that a chronic stimulus to release, such as dehydration, increases the rate of hormone synthesis, whereas an acute stimulus, such as hemorrhage, does not. Third, and most important, is that vasopressin appears to be initially synthesized in the form of a large precursor molecule. There are three pieces of evidence for this: (1) after infusion of cysteine-^{35}S into the third ventricle of dogs, the labeled vasopressin molecules are not found in association with ribosomes; (2) there is a lag period of about 90 minutes between the incorporation of label into peptide, and the appearance of labeled vasopressin; (3) if puromycin, which inhibits ribosomal peptide synthesis, is administered before the label, no labeled hormone appears. When puromycin is administered after the isotope, labeled vasopressin does appear. This evidence indicates that the active peptide originates as part of a larger peptide, which is broken down shortly after synthesis, probably as the neurosecretory granule is formed (Sachs and Takabatake, 1964).

Synthesis as part of a larger molecule is not confined to the neurohypophyseal peptides. It is also found with angiotensin II, which is formed by enzymatic action from an α_2-globulin via a decapeptide, angiotensin I; with kinins, including bradykinin, which are formed from α_2-globulin precursors by the action of a group of enzymes, the kallikreins; and with insulin, which arises from a large precursor molecule, proinsulin, in which the two chains of the final molecule are connected through a sequence of amino acids known as the C-peptide. A similar situation may hold with any polypeptide below a certain chain length, as there are theoretical arguments which dictate a minimum length of mRNA which can be accommodated within a ribosomal unit. Other biologically active peptides, including ACTH, calcitonin, parathormone, and glucagon, may be formed by similar mechanisms.

It is likely that the process by which oxytocin is synthesized is similar to that of vasopressin. Vogt (1953) showed that the vasopressin:oxytocin ratio decreases during progress down the hypothalamic–neurohypophyseal tract. Since most of the release of vasopressin from its precursor takes place in the neuronal cell body, this suggests that oxytocin may be dissociated at a site distal to the cell body, i.e., in the axon, or in the axon terminals of the posterior pituitary. Furthermore, if oxytocin can be transported as a precursor, then it is possible that it might be released into the circulation in this form. Peripheral release of the active peptide could then occur in a manner similar to that of angiotensin or bradykinin. It has recently been shown that "hormonogen" molecules, in which additional amino acids are linked to the amino terminus of vasopressin, can be activated *in vivo*, presumably by enzymatic action (Kyncl and Rudinger, 1970). The possibility that oxytocin might be released in precursor form will be considered further in the discussion of its physiological functions.

B. The Release of Oxytocin and Vasopressin from the Posterior Pituitary

Early studies on the release of oxytocin and vasopressin from the posterior pituitary suggested that there was a direct relationship between the amount of stainable material (neurosecretory granules) in the gland and its content of active peptides. Following a stimulus, both decreased in parallel. More recently, several workers have shown that the peptides occur in two forms in the gland: one associated with the neurosecretory granules, and one apparently free in the cytoplasm (Barer *et al.*, 1963). The relative proportions of these two forms can show considerable variation, particularly after acute stimuli. Thus, following injection of rats with formalin, stainable neurosecretory material decreases without any change in the vasopressin content of the gland (Moses *et al.*, 1963). This suggests a rapid conversion from the granular to the free form, and stands in contrast to chronic stimuli, such as lactation and water deprivation, in which depletion of stainable material and the hormone proceed in parallel. An increase in the "free" form of vasopressin has also been found following hemorrhage and anesthesia in the rat (Daniel and Lederis, 1966) coupled with the loss of granular material as shown by electron microscopy. Sachs and Haller (1968) have shown that the dog neurohypophysis can release only a small fraction of its contained vasopressin when subjected to stimulation *in vitro* or *in vivo*. In addition, they found using glands which had incorporated a cysteine-^{35}S label, that the specific activity of the hormone secreted in response to an acute stimulus was several times greater than that of the hormone remaining in the gland. This suggests that neurohypophyseal vasopressin is metabolically heterogeneous, with one fraction which has a relatively fast turnover.

Recent evidence suggests that material from the granules can be released directly into the circulation by the process of exocytosis (Herlant, 1967; Nagasawa *et al.*, 1970). It is not clear how the earlier data on the "free" and granular forms of vasopressin can be reconciled with this information, unless there are two processes occurring simultaneously. Furthermore, it is not known whether a stimulus to release would act at the level of the granular membrane, with release of its contents, or on the free peptide in the cytoplasm, with secondary release from the granules which act as a backing store.

The precise mode of secretion, direct or indirect release of the contents of the granules, could be of considerable physiological significance. In the granules themselves, the hormones are associated with the binding protein, neurophysin. Direct release of granular contents might be expected to increase circulating levels of bound physiologically inactive hormone. By contrast, indirect release through the cytoplasm would probably involve dissociation of the hormone from binding peptide so that it would be released into the circulation in its active form.

Another factor which might determine the nature of the material released is the site at which the release occurs. It is usually assumed that this is the axon terminals in the posterior pituitary. However, it has been pointed out (Bern and Knowles, 1966) that release could take place anywhere along the axon, and even from the neuronal cell body itself, since this is often in intimate contact with capillaries. Release at this level, if it is possible, would be particularly likely to include precursor material.

III. Neurophysin

In the 1920's it was argued whether the different activities of posterior pituitary extracts were associated with a single large molecule (Abel, 1924) or with several smaller molecules (Dudley, 1919). This appeared to be resolved by the studies of Kamm and his colleagues (Kamm *et al.*, 1928), who showed that there were two active principles, one oxytocic and the other pressor. However, the argument was continued by van Dyke and his co-workers (1942), who maintain that the separation of the activities as two small molecules was an artifact of the chemical procedures used. They isolated a large molecule, the so-called van Dyke protein, which has both oxytocic and pressor properties in the same proportions as the original extract. Some reconciliation of the two schools of thought was brought about by the work of Acher and his colleagues (1956), who showed that, in the posterior pituitary, the active peptides were associated with a binding protein to which they gave the name "neurophysin." The active principles could be separated from this protein by electrophoresis, dialysis against dilute acid, or precipitation with trichloroacetic acid, which would not be expected to break peptide bonds. The complex between neurophysin and the small peptides probably corresponds to the large molecule described by van Dyke. It is now thought that neurophysin is synthesized at a site adjacent to the small peptides in the cell bodies of the hypothalamus, and that it associates with the hormones in the Golgi apparatus to form the neurosecretory granules. Release of the active small peptides is associated with splitting of the neurophysin–hormone complex.

A. The Properties of Neurophysin

Neurophysin has been extensively investigated, with particular emphasis on its chemistry. To those not immediately involved with this subject, some of the published data can be confusing, especially as neurophysin is thought to exist in a number of forms, and each author has a separate system of nomenclature for the materials which he or she has prepared. The confusion is made no easier by the observation that several of the different types of neurophysin may represent artifacts of preparation (Hope, 1968; van Dyke, 1968). One critical factor is the pH at which the extractions are carried out, since this influences the activity of proteolytic enzymes.

Despite these difficulties, certain generalizations can be made about the properties of neurophysin.

1. Neurophysins extracted from the pituitaries of different species have a very similar amino acid composition (Pickering, 1969). The analysis shows a high proportion of glycine, glutamic acid, proline, and cystine. On a weight for weight basis, the number of disulfide links is similar to that of oxytocin and vasopressin.

2. The porcine posterior pituitary contains three types of neurophysin, distinguished by their mobility on starch-gel electrophoresis (Uttenthal and Hope, 1970). All can bind both oxytocin and lysine vasopressin.

3. The molecular weight has been estimated by several workers. The lowest values, which are the most likely to be correct, are of the order of 9000–10,000 for porcine materials (Wuu and Saffran, 1969; Uttenthal and Hope, 1970). As the protein concentration is raised, higher values are obtained due to polymerization.

4. The number of molecules of oxytocin and vasopressin which can be bound by a single molecule of neurophysin has been disputed. The estimates are influenced by the figure taken for the molecular weight of neurophysin. However, most authors agree that each molecule of neurophysin has not more than two or three combining sites, while in the intact state it seems likely that only one combining site per molecule is active (Hope, 1968; Wuu and Saffran, 1969).

5. Binding of the small peptides to neurophysin is optimal at pH

5.8 and is inhibited by concentrations of calcium greater than 10^{-6} M (Ginsburg et al., 1966).

6. Complexes of neurophysin and vasopressin can be crystallized (Hope, 1968), but not complexes of neurophysin and oxytocin. Crystalline structures have been observed by electron microscopy within the neurosecretory granules (Bargmann and von Gaudecker, 1969).

7. Binding of oxytocin or vasopressin to neurophysin is associated with extensive conformational changes in the neurophysin molecule (Breslow, 1970).

B. Neurophysin as a Precursor of Oxytocin and Vasopressin

It is normally assumed that neurophysin acts solely as a binding protein in the posterior pituitary, packaging the active hormone for transport down the axons, and subsequently retaining them in a nondiffusible form in the axon terminal until a physiological requirement for release arises. However, there is speculation, supported by some indirect evidence, that neurophysin represents the precursor postulated by Sachs and his group. First, the amino acid composition of neurophysin is similar to that of the active peptides, in particular in its high content of disulfide bonds. The protein isolated by Preddie (Preddie, 1965; Preddie and Saffran, 1965) from bovine posterior pituitaries, and considered as a possible precursor, also showed a high concentration of disulfide links and could have been a modified form of neurophysin. Second, neurophysin is secreted in the same area as the active peptides and in a proportion which suggests that there is one molecule of neurophysin to each oxytocin or vasopressin molecule (Hope, 1968). While it is always possible that neurophysin is formed separately from the small peptides, and at the same time a large segment of precursor molecule goes to waste, it is attractive to speculate that the large fragment of the precursor molecule has a continuing function as the physiological binder in the granules. Third, there is evidence from other systems that if a polypeptide chain is split by rupture of a peptide bond, the fragments can show a binding affinity for each other, since the complementarity of the segments is thermodynamically favored even in the absence of a covalent link between the two. One example of this is the affinity of the heavy and light chains of an immunoglobulin molecule, after reduction of the disulfide link. Other examples, and the type of bonds which might be involved, have been given by Smith (1963). Fourth, the similarity of the neurophysin from different species, as reflected by their amino acid composition and antigenicity, is reminiscent of the active peptides themselves which, with only occasional exceptions, are identical in all mammalian species.

C. Circulating Neurophysin

The posterior pituitary is depleted of neurophysin by prolonged dehydration (Friesen and Astwood, 1967). Fawcett and his colleagues (1968), using dogs in whom neurophysin had been labeled *in vivo* by the infusion of cysteine-^{35}S into the third ventricle, showed that there was a simultaneous release of both vasopressin and neurophysin into the circulation after hemorrhage. Similar results were obtained from *in vitro* studies. This evidence indicates that neurophysin can be released into the bloodstream.

1. The Measurement of Circulating Neurophysin

Direct measurement of neurophysin in the circulation is a very recent development. It depends entirely on the use of radioimmunoassay, since there is no sensitive biological assay. Radioimmunoassays for circulating neurophysin have been described by three groups (Cheng and Friesen, 1971; Legros *et al.*, 1969; Martin *et al.*, 1971). At the time of writing, the data are of a preliminary nature, as would be expected of an area so little explored. The most detailed work is that of Cheng and Friesen. They initially developed an assay for a highly purified preparation of porcine neurophysin, using this material for immunization, radioiodination, and standardization. It was then found that neurophysin from other species, including the dog, the rat, and the human, showed a complete cross-reaction with the porcine material. A similar cross-reaction between bovine and human neurophysin has been found by Legros *et al.* (1969) and Martin *et al.* (1971). An assay for either bovine or porcine neurophysin can therefore be applied to the detection of neurophysin in a number of species. This is not surprising in view of the chemical similarities between the neurophysins.

Cheng and Friesen (1970) have applied their assay to the measurement of circulating levels of neurophysin in the pig and rat. Prior to assay, neurophysin is concentrated and partially purified from plasma by means of differential precipitation with acetone. A striking rise in neurophysin levels was noted following hemorrhage in the pig, the levels falling when the blood loss was replaced. In the rat, a rise was found after stimuli such as dehydration, hemorrhage, and the infusion of hypertonic saline. The assay was also used to trace neurophysin in the posterior pituitary and its associated structures.

Legros *et al.* (1969) used an assay for bovine neurophysin. Using no extraction and concentration procedure, they found basal levels of neurophysin to be in the range 1–4 ng/ml in the serum of nonpregnant women. In pregnant women, the levels were considerably elevated. The possible significance of this material will be considered further in the discussion on the role of the posterior pituitary in parturition. Similar cross-reacting material was found also in human posterior pituitary, anterior pituitary, kidney, uterus, and breast; none was found in placenta, liver, lung, pylorus, or spleen.

Martin et al. (1971) also used an assay for bovine neurophysin. Using bentonite as an adsorbent, added neurophysin could be quantitatively recovered from human plasma. In the absence of added neurophysin a small amount (about 1–3 ng/ml) of cross-reacting material was found in the plasma of nonpregnant women and normal men. Provided that artifact can be eliminated, this represents the basal level of neurophysin in human plasma. The criteria for the exclusion of an artifact in radio-immunoassays for small peptide hormones have been described elsewhere (Chard, 1971). An interesting observation from this assay is the presence of neurophysin in tumors which are associated with ectopic secretion of vasopressin, oxytocin, or even ACTH. This indicates that neurophysin synthesis, like that of oxytocin and vasopressin, is not necessarily associated with the classical morphological type of neurosecretory system. Synthesis of a wide range of peptides by these tumors is more common than has previously been thought.

2. The Significance of Circulating Neurophysin

There is little doubt that neurophysin can be found in the circulation and is not confined to the hypothalamus and posterior pituitary. What is the significance of this finding? Four possibilities will be considered.

a. That it has no function in the circulation: this is the simplest theory and supposes that circulating neurophysin is merely a waste product of the process of neurosecretion, the bloodstream being the pathway of excretion. This theory must be assumed to be correct until firm evidence for any other function can be produced.

b. That neurophysin has a direct function of its own. This would assume that neurophysin had some systemic effect, independent of, but equivalent in importance to those of oxytocin and vasopressin. There is little evidence for such a function. A lipolytic peptide has been isolated from pig pituitaries, with a molecular weight of 8900 and an amino acid composition similar to that of neurophysin (Rudman et al., 1970).

c. That neurophysin is the precursor molecule. The evidence for this has been cited above. Nevertheless, it must remain speculative until further experimental data are available.

d. That it acts as a binder for the active peptides in the circulation: since this may be its function in the posterior pituitary, neurophysin might serve a similar function in the blood. Nevertheless, the situation in the circulation, where neurophysin is found in only low concentrations, will be different from that in the gland itself, where it is packaged with the hormones at high concentrations. Ginsburg and Thomas (1969) have shown that binding of vasopressin is dependent on the concentration of the neurophysin molecules and, furthermore, that binding of a molecule creates steric changes which favor the process. But for this to occur, high concentrations of the reactants are essential, and this situation is unlikely to hold in the circulation. Further arguments against a role of neurophysin as a plasma binder are the pH dependence of the reaction, which *in vitro* is optimal at pH 5.8, and the fact that binding is inhibited by a concentration of calcium two orders of magnitude less than that normally found in the circulation.

If neurophysin can bind the active peptides in the circulation, it should be possible to show such binding, even if it is not specifically identified with neurophysin itself. The question of plasma binding of oxytocin and vasopressin has been reviewed by Lauson (1967). Conflicting results have been obtained by different workers. Most experiments using ultrafiltration of plasma or serum have failed to show evidence of binding, either of exogenous or endogenous hormone. An exception is a recent study of human plasma, which showed that 30% of added vasopressin was nondialyzable (Fabian *et al.*, 1969). Since the percentage bound was independent of the hormone concentration over a wide range, it is difficult to attribute this to any familiar variety of peptide binding. A disadvantage of ultrafiltration methods is that they do not exclude the possibility that the binder itself is ultrafiltrable. This could apply to neurophysin if its molecular weight is less than 10,000. In contrast to the negative results obtained with ultrafiltration are the positive results of Smith and Thorn (1965). Using a gel-filtration technique, they claimed that, in the plasma of the rat, vasopressin is bound to a low molecular weight protein, the latter being eluted in the same position as a reference preparation of bovine neurophysin. Furthermore, this binding was inhibited in the presence of calcium, which can prevent binding of neurophysin to small peptides *in vitro* (Ginsburg *et al.*, 1966).

Legros and Franchimont (1971) have observed a component in the sera of pregnant women which binds iodine-labeled oxytocin, as judged by alteration of mobility of the latter on starch-gel electrophoresis. This component increases in amount throughout pregnancy and might, therefore, correspond to the material decribed by the same authors which cross-reacts with bovine neurophysin, and increases in amount during pregnancy. Equally, it should be rigorously excluded that the fast-moving component is not a breakdown product of oxytocin, due to the action of oxytocinase. Iodine-labeled oxytocin is more sensitive to the proteolytic action of this enzyme than is the native hormone (James et al., 1971). It has recently been shown (Martin, 1971) that patients treated with Pitressin, which is prepared from pituitary glands, often have circulating antibodies to neurophysin (Fig. 1). In such patients, exogenous synthetic lysine-vasopressin has an extended half-life. This suggests that the peptide is bound to neurophysin, and that the resulting complex is in turn bound by γ-globulin molecules and thus protected from the normal clearance mechanisms.

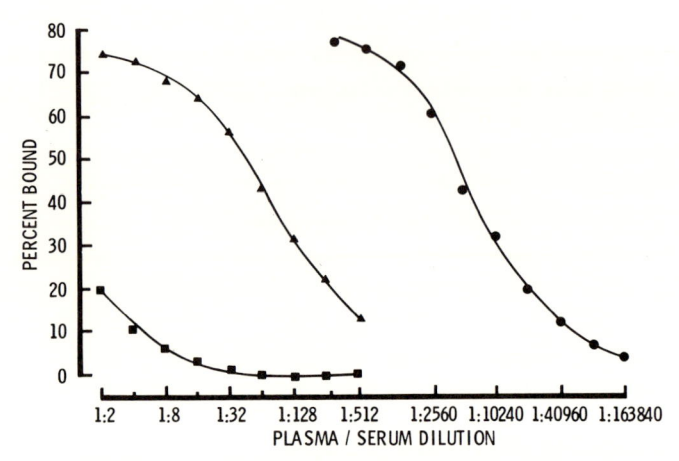

Fig. 1. The binding of ^{125}I-labeled neurophysin by control human plasma (■——■), plasma from a patient treated with Pitressin (▲——▲), and a rabbit antiserum to bovine neurophysin (●——●).

The question whether or not circulating neurophysin can bind the hormones must remain open until further evidence is available. Even if it is a circulating binder, the physiological role which this might play is not immediately obvious. For instance, if the situation is to be compared with the binding of steroids, or of certain drugs, then a proportion of circulating oxytocin or vasopressin would be physiologically inactive. There is no firm evidence for or against such a fraction. Furthermore, binding is usually assessed by the addition of exogenous peptide to plasma either *in vitro* or *in vivo*. It is always possible, as with vitamin B$_{12}$ (Hall, 1962), that the binding of exogenous and endogenous material is quite different. A further possibility, which will be discussed later, is that neurophysin binds the peptides in the tissues.

The development of radioimmunoassays for neurophysin, oxytocin, and vasopressin raises the possibility of further investigation of some of these roles of neurophysin. An immunoassay detects the hormone by its chemical properties, and it is possible to trace the peptide independently of its biological activities, which may become manifest only after their release from binding or after the precursor has reached the target organ. Such procedures have been applied to the study of the renin–angiotensin system (Boyd et al., 1969). Experiments of this type have also been performed using human late pregnancy plasma, and extracts of myometrium obtained during cesarean section. Using a wide variety of conditions, it was not possible to demonstrate any formation of oxytocin within the system (Chard and Boyd, unpublished observations). Very recently, it has been shown that there is a simultaneous release of vasopressin and neurophysin, following stimuli such as hemorrhage (Burton et al., 1971). This, again, does not support the view that circulating neurophysin is a precursor of the active hormones.

IV. Vasopressin

Three topics will be discussed here: the mechanisms controlling vasopressin release; the role of vasopressin as a corticotropin-releasing factor; and the release of vasopressin by the fetal pituitary at the time of delivery.

A. The Control of Vasopressin Release

The basic mechanisms are well known: (1) receptors in the hypothalamus sensitive to osmotic stimuli; (2) receptors in the large vessels of the thorax which are sensitive to changes in blood volume, the stimuli being mediated via the vagus and the midbrain to the hypothalamus.

1. THE CONTROL OF VASOPRESSIN RELEASE BY OSMORECEPTORS

The classical work of Verney (1947) demonstrated that an increase in the tonicity of the blood entering the carotid circulation could lead to the release of vasopressin. As a result of these and subsequent studies, it is widely assumed that the physiological control of vasopressin release in relation to salt and water metabolism is mediated by osmoreceptors situated in the distribution of the carotid artery. These receptors appear to lie in the diencephalon (Saito et al., 1969). Recent studies using microelectrodes implanted in single cells of the hypothalamus have indicated that the osmosensitive neurons are situated at the periphery of the supraoptic nucleus (Hayward and Vincent, 1970). The connections between these neurons and the neurosecretory cell bodies include both adrenergic and cholinergic synapses (Bridges and Thorn, 1970).

However, it should be noted that much of this experimental work has been carried out with grossly unphysiological stimuli. The osmoreceptors have been located by the infusion of hypertonic solutions, often directly into the carotid artery. Normal water and electrolyte balance does not involve such dramatic variations, and plasma osmolality in the human shows very little variation under physiological conditions. The intracarotid infusion of hypertonic solutions can stimulate a number of intracranial structures in which the blood–brain barrier does not prevent the passage of ions (Clemente et al., 1957; Holland et al., 1959). The response to such solutions might, therefore, be nonspecific. In this respect, it is notable that they seem to cause parallel release of both oxytocin and vasopressin (Abrahams and Pickford, 1954; Holland et al., 1959), whereas a specific release would be expected to consist of vasopressin alone.

It is possible that other mechanisms might be involved in the finer changes of the nonexperimental situation. The infusion of small quantities of angiotensin into conscious dogs can stimulate vasopressin release equivalent to that found after 24 hours of dehydration (Bonjour and Malvin, 1970). Intracarotid injections are more efficient than intravenous (Mouw et al., 1971), suggesting that the receptors are somewhere in the brain. These results indicate that there may be a physiological relationship between the renin–angiotensin–aldosterone system and the secretion of vasopressin. Angiotensin, itself, when applied directly to the brain, is the most potent dipsogenic substance known (Epstein et al., 1970). A mechanism involving angiotensin release by the kidney, with subsequent effects on the brain and hypothalamus, might be highly sensitive to small variations in water and electrolyte metabolism.

2. The Control of Vasopressin Release by Volume Receptors

Increasing emphasis is being placed on the role of intrathoracic volume receptors in the control of vasopressin release. Most experiments have involved the comparatively unphysiological stimulus of hemorrhage, but changes have also been demonstrated in response to small variations in left atrial pressure (Johnson et al., 1969). There has been some argument, however, as to whether the fluid and electrolyte changes found in this type of experiment are actually due to altered release of vasopressin or to some other mechanism (Goetz et al., 1970). It seems likely that both osmotic and volume receptors are important in the control of vasopressin secretion, and that neither is dominant over the other (Johnson et al., 1970). Osmotic stimuli can be overridden in the presence of a water diuresis (Olsson and McDonald, 1970). The parallel activity of these two systems may explain why there has been confusion over the role of vasopressin in the fluid and electrolyte changes which accompany acute adrenal insufficiency. Thus, whether or not there is a change in vasopressin levels may be determined by variations in maintenance therapy (Share and Travis, 1970). A dissociation between the two systems, with a relative impairment of osmotic control, has been indicated as a cause of "essential" hypernatremia (De Rubertis et al., 1971).

Although acute stimuli from the volume receptors can cause vasopressin release, it is doubtful if the peptide plays a role in the normal control of the circulation, despite some recent suggestions to the contrary (Traber et al., 1968; Rocha et Silva and Rosenberg, 1969). The levels found by specific assays in normal subjects are considerably below those which would be expected to have a pressor effect.

3. The Relation of Vasopressin Release to Higher Centers in the Brain

An aspect of vasopressin function which has received little attention is its relationship to higher levels of the central nervous system, in particular the thirst center. Miller et al. (1968) have shown that water-loaded rats could be trained to choose the arm of a T-maze in which they did not receive an injection of vasopressin. By contrast, rats with diabetes insipidus and a salt load chose the arm in which they received vasopressin, thus helping them to excrete excess NaCl. An excess of water or NaCl can therefore act as a drive, and the return to normal levels produced by an endocrine response can act as a reward. Chiaraviglio and Taleisnik (1969) showed that the introduction of cholinergic or adrenergic agents into the third ventricle of rats determined their choice between the consumption of distilled water or 1% NaCl. Vasopressin and oxytocin do not, themselves, appear to affect the thirst center, while angiotensin has a very potent effect (Epstein et al., 1970).

B. Vasopressin as a Corticotropin-Releasing Factor (CRF)

The hypothalamic–neurohypophyseal system is a specialized subsection of a much broader hypothalamic–neurosecretory system, which includes the releasing factors for the anterior pituitary. The major difference is that the neurohypophyseal system discharges its products into the systemic circulation, whereas the hypothalamic releasing factors are secreted into the small-volume pituitary portal circulation, or possibly into the cerebrospinal fluid. Both types of peptide are synthesized within neuronal cell bodies of the hypothalamus, and both are released into the blood stream through a virtually identical neurohemal organ. The importance of this similarity between the two systems is 2-fold. First, the posterior pituitary is much more accessible for experimental work, and may provide a useful model for the physiology of the releasing factors. Second, the neurohypophyseal principles may themselves be releasing factors. Anatomically this is quite possible. Fibers from the supraoptic and paraventricular nuclei, indistinguishable from those proceeding to the posterior pituitary itself, are traceable to the capillaries of the pituitary portal system (Daniel, 1966). In addition, the system of "short" portal vessels which arises from the arterial ring supplying the posterior pituitary, represent a direct connection between the anterior and posterior lobes.

Since the demonstration by Nagareda and Gaunt (1951) that vasopressin could stimulate the pituitary–adrenal axis, there has been extensive argument as to whether this is a physiological role of the peptide (reviewed by Ratcliffe and Knight, 1971). The chief protagonists of the view that vasopressin can act as a releasing factor are McCann and Dhariwal (1966). They have concluded that vasopressin acts by potentiating a specific corticotropin-releasing factor (Yates et al., 1971). Studies on homozygous Brattleboro rats, which have a hereditary absence of vasopressin, have shown partial deficiencies in pituitary–adrenal function (McCann et al., 1966), further indicating that although vasopressin may not be the main corticotropin-releasing factor, it nevertheless has a subsidiary role in the pituitary–adrenal response to stress.

Although attractive, the concept of vasopressin as a releasing factor is not easy to either prove or disprove. For instance, observation of the effects of administered vasopressin, either systemic or local, is likely to be confusing, since it will have potent side effects such as vasoconstriction, which might cause a secondary "stress" release of ACTH. However, Brostoff and his colleagues (1968) showed that the infusion of LVP in man is a relatively specific stimulus to the pituitary–adrenal axis, since a parallel release of growth hormone was only seen when the subject experienced side effects. Arimura and his colleagues (1969) have shown that the corticotropin-releasing activity of lysine-vasopressin analogs is not related to their pressor or antidiuretic activity.

If vasopressin does have a role in ACTH release, the neurons in which the pathways originate might be under separate control from those involved in the systemic release of vasopressin. The quantity of hormone liberated at these terminals, since the target organ is only a few millimeters downstream in a capillary bed, could be so minute as to be insignificant in the general circulation and undetectable by classical plasma assays.

C. The Release of Vasopressin by the Human Fetal Pituitary during Parturition

The presence of vasopressin in umbilical cord blood, at levels higher than those normally encountered in adult plasma, was shown by Hoppenstein et al. (1968). Raised levels were found at spontaneous delivery (average 35 μU/ml) and lower levels when the child was delivered by cesarean section (average 0.83 μU/ml). The levels decreased rapidly after birth, and remained at subnormal values for some days, suggesting pituitary exhaustion. These findings have been confirmed and extended using a highly specific radioimmunoassay for arginine-vasopressin (Chard et al., 1971).

Two features of this situation merit further comment. First, when simultaneous samples are available from the umbilical artery and vein, the levels in the artery are almost invariably found to be the higher. This arteriovenous difference indicates that the peptide originates in the fetal neurohypophysis, and is partly cleared during its passage through the placental circulation. Second, the levels in the umbilical artery are sometimes as high as 3–4 ng (1.5–2 mU) per milliliter. These levels are among the highest recorded in human physiology and could well have a vasopressor action. Such an effect on the umbilical and placental circulation would be detrimental to the well-being of the child. However, no correlation has been found between the condition of the fetus at the time of delivery and the cord levels of vasopressin, so that the clinical significance of this finding is unclear. Furthermore, on isolated umbilical cord vessels, oxytocin is a much more effective vasoconstrictor than is vasopressin (Somlyo and Somlyo, 1970).

The cause and significance of this release of vasopressin will be considered in the discussion on fetal release of oxytocin (Section V, E). It should be noted that one group of workers consider that the neurohypophysis of fetuses from certain mammals may secrete large amounts of arginine-vasotocin (Vizsolyi and Perks, 1969). The possibility that this is the material which is being measured in cord blood has been excluded by radioimmunological studies using antisera of defined specificity.

In view of the earlier comments on the possible role of vasopressin as a releasing factor for ACTH, it is of interest that the cord blood levels of ACTH are almost invariably within the normal range for the adult under resting conditions (Ratcliffe and Chard, unpublished observations). If the fetal anterior pituitary at the time of delivery is capable of releasing ACTH, then this presents a situation in which the release of endogenous vasopressin does not affect ACTH secretion. However, the pituitary–adrenal system may not be fully responsive at this period of life (Milkovic and Milkovic, 1966).

V. Oxytocin

Oxytocin is the "orphan" hormone of general endocrinology. Apart from its role in parturition and lactation, it has no very clearly defined functions. Thus, in the case of the female, it has to be assumed that the peptide operates for only a few hours in a lifetime. In the male, it may have no function at all. Yet oxytocin is found in both male and female pituitaries in quantities equivalent to those of vasopressin (Currie et al., 1960). Furthermore, there is no evidence that oxytocin synthesis is any less active than that of vasopressin, as judged by comparison of activity in the supraoptic and paraventricular nuclei.

It is difficult to believe that the functions of oxytocin are as circumscribed as this. In this section the traditional functions of the peptide in parturition and lactation will be discussed. Other possible roles will also be considered, including the control of anterior pituitary function (as a releasing factor), the stimulation of sperm transport, some general metabolic effects, and a role in the control of salt and water metabolism.

A. *The Measurement of Circulating Oxytocin*

It was pointed out above that studies of the functions of oxytocin and vasopressin have been retarded by the lack of specific and sensitive assays for the circulating levels of the hormone. This applies with even more force to oxytocin than to vasopressin. Assays for the former depend on muscle contraction: either the uterus, or the myoepithelial tissue of the breast. Numerous biological substances can mimic this effect and, as a result, the conditions for a satisfactory assay of oxytocin are even more exiguous than those for vasopressin. Indeed, there are those who would argue that oxytocin as such is hardly ever measured (Theobald, 1968). Examination of the literature on oxytocin levels in the human shows that the viewpoint is not exaggerated. It is rare to find reports in which oxytocin has been sought but not found, and it is remarkable how often levels lie in the lower range of sensitivity of the assay used, whether this be 5 or 500 μU/ml. Similar observations can also be made about some work with vasopressin.

There are few ways in which to improve the specificity of biological assays for oxytocin, beyond those which have already been described. But if the assay itself cannot be improved, it is still possible to achieve specificity by the application of preliminary extraction and purification procedures. A number of such techniques have been described (Bisset and Walker, 1954; Ginsburg and Smith, 1959; Folley and Knaggs, 1965; Coch *et al.*, 1965; Chard *et al.*, 1970) though none are perfect.

The Measurement of Oxytocin by Radioimmunoassay

A recent approach to the problem of specificity in the measurement of oxytocin has been the application of radioimmunoassay techniques (Glick *et al.*, 1969; Chard *et al.*, 1969). None of the identifiable substances which are known to interfere with a biological assay have any

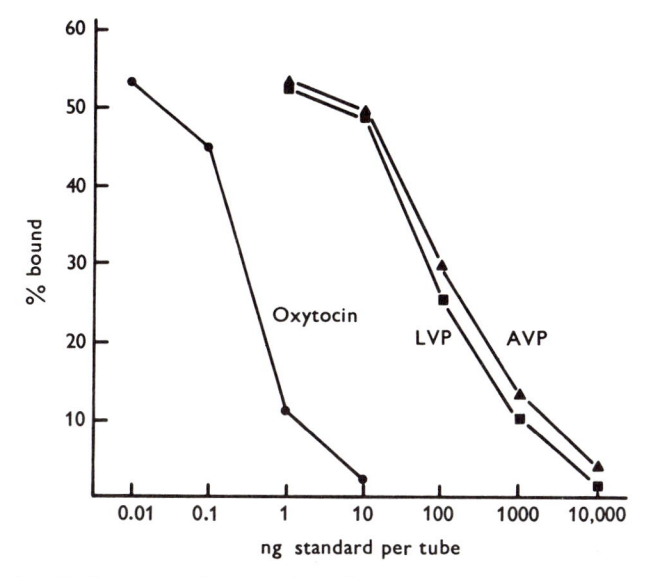

Fig. 2. Standard curves, showing the inhibition of the binding of oxytocin-^{131}I and a rabbit antioxytocin serum, by oxytocin, arginine-vasopressin (AVP), and lysine-vasopressin (LVP).

effect on the antigen-antibody reaction of the radioimmunoassay. Not surprisingly, arginine-vasopressin shows some cross-reaction with oxytocin, but its activity in this respect is only 0.1% of that of oxytocin itself (Fig. 2), which compares favorably with the minimum of 5% interference found with biological assays. Using a radioimmunoassay which, when combined with an extraction procedure, has a sensitivity of 1 μU/ml of plasma, negative results are the rule rather than the exception (Chard *et al.*, 1970). This is reassuring, since if nothing is measured, the problem of nonspecificity does not arise. Set against a background of negative "blank" values, positive results are easier to interpret.

Some mention should be made of the disadvantages of a radioimmunoassay. The assay may measure fragments of the hormone which are not biologically active (Besser *et al.*, 1969; Franchimont, 1971). Such a dissociation between biological and immunological activity can occur with oxytocin (Forsling *et al.*, 1971; James *et al.*, 1971). However, the difference between estimates by the two methods is not great. A study of endogenous levels of oxytocin in goat plasma collected at the time of delivery has shown almost identical results by radioimmunoassay and bioassay (McNeilly *et al.*, 1971). Another possibility with a radioimmunoassay is that apparent levels may be found which are due to nonspecific inhibition of the antigen-antibody reaction, unrelated to any biological activity in the plasma. As noted above, the finding of negative results in blank samples goes some way to excluding this possibility. However, it cannot be totally excluded because the very situation which is being investigated may be associated with the release of such nonspecific inhibitors. With most hormones, the study of well-defined physiological situations will provide the answer to the problem of nonspecificity. For instance, the suppression of ACTH secretion by dexamethasone administration should be reflected in the plasma levels of the hormone as measured by the assay. With oxytocin in the human, there are no such well defined situations and specificity can be proved only when there is confirmation from bioassay, and from indirect studies on the function involved.

B. Oxytocin and Lactation

The galactokinetic effect of posterior pituitary extracts was described by Ott and Scott (1910), and the role of oxytocin in normal lactation by Ely and Petersen (1941). There is evidence, both from assays of circulating hormone and from a variety of experimental manipulations, that oxytocin release is the result of a neuroendocrine reflex originated by stimulation of the breast or nipple. Circulating oxytocin then produces milk letdown by stimulating the myoepithelial elements of the mammary gland to contract. However, there are several details of this simple process which are not entirely clear, such as the nature and timing of oxytocin release in relation to milk letdown, and this can be studied only by direct assay of circulating hormone. An important observation from such studies is that oxytocin release does not invariably occur at the time of suckling. Cleverley and Folley (1970) were able to find oxytocin in only 17 out of 24 experiments on cows from whom serial samples were taken. There was no difference in milk yield between those animals in which oxytocin was detected and those in which it was not. Studies in women show that oxytocin release with normal lactation is the exception rather than the rule (Fox and Knaggs, 1969; Fox and Chard, unpublished observations). Thus, milk letdown can occur without detectable oxytocin release. Another observation, arising from studies in both animals (Knaggs, 1963; Cleverley and Folley, 1970) and man (Fox and Knaggs, 1969), is that the release of oxytocin is usually transient. This "spurt" release is of considerable significance in relation to the physiological function of the hormone. First, it may explain why oxytocin cannot be uniformly detected at the time of suckling. Second the circulating levels of the hormone are often unrelated to the effect on the target organ. The same level of activity, in terms of intramammary pressure, may be associated with widely differing and even undetectable levels of oxytocin in the bloodstream. It is possible that supplementary mechanisms may operate, such as direct mechanical stimulation or intrinsic neural reflexes. An alternative explanation of constant end-organ activity in the face of fluctuating levels of a circulating stimulant is local binding of the hormone. This possibility is considered below in the discussion on human parturition.

The timing of the release of oxytocin has been studied in detail. The spurt release can be initiated by stimulation of the nipple either by the young or artificially by a teat-cup (Knaggs, 1963) and is often followed by a second release. However, analysis of data accumulated over a period of several years on animal lactation has shown that the release of oxytocin cannot be precisely related to any one event in the suckling or milking process. Using this information, McNeilly (personal communication, 1970) has suggested that the concept of oxytocin release as a conditioned reflex must be discarded, and replaced with the concept of a period, which may embrace the whole suckling process, and during which oxytocin release is likely to occur. This concept of a specific period during which the threshold for oxytocin release is lowered may be a considerable advance in thinking about oxytocin release in lactation, and also possibly under other circumstances.

It is of interest, in view of the apparent inactivity of oxytocin in the male, that transient oxytocin release has been found in a man with galactorrhea following stimulation with a breast pump (Edwards and Besser, unpublished observations).

C. Oxytocin as a Releasing Factor

The role of oxytocin as a releasing factor for prolactin has been argued since the concept was suggested by Petersen (1942). The idea is attractive, since there is a close relationship between oxytocin and prolactin in the control of lactation, and there are morphological features, discussed above (Section IV, C) which suggest pathways between the anterior and posterior pituitary. The first experimental evidence came from Benson and Folley (1957), who showed that oxytocin can prevent mammary involution in lactating rats deprived of their litters. However, the interpretation of this work has been attacked, notably by Meites and Hopkins (1961) who attribute the stimulation of milk secretion by oxytocin to the periodic emptying of the alveoli. The increase in milk yield in cattle given oxytocin is also known to be due to a simple mechanical effect on milk letdown.

A second line of evidence for the role of oxytocin as a releasing factor is its effect on luteotropic activity, which is a known function of prolactin. Oxytocin can induce alterations in the length of the luteal phase in cattle (Armstrong and Hansel, 1958; Donaldson and Takken, 1968), but not in rats (Rothchild and Quilligan, 1960). It has also been shown that the corpora lutea of heifers treated with oxytocin have a decreased ability to synthesize progesterone (Wilks *et al.*, 1969). However, it is possible that release of the uterine luteolytic factor might be responsible for some of these results. Huntingford (1963) studied intrasplenic ovarian grafts in castrated rats, and demonstrated that luteinization could be produced by oxytocin, although a direct effect on the graft was not excluded. Huntingford noted a number of points that might explain the contradictory results of previous workers, such as species differences, and the dose and duration of treatment with oxytocin. For instance, he found that high doses of oxytocin would inhibit luteinization, while lower doses were stimulating. Donaldson and Takken (1968) also showed that low doses of oxytocin could stimulate the corpus luteum in cattle, while higher doses were inhibitory. Similar results were noted by Saffran (1959) when investigating vasopressin as a corticotropin-releasing factor; low doses caused release while high doses had no effect.

A notable feature of prolactin and its control by the hypothalamus, is that, in contrast to the other anterior pituitary hormones, the effect of its releasing factor is inhibitory. The anterior pituitary deprived of its connections with the hypothalamus, either *in vitro* or *in vivo,* secretes prolactin at a high rate (reviewed by Chard, 1964). This fact throws some doubts on experimental work which indicates a stimulating rather than an inhibitory effect on luteal function. Indeed, Haun and Sawyer (1960) have suggested that the function of oxytocin is to release the inhibition. However, this criticism of earlier work does not take into account the quantitative factors emphasized by Huntingford. Furthermore, it is difficult to investigate the possible effects of compounds which may be highly active in the pituitary portal circulation by systemic administration. Under these circumstances, nonspecific effects may be the rule rather than the exception. Such effects are also seen when large amounts of material are applied to *in vitro* preparations. For instance, both oxytocin and vasopressin can elicit thyrotropin release from the cultured bovine anterior pituitary (Krass et al., 1968).

There is evidence for an effect of oxytocin on other aspects of gonadotropic function (Franchimont and Legros, 1969), though others have not been able to confirm this (Ditlove and Faiman, 1970).

D. Oxytocin and Sperm Transport

That oxytocin might play a role in sperm transport was noted by Harris (1947). He suggested that a release of the peptide at the time of coitus would augment uterine mobility and thus accelerate the ascent of spermotozoa. Despite careful experimental work in the intervening years, the evidence for this function is circumstantial and incomplete. In particular, as with other branches of oxytocin physiology, there is a paucity of data from specific assays of plasma levels.

1. Oxytocin and Sperm Transport in the Female

There are three lines of evidence for a role of oxytocin in sperm transport in the female: (1) An increase in uterine motility is associated with coitus. This increase has been shown in response to genital stimulation in cattle (van Demark and Hays, 1952), and a similar response has been shown during orgasm in the human (Fox and Fox, 1969). It has been argued by Cross (1958) that the increase of uterine motility observed under these circumstances could be due to a spinal reflex. (b) An increase in milk-ejection pressure follows genital stimulation in cattle (Hays and van Demark, 1953; Debackere and Peeters, 1960). This was assumed to reflect elevated levels of circulating oxytocin, and was equivalent to that following injection of 50–100 mU of oxytocin intravenously. That the effect was due to a circulating substance, and not to a nervous reflex, was shown by cross-circulation experiments (Debackere et al., 1961). Milk ejection has been observed in association with orgasm in the human (Harris and Pickles, 1953). (c) Fitzpatrick (1957) showed a considerable increase in circulating oxytocin following genital stimulation in cows, but in the light of subsequent data the levels seem remarkably high. McNeilly and Folley (1970) studied 26 matings in goats. Oxytocin was found in the circulating blood of the female in 19 of these, the levels ranging from 2 to 190 μU/ml. In most experiments, oxytocin was found before intromission, often as the male entered the mating room. Fox and Knaggs (1969) have found oxytocin in the plasma of women at the time of orgasm. However, as with other aspects of oxytocin physiology, this seems to be a sporadic occurrence (Fox and Chard, unpublished observations), and it should be noted that the human nonpregnant uterus is relatively insensitive to oxytocin.

Against a role of oxytocin in sperm transport is the fact that sperm migration is normal in female rats with experimental diabetes insipidus (Manabe, 1969).

2. Oxytocin and Sperm Transport in the Male

Cross-circulation experiments using a ram and a lactating ewe (Debackere et al., 1961) have shown that an increase in milk ejection is associated with stimulation of the internal genitalia of the ram. Further evidence for a role of oxytocin in sperm transport in the male is reviewed by Cross (1966). He concludes that a reflex release of oxytocin after ejaculation might accelerate the passage of sperm to the epididymis in readiness for subsequent ejaculation. In male rabbits, administered oxytocin is said to raise the motivation for copulation, and to increase the output of fluid from the accessory glands (Fjellstrom et al., 1968). Assays for oxytocin in human male plasma collected at the time of orgasm have been negative (Fox and Knaggs, 1969).

E. Oxytocin and Salt and Water Metabolism

In contrast to vasopressin, the functions of oxytocin in salt and water metabolism are ill-defined, although there is evidence that it may play an important role. This evidence is 2-fold: that based on observations of the effects of administered oxytocin, and that based on measurement of oxytocin levels in plasma and urine.

1. The Effect of Exogenous Oxytocin on Salt and Water Metabolism

Most of the work on the effects of exogenous oxytocin was carried out using partially or highly purified pituitary extracts (reviewed by Thorn, 1968). Such extracts are likely to contain material other than oxytocin, and although the work was excellent, there must be doubts on the specificity of the results. Since highly purified synthetic oxytocin became available, this problem of specificity has been largely eliminated. Two effects of exogenous synthetic oxytocin have been described: a diuretic-antidiuretic effect and a natriuretic effect.

The data in experimental animals, mainly dogs and rats, are summarized in Table I. In high doses, oxytocin causes antidiuresis, which in the case of the rat represents 1% of the effect of an equivalent dose of arginine-vasopressin. In smaller doses it can have a diuretic effect. Several workers have observed a natriuretic effect of oxytocin, particularly at low rates of urinary flow. Lees and Allsup (1969) studied the interaction of oxytocin and aldosterone in rats and showed that the natriuretic effect was less after adrenalectomy. In contrast to these results

Table I
The Effects of Synthetic Oxytocin on Salt and Water Metabolism in Experimental Animals

Effect studied	Species	Result	Authors
Antidiuresis	Rat	+	Chan (1965)
Antidiuresis	Rat	+	Berde and Boissonas (1968)
Antidiuresis	Dog	+	Brooks and Pickford (1958)
Diuresis	Rat	+	Chan (1965)
Diuresis	Rat	+	Barnafi et al. (1960)
Diuresis	Rat	+	Brunner et al. (1957)
Increased Na excretion	Rat	+	Croxatto and Labarca (1958)
Increased Na excretion	Rat	+	Barnafi et al. (1960)
Increased Na excretion	Rat	+	Chan (1965)
Increased Na excretion	Rat	+	Brunner et al. (1957)
Increased Na excretion	Dog	+	Chan and Sawyer (1961)
Increased Na excretion	Dog	−	Massry et al. (1969)

Massry and his colleagues (1969) were unable to find an effect of oxytocin on the natriuresis associated with extracellular volume expansion. However, under these circumstances, urinary flow would tend to be high and, therefore, oxytocin would be less effective as a natriuretic agent. Another group (Sadowski et al., 1968) have shown that infusions of oxytocin into a renal artery have a sodium-retaining effect, in both the infused and the opposite kidney. This would suggest an indirect effect of oxytocin on sodium handling. The method of administration does not allow a comparison of these results with those of other workers. At very high doses, oxytocin has an effect on renal plasma flow and glomerular filtration rate, but this is not apparent when more physiological doses are used (Chan and Sawyer, 1961).

In the human, as in animals, an antidiuretic effect has been found at high doses (Thomson, 1960; Saunders and Munsick, 1966; Munsick and Gresham, 1970) though one group, surprisingly, could not find this (Cross et al., 1960). Natriuresis has not been convincingly demonstrated (Cross et al., 1960; Thomson, 1960; Saunders and Munsick, 1966; Goodwin et al., 1970). However, as the doses used were grossly unphysiological, the evidence does not exclude an effect at lower levels. Furthermore, experiments of this type should be carried out with close attention to the salt and water balance of the subjects studied and, in particular, to the rate of urinary flow. The actions of oxytocin on the toad bladder and the frog skin *in vitro* have also been examined. The effects are identical with those of vasopressin, although higher concentrations are required.

2. The Measurement of Oxytocin Levels in Relation to Salt and Water Metabolism

Massry and his colleagues (1969) measured jugular oxytocin in dogs during the natriuresis associated with extracellular volume expansion. In 5 out of 8 cases no significant rise was found. Schrier and his colleagues (1968) found no increase of oxytocin in the plasma of dogs excreting sodium following an infusion of 0.9% saline. Jones and Pickering (1969) compared rats given 2% saline to drink, or deprived of water for 5 days. Depletion of vasopressin from the neurohypophysis was the same in both groups, whereas depletion of oxytocin was greater in the saline-treated animals.

Studies using a highly specific radioimmunoassay have shown that oxytocin levels in the peripheral venous blood of normal males are usually below the sensitivity of the assay, 1 μU/ml (Chard et al., 1970). This method cannot, therefore, be applied to the detection of variations in circulating levels in relation to salt and water metabolism. However, oxytocin can be detected in normal male urine (Boyd and Chard, 1971) at levels which would correspond to a plasma concentration below the sensitivity of the assay. The finding of oxytocin in male urine demonstrates two important points: (1) that the male posterior pituitary, which is known to contain oxytocin, can release the peptide and (2) that this release, over the time scale of a typical urine collection, is continuous rather than intermittent.

Measurement of oxytocin in urine, in amounts which reflect the secretion of only a few milliunits from the gland, presents a new opportunity for the study of the nonobstetric functions of the peptide. At the time of writing, experimental evidence in this area is limited. In a normal male subject, studied over 5 days, and secreting persistently hypertonic urine, urinary oxytocin levels were closely correlated with those of vasopressin. It is not possible to say whether this represents a specific physiological release of the hormone, or simply an overspill of the peptide from the pituitary gland, nonspecifically related to the output of vasopressin. The amounts of oxytocin are very small, and correspond to plasma levels below those at which oxytocin might be expected to have any effect on salt and water metabolism.

If the urinary levels of oxytocin are to be used as an indication of endogenous hormone release, it is essential that the urinary clearance rate of this hormone be accurately known. A recent study has shown that, contrary to expectation, the urinary clearance of oxytocin is directly related to the rate of urinary flow (Boyd et al., 1972). Thus, oxytocin appears to be handled by the kidney in exactly the same manner as water. This has the important implication that the urinary concentration reflects the plasma concentration, regardless of the rate of urine output. There is some evidence that the urinary excretion of vasopressin may follow a similar pattern (Fabian et al., 1969).

F. Other Functions of Oxytocin

Since so little is known about oxytocin, it is not surprising that a wide variety of functions has been suggested. Most of these suggestions are based on the effects of synthetic oxytocin, often at concentrations more than one million times those known to be physiological. Nevertheless, in view of the possibility of local concentration of peptide hormones, such functions cannot be totally excluded. The following is an incomplete list: (1) an "insulinlike" metabolic effect, stimulating the uptake of glucose and the formation of free fatty acids by adipose tissue (Mirsky, 1969); (2) antiarrhythmic effect on the myocardium (Panisset and Beaulnes, 1961); (3) a vasodilator effect (Kitchin et al., 1959).

Oxytocin has been described in a tumor associated with ectopic hormone secretions (Marks et al., 1968). Using a radioimmunoassay, oxytocin has been found recently in a number of such tumors, the clinical presentation being either ectopic ACTH secretion, or ectopic vasopressin secretion (Chard, unpublished observations).

G. Oxytocin and Parturition in Animals

Since the original observations by Dale (1906) and Blair-Bell (1909) that extracts of the posterior pituitary have a potent stimulating effect on the uterus, it has been assumed that this gland plays a role in normal parturition, and particularly in the ejection of the fetus. This was confirmed by the demonstration in sheep, cows, and goats that circulating levels of oxytocin were raised during labor, being highest at the time of delivery (Fitzpatrick, 1961; Fitzpatrick and Walmsley, 1962; Knaggs, 1963; Folley and Knaggs, 1965; Chard et al., 1970). Release is thought to be mediated by a nervous reflex from stretching of the cervix and vagina. A rise in circulating oxytocin levels in response to vaginal stimulation has been shown in cows (Roberts and Share, 1968). This response is enhanced by estrogen administration, and depressed by progesterone (Roberts and Share, 1969, 1970), an observation which suggests that the steroid environment in pregnancy may have an important central influence on oxytocin release.

H. Oxytocin and Parturition in the Human

By contrast to the situation in animals, the role of endogenous oxytocin in human labor has been much argued. There have been a number of studies on the circulating levels of oxytocin in normal human labor using either bioassay or immunoassay (Table II), which have shown the presence of oxytocin in amounts exceeding 100 μU per milliliter of plasma. In the light of the data obtained from animals, these findings would occasion no surprise, were it not that indirect evidence suggests that levels of endogenous hormone do not exceed 10 μU/ml (Table II). Most of this indirect evidence comes from studies in which oxytocin is given by continuous intravenous infusion for the induction of labor. Two authors have calculated the plasma levels achieved by infusions at a rate sufficient to produce uterine contractions which mimic those

Table II
The Circulating Levels of Oxytocin in Spontaneous Human Labor

Type of assay	Levels (μU/ml)	References
Bioassay	1390	Hawker et al. (1961)
Bioassay	80–200	Fitzpatrick and Walmsley (1965)
Bioassay	300–900 (internal jugular) 100–300 (peripheral)	Coch et al. (1965)
Immunoassay	7500	Bashore (1967)
Immunoassay	10–75 (1st stage) 100–200 (2nd stage)	Glick et al. (1969)
Indirect estimate	3	Saameli (1963)
Indirect estimate	0.07	Theobald (1968)

of spontaneous labor. The estimates made on this basis have been 3 μU/ml (Saameli, 1963) and 0.07 μU/ml (Theobald, 1968). In addition, Caldeyro-Barcia and Poseiro (1959) have suggested that the rate of infusion of oxytocin which corresponds to endogenous release at the beginning of labor is 2 mU per minute; this would yield plasma levels less than 10 μU/ml. In another indirect approach, Cobo (1968) measured intrammary pressure in several women throughout spontaneous labor. He was unable to find an increase in pressure at any stage, despite the fact that such an increase could be produced by exogenous oxytocin at an infusion rate of as little as 2 mU per minute. This provides further evidence that physiological levels of endogenous oxytocin do not exceed 10 μU/ml.

1. MEASUREMENT OF CIRCULATING OXYTOCIN IN HUMAN PARTURITION BY RADIOIMMUNOASSAY

The circulating levels of oxytocin in human labor have been reexamined by means of a highly specific radioimmunoassay (Chard et al., 1970, 1971). Some of the characteristics of the assay have been noted above. This study showed that oxytocin can be detected only sporadically during labor (Table III). If oxytocin is present at all in the maternal circulation, it is usually at levels below 1 μU/ml, the sensitivity limit of the assay. No correlation has been found between the intermittent appearance of oxytocin and individual uterine contractions. When positive levels have been found in serial bleeds, considerable variation has been noted in the successive samples. This is strongly suggestive of a "spurt" release, similar to that described in lactation.

Table III
Plasma Levels of Oxytocin in Venous Samples Obtained from Women during Labor

Stage of labor	Number of subjects	Number of samples	Samples containing detectable oxytocin		
			Number	% of Total	Oxytocin levels (μU/ml)
1st	24	50	14	28	2–12 (mean 7)
2nd	74	74	9	13	2–18 (mean 9)

2. TECHNICAL ASPECTS OF MEASUREMENT OF OXYTOCIN IN THE MATERNAL CIRCULATION

There are a number of possible criticisms of these findings: (a) That the assay cannot measure endogenous oxytocin in plasma. But the radioimmunoassay yields results which are statistically identical to those of simultaneous bioassays in the goat during parturition (Chard et al., 1970). (b) That oxytocin is too rapidly destroyed by oxytocinase in human late pregnancy plasma for it to be measured. This point has been studied in some detail (James et al., 1971). With care in the collection of samples, there is no significant destruction of oxytocin in either plasma or whole blood from pregnant subjects. Furthermore, circulating oxytocin can be detected in the plasma of pregnant subjects receiving intravenous oxytocin for the induction of labor. (c) That since endogenous oxytocin is released from the pituitary, it will be diluted in the circulation to levels below the sensitivity of the assay. This might explain why positive results can be obtained in jugular samples from the goat. However, it would not explain why clinical infusions of oxytocin into an antecubital vein are effective at exceptionally low rates, and that oxytocin can be detected in the circulation during such infusions.

3. The Significance of Oxytocin in the Maternal Circulation during Human Parturition

The significance of these findings in human labor may be looked at in two ways: (a) the results are valid as presented, and the situation in normal labor consists of intermittent release of oxytocin by the maternal pituitary; (b) the results are invalid because oxytocin is in some way inaccessible to the assay.

a. Assuming that the results are valid, the data agree with the indirect information on the role of endogenous oxytocin in human labor (Theobald, 1968). Thus, there is no evidence that endogenous oxytocin plays a prime role in the initiation or maintenance of labor, since in most samples studied, the levels are lower than those achieved by the so-called "physiological" infusion rates. Equally, the data would in no way disagree with Theobald's concept of the role of oxytocin, which is that a low fixed level (possibly of the order of 0.07 μU/ml) plays a permissive role; its presence is essential for the functional organization of uterine activity, but labor is not triggered by a rise in this level.

This argument assumes that the plasma levels reflect not only pituitary release, but also the biologically effective levels of the hormone. An alternative concept is that oxytocin is bound at its target organ, the myometrium. Neurophysin-like material has been found in the myometrium of both the pig (Ginsburg and Jayasena, 1968) and the human (Legros and Franchimont, 1971). Localization of oxytocin in the myometrium has been shown by immunofluorescence (Gusdon, 1967) and by the tracing of tritium-labeled peptide (Sjoholm and Ryden, 1969). If bound oxytocin is the active form, or an essential intermediate for the active form, circulating oxytocin would be trapped and held by the myometrium, thus smoothing out the effects of a discontinuous release from the pituitary.

b. The data may be invalid because oxytocin is inaccessible to the assay. There are two possibilities: first that the hormone might be bound in the circulation, and second, that it might be present in precursor form. The evidence for plasma binding is equivocal, although a specific binder occurring during pregnancy has been described (Legros and Franchimont, 1971). However, oxytocin is extracted from plasma after acidification, and it is unlikely that any protein–peptide interaction would survive under these conditions. Furthermore, both added and infused oxytocin are recovered identically from the plasma of both pregnant and nonpregnant subjects. The myometrium is well stocked with enzymes, including reninlike material (Ferris et al., 1967) which might activate a precursor, and might explain why oxytocin cannot usually be found by radioimmunoassay, whereas it might be detected by a bioassay, which uses an end organ as the indicator. The intermittent appearance of oxytocin in the circulation could be attributed to an overflow from an activation system.

Finally, neither a precursor theory, nor binding in plasma or tissues would explain the results of Cobo (1968), who was unable to find an increase in intramammary pressure during spontaneous labor. Like the uterus, the breast contains binding material (Ginsburg and Jayasena, 1968), and would presumably also have a precursor activating system. It should be emphasized that the only ground for considering precursor or binding theories are the surprising results of oxytocin assays in human labor, coupled with the deeply held belief that oxytocin levels should be raised at this time. If the latter is incorrect, and there is considerable evidence against it (Csapo and Wood, 1968), then negative findings can be accepted at their face value, without any need for elaborate speculation.

I. Oxytocin Release by the Human Fetus

1. Measurement of Oxytocin in the Umbilical Circulation

By contrast to the situation in the mother, oxytocin can be found consistently in the fetal umbilical circulation at the time of delivery (Chard et al., 1970; Chard et al., 1971) (Fig. 3). In most cases, the levels are higher in the umbilical artery than the umbilical vein, which suggests that the origin is the fetal posterior pituitary. Samples of umbilical cord plasma have also been collected at the time of cesarean section, but the situation is complicated by the appearance of oxytocin in the maternal circulation at this time. Release of oxytocin during surgery has been reported by other workers (Bisset et al., 1956) and may represent a nonspecific stress response. In operations performed with the patient not in labor, oxytocin is found in the umbilical circulation, but with higher levels in the vein than the artery. This is consistent with placental transfer of oxytocin from the maternal circulation, in the absence of any release from the fetal pituitary. In operations performed with the patient in labor, there was almost invariably a higher level in the umbilical artery than the umbilical vein, even in the presence of positive maternal levels.

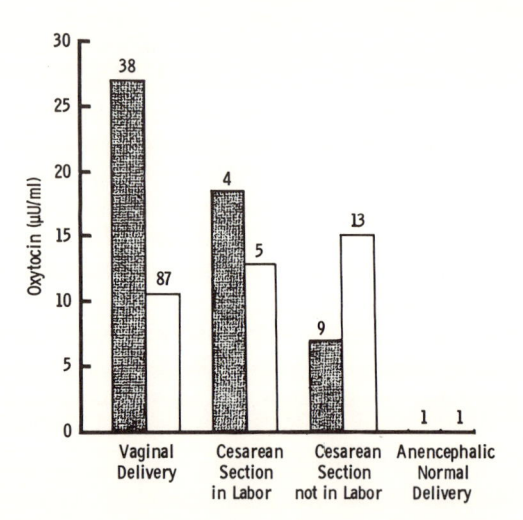

Fig. 3. Plasma levels of oxytocin in arterial (hatched areas) and venous (clear areas) umbilical cord blood. Figures refer to number of subjects studied.

2. Technical Aspects of the Measurement of Oxytocin Levels in the Umbilical Circulation

The occurrence of oxytocin in the fetal circulation, at a time when none can be found in the mother, is not in doubt. It is rather more difficult to assess the validity of the different levels found in the umbilical artery and vein. First, separate identification of the two types of vessel may not always be accurate. This is a source of error which may explain why, although most paired samples obtained at the time of vaginal delivery show a positive arteriovenous difference, occasional cases show the opposite. Second, the conditions of sampling are somewhat artificial, and may vary considerably between cases. Blood is collected from the umbilical cord vessels on the placental side of the clamp, the arterial sample being collected first. However, it cannot be assumed that the umbilical circulation is static under these conditions, since the arteries will tend to constrict, leading to a redistribution of blood toward the venous side of the circulation. This redistribution, the extent of which is determined by the ease and rapidity with which the samples are obtained, may affect the results. Thus, in those cases where only venous blood could be obtained, because the artery had constricted, the levels were higher than in those cases where both types of samples were obtained. An additional technical problem is the limitation on the timing of sample collection. The present data are based on material taken at the time of delivery, either vaginal or by cesarean section. The latter provide a limited view of events actually before or during labor, and suggests that fetal release of oxytocin is only found during labor. However, the numbers are small, and this conclusion could be negated by further evidence. With respect to the timing of the second stage samples, it is probable that oxytocin release is a continuous process, since the precise timing of delivery is a random event, determined by many factors including the skill of the accoucheur and the cooperation of the mother. It is unlikely, therefore, that oxytocin release is related to any specific event in the second stage. A final possibility is that oxytocin release is an acute phenomenon associated with the transition from intra- to extrauterine life. If this is so, it is difficult to see why it should not occur when the fetus is delivered by elective cesarean section.

3. The Significance of Circulating Oxytocin in the Human Fetus

The levels of oxytocin found in umbilical arterial blood would, if they were delivered directly to the myometrium, produce uterine contractions equivalent to those achieved by the highest rates of clinical infusion. Since the evidence from cesarean sections indicates that oxytocin can cross the placenta, and since the peptide is being directed to the myometrium overlying the placental site, the area responsible for the normal quiescence of the pregnant uterus (Csapo and Wood, 1968), it is possible that fetal release of oxytocin has some physiological significance in normal labor. This is further emphasized by the almost complete absence of oxytocin in the maternal circulation. It is also possible that oxytocin release by the fetus has a vasoconstrictor effect on the umbilical vessels (Somlyo and Somylo, 1970).

The concept that the fetus plays a role in its own delivery is not new. Most investigations have emphasized the importance of the fetal pituitary–adrenal axis in this function (Liggins *et al.*, 1967; Liggins, 1968). Some of the experimental data could be reinterpreted as showing the hypothalamic–neurohypophyseal axis to be the critical area. In addition, anatomical abnormalities of the central nervous system, such as anencephaly, are often associated with prolonged pregnancy. These abnormalities involve the hypothalamus, which is the site of synthesis of oxytocin, and the anterior pituitary is only secondarily affected. It is of interest that small quantities of both oxytocin and vasopressin have been extracted from the pituitary and adjacent structures of an anencephalic, in whom there was no histological evidence of nervous tissue (Boyd *et al.*, unpublished observations).

The stimulus for the fetal release of oxytocin is not known. The response is nonspecific, since vasopressin is released at the same time, although in larger quantities. In those cases where both hormones have been estimated, the ratio of vasopressin to oxytocin is highly variable. A common denominator of the response might be anoxia due to the reduction of placental blood flow with uterine contractions. Alternatively, the anoxia may precede labor, and be responsible for its initiation via neurohypophyseal hormone release. Thus, there is evidence that the mature human fetus has virtually outgrown its placental reserve and is, therefore, subject to a precarious nutritional state (McKeown, 1970).

VI. The Natriuretic Hormone

The evidence for and against the existence of a natriuretic hormone or "third factor" will not be considered here. Assuming that it does exist, there is evidence that it arises in the central nervous system, probably in the hypothalamus (Cort et al., 1968). If this is so, then it is likely that systemic release occurs by neurosecretion, since this is the common pathway for all other hypothalamic products, including the releasing factors and the neurohypophyseal peptides. As neurosecretion implies the presence of a neurohemal organ, the natriuretic hormone would have to emerge either through one of the known neurohemal areas (posterior pituitary or median eminence), or through a separate and as yet unidentified area. On conceptual grounds, the posterior pituitary would seem to be the most likely, and it has been suggested that the natriuretic hormone is an analogue, such as 4-leucine vasotocin, of the known hormones (Cort et al., 1969). However, until the hormone can be purified and specifically identified, its isolation from extracts of the posterior pituitary is likely to prove difficult, since such extracts contain a wide variety of peptides and peptide fragments, and the potent effects of oxytocin and vasopressin would have to be excluded. It should also be considered whether the "natriuretic hormone" is simply a combination of known pituitary peptides. Thus the characteristics of the material isolated by Sealey and his colleagues (1969) are remarkably similar to those of the bound form of vasopressin described by Smith and Thorn (1965).

VII. Summary and Conclusions

This chapter has attempted a critical review of some aspects of posterior pituitary function in which further progress can be anticipated.

Recent work has clarified some details of the mechanism of neurosecretion, although the precise nature of the process of release requires further investigation. Oxytocin and vasopressin are synthesized in the form of a large precursor molecule, the nature and fate of which remains to be determined. It is possible that neurophysin is the precursor, and that it is released into the blood stream in parallel with the active peptides. In the circulation, neurophysin may have additional functions. These include binding of oxytocin and vasopressin; a separate but identified function of its own; or circulation of the intact precursor molecule with release at the target organ.

The control mechanisms for vasopressin release are well defined, but it is possible that additional mechanisms may be involved in the fine control of this release in relation to salt and water metabolism. The role of vasopressin and oxytocin as releasing factors for corticotropin and prolactin continues to be argued. Such is the problem of distinguishing the local effects of these peptides from their systemic effects, that it is unlikely that a clear answer will be obtained until specific and sensitive assays are available for corticotropin-releasing factor and prolactin-inhibiting factor.

Oxytocin has, in the past, been relegated to a role in lactation and parturition. These events take up only a few hours in the life of most mammals, and none in the males of the species. It is possible that it may have other functions; prime among these would be a role in salt and water metabolism, if only because it so closely relates phylogenetically to vasopressin. Meanwhile, the traditional functions of oxytocin have come under the spotlight of specific and sensitive assays. These have confirmed its role in lactation and animal parturition. In human parturition, the situation is confusing, and release by the fetus may turn out to be equal in importance, if not more so, than release by the mother. Further advances in the field of oxytocin physiology demand a better understanding of the relationship between its release and its peripheral action.

References

Abel, J. J. (1924). *Bull. Johns Hopkins Hosp.* 35, 305.
Abrahams, V. A., and Pickford, M. (1954). *J. Physiol. (London)* 126, 320.
Acher, R., Chauvet, J., and Olivry, G. (1956). *Biochim. Biophys. Acta* 22, 421.
Arimura, A., Schally, A. V., and Bowers, C. Y. (1969). *Endocrinology* 84, 579.
Armstrong, D. T., and Hansel, W. (1958). *Fed. Proc. Fed. Amer. Soc. Exp. Biol.* 17, 6.
Barer, R., Heller, H., and Lederis, K. (1963). *Proc. Roy. Soc., Ser. B* 158, 388.
Bargmann, W., and Scharrer, E. (1951). *Amer. Sci.* 39, 255.
Bargmann, W., and Von Gaudecker, B. (1969). *Z. Zellforsch. Mikrosk. Anat.* 96, 495.

Barnafi, L., Rosas, R., de la Lastra, M., and Croxatto, H. (1960). *Amer. J. Physiol.* **198**, 255.
Bashore, R. A. (1967). *Obstet. Gynecol.* **29**, 431.
Beleslin, D., Bisset, G. W., Haldar, J., and Polak, R. L. (1967). *Proc. Roy. Soc., Ser. B* **166**, 443.
Benson, G. K., and Folley, S. J. (1957). *J. Endocrinol.* **16**, 189.
Berde, B., and Boissonas, R. A. (1968). In "Neurohypophysial Hormones & Similar Polypeptides" (B. Berde, ed.), pp. 802–870. Springer-Verlag, Berlin and New York.
Bern, H. A., and Knowles, F. G. W. (1966). In "Neuroendocrinology" (L. Martini and W. F. Ganong, eds.), Vol. 1, pp. 139–186. Academic Press, New York.
Besser, G. M., Orth, D. N., Nicholson, W. E., and Woodhan, J. (1969). *J. Endocrinol.* **46**, i.
Bisset, G. W., and Walker, J. M. (1954). *J. Physiol. (London)* **126**, 588.
Bisset, G. W., Lee, J., and Bromwich, A. F. (1956). *Lancet* **ii**, 1129.
Blair-Bell, W. (1909). *Brit. Med. J.* **ii**, 1609.
Bonjour, J.-P., and Malvin, R. L. (1970). *Amer. J. Physiol.* **218**, 1555.
Boyd, G. W., Adamson, A. R., Fitz, A. E., and Peart, W. S. (1969). *Lancet* ***i***, 213.
Boyd, N. R. H., Jackson, D. B., Forsling, M. L., Hollingsworth, S. A., and Chard, T. (1972). *J. Endocrinol.* In press.
Boyd, N. R. H., and Chard, T. (1971). In "Radioimmunoassay Methods" (K. E. Kirkham and W. M. Hunter, eds.), p. 52. Livingstone, Edinburgh.
Breslow, F. (1970). *Proc. Nat. Acad. Sci.* **67**, 493.
Bridges, T. E., and Thorn, N. A. (1970). *J. Endocrinol.* **48**, 265.
Brooks, F. P., and Pickford, M. (1958). *Endocrinology* **78**, 779.
Brostoff, J., James, V. H. T., and Landon, J.(1968). *J. Clin. Endocrinol. Metab.* **28**, 511.
Brunner, H., Kuschinsky, G., Munchow, O., and Peters, G. (1957). *Naunyn-Schmiedebergs Arch. Exp. Pathol. Pharmakol.* **230**, 80.
Burton, A. M., Forsling, M. L., and Martin, M. J. (1971). *J. Physiol.* In press.
Caldeyro-Barcia, R., and Poseiro, J. J. (1959). *Ann. N.Y. Acad. Sci.* **78**, 813.
Chan, W. Y. (1965). *Endocrinology* **77**, 1097.
Chan, W. Y., and Sawyer, W. H. (1961). *Amer. J. Physiol.* **201**, 799.
Chard, T. (1964). *J. Obstet. Gynaecol. Brit. Commonw.* **7**, 624.
Chard, T. (1971). In "Radioimmunoassay Methods" (K. E. Kirkham and W. M. Hunter, eds.), p. 491. Livingstone, Edinburgh.
Chard, T., Forsling, M. L., and Kitau, M. J. (1969). *J. Endocrinol.* **43**, lxi.
Chard, T., Boyd, N. R. H., Forsling, M. L., McNeilly, A. S., and Landon, J. (1970). *J. Endocrinol.* **48**, 223.
Chard, T., Boyd, N. R. H., Edwards, C. R. W., and Hudson, C. N. (1971). *Nature (London)*. In press.
Cheng, K. W., and Friesen, H. G. (1970). *Metabolism* **19**, 876.
Cheng, K. W., and Friesen, H. (1971). *Endocrinology* **88**, 608.
Chiaraviglio, E., and Taleisnik, S. (1969). *Amer. J. Physiol.* **216**, 1418.
Clemente, C. D., Sutin, J., and Silverstone, J. T. (1957). *Amer. J. Physiol.* **188**, 193.
Cleverley, J. D., and Folley, S. J. (1970). *J. Endocrinol.* **46**, 347.
Cobo, E. (1968). *J. Appl. Physiol.* **24**, 317.
Coch, J. A., Brovetto, J., Cabot, H. M., Fielitz, C. A., and Caldeyro-Barcia, R. (1965). *Amer. J. Obstet. Gynecol.* **91**, 10.

Cort, J. H., Pliska, V., and Dousa, T. (1968). *Lancet* **i**, 230.
Cort, J. H., Sedlakova, E., Lichardus, B., and Dousa, T. (1969). *Proc. Int. Congr. Nephrol., 4th, 1968* **2**, 107.
Cross, B. A. (1958). *J. Endocrinol.* **16**, 237.
Cross, B. A. (1966). In "Neuroendocrinology" (L. Martini and W. F. Ganong, eds.), Vol. 1, pp. 217–259. Academic Press, New York.
Cross, R. B., Dicker, S. E., Kitchin, A. H., Lloyd, S., and Pickford, M. (1960). *J. Physiol. (London)* **153**, 553.
Croxatto, H., and Labarca, E. (1958). *Experientia (Basel)* **14**, 339.
Csapo, A., and Wood, E. C. (1968). In "Recent Advances in Endocrinology" (V. H. T. James, ed.), 8th Ed., p. 207. Churchill, London.
Currie, A. R., Adamsons, H., and van Dyke, H. B. (1960). *J. Clin. Endocrinol. Metab.* **20**, 947.
Dale, H. H. (1906). *J. Physiol. (London)* **34**, 163.
Daniel, A. R., and Lederis, K. (1966). *J. Endocrinol.* **34**, 91.
Daniel, P. M. (1966). In "Neuroendocrinology" (L. Martini and W. F. Ganong, eds.), Vol. 1, pp. 15–80. Academic Press, New York.
Debackere, M., and Peeters, G. (1960). *Arch. Int. Pharmacodyn. Ther.* **123**, 462.
Debackere, M., Peeters, G., and Tuyttens, N. (1961). *J. Endocrinol.* **22**, 321.
DeRubertis, F. R., Michelis, M. F., Beek, N., Field, J. B., and Davis, B. B. (1971). *J. Clin. Invest.* **50**, 97.
Ditlove, J., and Faiman, C. (1970). *J. Clin. Endocrinol. Metab.* **30**, 672.
Donaldson, L. E., and Takken, A. (1968). *J. Reprod. Fert.* **17**, 373.
Dudley, H. W. (1919). *J. Pharmacol. Exp. Ther.* **14**, 295.
du Vigneaud, V. (1956). *Harvey Lect.* **50**, 1.
Ely, F., and Petersen, W. E. (1941). *J. Dairy Sci.* **24**, 211.
Epstein, A. N., Fitzsimons, J. T., and Rolls, B. J. (1970). *J. Physiol. (London)* **210**, 457.
Fabian, M., Forsling, M. L., Jones, J. J., and Pryor, J. S. (1969). *J. Physiol. (London)* **204**, 653.
Fawcett, C. P., Powell, A. E., and Sachs, H. (1968). *Endocrinology* **83**, 1299.
Ferris, T. F., Gorden, P., and Mulrow, P. J. (1967). *Amer. J. Physiol.* **212**, 698.
Fitzpatrick, R. J. (1957). In "The Neurohypophysis" (H. Heller, ed.), pp. 203–217. Butterworth, London.
Fitzpatrick, R. J. (1961). In "Oxytocin" (R. Caldeyro-Barcia and H. Heller, eds.), p. 360. Pergamon, London.
Fitzpatrick, R. J., and Walmsley, C. F. (1962). *J. Physiol. (London)* **163**, 13P.
Fitzpatrick, R. J., and Walmsley, C. F. (1965). In "Advances in Oxytocin Research" (J. H. M. Pinkerton, ed.), p. 51. Pergamon, London.
Fjellstrom, D., Kihlstrom, J. E., and Melin, P. (1968). *J. Reprod. Fert.* **17**, 207.
Folley, S. J., and Knaggs, G. S. (1965). *J. Endocrinol.* **33**, 301.
Forsling, M. L., Boyd, N. R. H., and Chard, T. (1971). In "Radioimmunoassay Methods" (K. E. Kirkham and W. M. Hunter, eds.), p. 549. Livingstone, Edinburgh.
Fox, C. A., and Fox, B. (1967). *Brit. Med. J.* **i**, 300.
Fox, C. A., and Knaggs, G. S. (1969). *J. Endocrinol.* **45**, 145.
Franchimont, P. (1971). In "Radioimmunoassay Methods" (K. E. Kirkham, and W. M. Hunter, eds.), p. 535. Livingstone, Edinburgh.
Franchimont, P., and Legros, J. J. (1969). *Ann. Endocrinol.* **30**, 125.
Friesen, H. G., and Astwood, E. B. (1967). *Endocrinology* **80**, 278.
Ginsburg, M., and Jayasena, K. (1968). *J. Physiol. (London)* **197**, 65.

Ginsburg, M., and Smith, M. W. (1959). *Brit. J. Pharmacol. Chemother.* **14**, 327.
Ginsburg, M., and Thomas, P. J. (1969). *J. Physiol. (London)* **201**, 181.
Ginsburg, M., Jayasena, K., and Thomas, P. J. (1966). *J. Physiol. (London)* **184**, 387.
Glick, S. M. (1969). In "Protein and Polypeptide Hormones" (M. Margoulis, ed.), pp. 660–661. Excerpta Med. Found., Amsterdam.
Glick, S. M., Kumaresan, P., Kagan, A., and Wheeler, M. (1969). In "Protein and Polypeptide Hormones" (M. Margoulies, ed.), p. 81–83. Excerpta Med. Found., Amsterdam.
Goetz, K. L., Bond, G. C., Hernreck, A. S., and Trank, J. W. (1970). *Amer. J. Physiol.* **219**, 1424.
Goodwin, F. L., Ledingham, J. G. G., and Laragh, J. H. (1970). *Clin. Sci.* **39**, 641.
Gusdon, J. P. (1967). *Amer. J. Obstet. Gynecol.* **98**, 526.
Hall, C. A. (1962). *Brit. J. Haematol.* **16**, 429.
Harris, G. W. (1947). *Phil. Trans. Roy. Soc. London, Ser. B* **232**, 385.
Harris, G. W., and Pickles, V. R. (1953). *Nature (London)* **172**, 1049.
Haun, C. K., and Sawyer, W. H. (1960). *Endocrinology* **67**, 270.
Hawker, R. W., Walmsley, C. F., Roberts, V. S., Blackshawe, J. K., and Downes, J. C. (1961). *J. Clin. Endocrinol. Metab.* **21**, 985.
Hays, R. L., and van Demark, N. L. (1953). *Amer. J. Physiol.* **172**, 557.
Hayward, J. N., and Vincent, J. D. (1970). *J. Physiol. (London)* **210**, 947.
Herlant, M. (1967). In "Neurosecretion" (F. Stutinsky, ed.), Vol. IV, pp. 20–35. Springer-Verlag, Berlin and New York.
Holland, R. C., Cross, B. A., and Sawyer, C. H. (1959). *Amer. J. Physiol.* **196**, 796.
Hope, D. B. (1968). In "Pharmacology of Hormonal Polypeptides and Proteins" (N. Back, L. Martini, and R. Paoletti, eds.), pp. 73–83. Plenum, New York.
Hoppenstein, J. M., Miltenberger, F. W., and Moran, W. H. (1968). *Surg. Gynecol. Obstet.* **127**, 966.
Howell, W. H. (1898). *J. Exp. Med.* **3**, 245.
Huntingford, P. J. (1963). *J. Obstet. Gynaecol. Brit. Commonw.* **70**, 929.
James, M. A. R., Forsling, M. L., and Chard, T. (1971). In "Radioimmunoassay Methods" (K. E. Kirkham and W. M. Hunter, eds.), p. 545. Livingstone, Edinburgh.
Johnson, J. A., Moore, W. W., and Segar, W. E. (1969). *Amer. J. Physiol.* **217**, 210.
Johnson, J. A., Zehr, J. E., and Moore, W. W. (1970). *Amer. J. Physiol.* **218**, 1273.
Jones, C. W., and Pickering, B. T. (1969). *J. Physiol. (London)* **203**, 449.
Kamm, C., Aldrich, T. B., Grote, I. W., and Bugbee, E. P. (1928). *J. Amer. Chem. Soc.* **50**, 573.
Kitchin, A. H., Konzett, H., and Pickford, M. (1959). *Brit. J. Pharmacol. Chemother.* **14**, 567.
Knaggs, G. S. (1963). *J. Endocrinol.* **26**, xxiv.
Krass, M. E., La Bella, F. S., and Vivian, S. R. (1968). *Endocrinology* **82**, 1183.
Kyncl, J., and Rudinger, J. (1970). *J. Endocrinol.* **48**, 157.
Lauson, H. D. (1967). *Amer. J. Med.* **42**, 713.
Lees, P., and Allsup, F. C. (1969). *Arch. Int. Pharmacodyn. Ther.* **177**, 457.
Legros, J. J., and Franchimont, P. (1971). In "Radioimmunoassay Methods" (K. E. Kirkham and W. M. Hunter, eds.), p. 156. Livingstone, Edinburgh.
Legros, J. J., Franchimont, P., and Hendrick, J. C. (1969). *C. R. Soc. Biol.* **163**, 2273.

Liggins, G. C. (1968). *J. Endocrinol.* **42**, 323.
Liggins, G. C., Kennedy, P. C., and Holm, L. W. (1967). *Amer. J. Obstet. Gynecol.* **98**, 1080.
McCann, S. M., and Dhariwal, A. P. S. (1966). In "Neuroendocrinology" (L. Martini and W. F. Ganong, eds.), Vol. 1, pp. 261–296. Academic Press, New York.
McCann, S. M., Antunes-Rodrigues, J., Nallar, R., and Valtin, H. (1966). *Endocrinology* **79**, 1058.
McKeown, T. (1970). *Brit. Med. J.* ii, 63.
McNeilly, A. S., and Folley, S. J. (1970). *J. Endocrinol.* **48**, lx.
McNeilly, A. S., Forsling, M. L., and Chard, T. (1971). In "Radioimmunoassay Methods" (K. E. Kirkham and W. M. Hunter, eds.), p. 558. Livingstone, Edinburgh.
Manabe, Y. (1969). *J. Reprod. Fert.* **18**, 371.
Marks, L. J., Berde, B., Klein, L. A., Roth, J., Goonan, S. R., Blumen, D. and Nabseth, D. C. (1968). *Amer. J. Med.* **45**, 967.
Martin, M. J. (1971). *J. Endocrinol.* **49**, 553.
Martin, M. J., Chard, T., and Landon, J. (1971). *J. Endocrinol.* In press.
Massry, S. G., Vorherr, H., and Kleeman, C. R. (1969). *Proc. Soc. Exp. Biol. Med.* **130**, 1276.
Meites, J., and Hopkins, T. F. (1961). *J. Endocrinol.* **22**, 207.
Milkovic, K., and Milkovic, S. (1966). In "Neuroendocrinology" (L. Martini and W. F. Ganong, eds.), Vol. 1, pp. 371–407. Academic Press, New York.
Miller, N. E., Dicara, L. V., and Wolf, G. (1968). *Amer. J. Physiol.* **215**, 684.
Mirsky, I. A. (1969). In "Handbook of Experimental Pharmacology" (B. Berde, ed.), Vol. XXIII, pp. 613–624. Springer-Verlag, Berlin and New York.
Mouw, V., Bonjour, J.-P., Maluin, R. L., and Vander, A. (1971). *Amer. J. Physiol.* **220**, 239.
Moses, A. M., Leveque, T. F., Giambattista, M., and Lloyd, C. W. (1963). *J. Endocrinol.* **26**, 273.
Munsick, R. A., and Gresham, E. M. (1970). *Amer. J. Obset. Gynecol.* **108**, 729.
Nagareda, C. S., and Gaunt, R. (1951). *Endocrinology* **48**, 560.
Nagasawa, J., Douglas, W. W., and Schulz, R. A. (1970). *Nature (London)* **227**, 409.
Oliver, G., and Schäfer, E. A. (1895). *J. Physiol. (London)* **18**, 277.
Olsson, K., and McDonald, I. R. (1970). *J. Endocrinol.* **48**, 301.
Ott, I., and Scott, J. C. (1910). *Proc. Soc. Exp. Biol. Med.* **8**, 48.
Panisset, J. C., and Beaulnes, A. (1961). *Rev. Can. Biol.* **20**, 47.
Petersen, W. E. (1942). *Proc. Soc. Exp. Biol. Med.* **50**, 298.
Pickering, B. T. (1969). In "Protein and Polypeptide Hormones" (M. Margoulies, ed.), pp. 780–781. Excerpta Med. Found., Amsterdam.
Portanova, R., and Sachs, H. (1967). *Endocrinology* **80**, 527.
Preddie, E. C. (1965). *J. Biol. Chem.* **240**, 4194.
Preddie, E. C., and Saffran, M. (1965). *J. Biol. Chem.* **240**, 4189.
Ratcliffe, J. G., and Knight, R. A. (1971). *Mod. Trends Endocrinol.* In press.
Rauch, R., Hollenberg, M. D., and Hope, D. B. (1968). *Biochem. J.* **110**, 38p.
Roberts, J. S., and Share, L. (1968). *Endocrinology* **83**, 272.
Roberts, J. S., and Share, L. (1969). *Endocrinology* **84**, 1076.
Roberts, J. S., and Share, L. (1970). *Endocrinology* **87**, 812.
Rocha e Silva, M., and Rosenberg, M. (1969). *J. Physiol. (London)* **202**, 535.

Rothchild, I., and Quilligan, E. J. (1960). *Endocrinology* **67,** 122.
Rudman, D., Del Rio, A. E., Garcia, L. A., Barnett, J., Howard, C. H., Walker, W., and Moore, G. (1970). *Biochemistry* **9,** 99.
Saameli, K. (1963). *Amer. J. Obstet. Gynecol.* **85,** 186.
Sachs, H. (1967). *Amer. J. Med.* **42,** 687.
Sachs, H., and Haller, E. W. (1968). *Endocrinology* **83,** 251.
Sachs, H., and Takabatake, Y. (1964). *Endocrinology* **75,** 943.
Sadowski, J., Szreder, I., and Sternik-Sagalara, K. (1968). *Proc. Soc. Exp. Biol. Med.* **123,** 294.
Saffran, M. (1959). *Can. J. Biochem. Physiol.* **27,** 319.
Saito, T., Yoshida, S., and Nakao, K. (1969). *Endocrinology* **85,** 72.
Saunders W. G., and Munsick, R. A. (1966). *Amer. J. Obstet. Gynecol.* **95,** 5.
Schrier, R. W., Verroust, P. J., and Jones, J. J. (1968). *Clin. Sci.* **35,** 433.
Sealey, J. E., Kirkham, J. P., and Laragh, J. H. (1969). *J. Clin. Invest.* **48,** 2210.
Segar, W. E., and Moore, W. W. (1968). *J. Clin. Invest.* **47,** 2143.
Share, L., and Travis, R. H. (1970). *Endocrinology* **86,** 196.
Sjoholm, I., and Ryden, J. (1969). *Acta Endocrinol.* **61,** 432.
Smith, M. W., and Thorn, N. A. (1965). *J. Endocrinol.* **32,** 141.
Smith, S. W. (1963). *Advan. Neuroendocrinol., Proc. Symp., Miami, 1961,* pp. 86–89.
Somlyo, A. P., and Somlyo, A. V. (1970). *Pharmacol. Rev.* **22,** 249.
Theobald, G. W. (1968). *Obstet. Gynecol. Surv.* **23,** 109.
Thomson, W. B. (1960). *J. Physiol.* (*London*) **150,** 284.
Thorn, N. A. (1968). *In* "Handbook of Experimental Pharmacology" (B. Berde, ed.), Vol. XXIII, pp. 372–442. Springer-Verlag, Berlin and New York.
Traber, D. L., Wilson, R. D., and Gardier, R. W. (1968). *Arch. Int. Pharmacodyn. Ther.* **176,** 360.
Uttenthal, L. S., and Hope, D. B.(1970). *Biochem. J.* **116,** 899.
van Demark, N. L., and Hays, R. L. (1952). *Amer. J. Physiol.* **170,** 518.
van Dyke, H. B. (1968). *Proc. Roy. Soc., Ser. B* **170,** 3.
van Dyke, H. B., Chow, B. P., Greep, R. O., and Rothen, A. (1942). *J. Pharmacol. Exp. Ther.* **74,** 190.
Verney, E. B. (1947). *Proc. Roy. Soc. Ser. B* **135,** 25.
Vogt, M. (1953). *Brit. J. Pharmacol. Chemother.* **8,** 193.
von Konschegg, A., and Schuster, E. (1915). *Deut. Med. Wochenschr.* **41,** 1091.
Vizsolyi, E., and Perks, A. M. (1969). *Nature* (*London*) **223,** 1169.
Wilks, J. W., Hansel, W., and Armstrong, D. T. (1969). *Endocrinology* **84,** 1032.
Winnick, T., Winnick, R. E., Acher, R. ,and Fromageot, C. (1955). *Biochim. Biophys. Acta* **18,** 488.
Wuu, T. C., and Saffran, M. (1969). *J. Biol. Chem.* **244,** 482.
Yates, F. E., Russell, S. M., Dallman, M. F., Hedge, G. A., McCann, S. M., and Dhariwal, A. P. S. (1971). *Endocrinology* **88,** 3.

ROLE OF THYMOSIN AND OTHER THYMIC FACTORS IN THE DEVELOPMENT, MATURATION, AND FUNCTIONS OF LYMPHOID TISSUE*

Allan L. Goldstein[†] *and Abraham White*

DEPARTMENT OF BIOCHEMISTRY
ALBERT EINSTEIN COLLEGE OF MEDICINE
YESHIVA UNIVERSITY, BRONX, NEW YORK

I. Introduction 122
II. Embryonic Development and Differentiation of the Thymus Gland 123
   A. Embryonic Development 123
   B. Origin of Thymic Lymphocytes 124
   C. Epithelial Secretory Cells 125
   D. Postnatal Development 125
III. Role of the Thymus in the Development, Maturation, and Function of the Lymphoid System 125

---

* The data referred to from our own laboratory are derived from studies which have been supported by Public Health Service Research Grant No. CA-07470 from the National Cancer Institute, and by grants from the American Cancer Society (E-613 and P-68), the National Science Foundation (GB-6616X), and the Damon Runyon Fund for Cancer Research (DRG-920).

† Recipient of a Career Scientist Award of the Health Research Council of the City of New York under Contract I-519.

       A. Early Experiences with Adult Thymectomy 125
       B. Recent Experience with Thymectomy of the Newborn . 126
  IV. Thymic Malfunction; Clinical Disorders 128
       A. Recent Recognition of Thymic Involvement in Disease in Man 128
   V. Mechanism of Action of the Thymus 130
       A. Progenitor of Cells 130
       B. Endocrine Function 131
  VI. Concluding Comments 142
       References 145

I. Introduction

The inclusion of a contribution on the thymus gland in a volume entitled "Current Topics in Experimental Endocrinology" may be questioned by some readers and surprising to others. The requisite evidence to permit addition of the thymus to the established list of endocrine glands has rapidly accumulated within recent years. On the basis of the available experimental and clinical data, it is apparent that the thymus is an endocrine gland and that this anatomical structure exerts a number of important biological influences, some of which can be mimicked by cell-free preparations of thymic tissue.

The concept that the thymus gland may have an endocrine role has arisen to a major degree from clinical evidence and from recent studies in experimental immunology. The data have established that the thymus gland influences the development and modulation of host resistance in a number of species, including the human. This influence is primarily on the maturation and proliferation of lymphoid cells involved in cell-mediated immunological reactions. The mechanism by which the thymus exerts these functions is not fully established. However, the evidence available permits the conclusion that the thymus is a major source of lymphoid cells which leave the gland and seed the peripheral lymphoid organs to become cells of potential immunological competence. In addition, the thymus gland is the source of one or more humoral factors which influence lymphoid tissue structure and function, including immunological phenomena. Finally, it has been suggested that cells derived from other anatomical sites, e.g., bone marrow, spleen, and lymph nodes, may return to the thymus and there acquire the prerequisites for becoming immunologically competent.

In addition to the more recently indicated prime role of the thymus gland in immunological phenomena, other possible functions of the thymus have been sought, claimed, and refuted and/or substantiated in the past 150 years. These roles include phenomena of normal and malignant growth, reproduction, and a number of diverse metabolic influences, e.g., calcium and phosphorus metabolism.

In this chapter we shall present primarily the results of more recent studies which have explored the role of the thymus in the regulation of lymphoid tissue structure and function. Inasmuch as lymphoid cells participate in a wide variety of processes contributing to the broad area of host resistance, it is evident that the thymus gland may influence a wide variety of phenomena. Among these, we shall consider (1) the proliferation and development of lymphoid tissue, (2) cell-mediated immune phenomena, including immunological tolerance, and (3) aberrant cellular proliferation induced by chemicals, ionizing radiation, or viruses. Finally, we shall present the more recent evidence for the mode of action of the thymus gland in the above processes, including a description of the preparation and properties of cell-free thymic extracts which have been reported to be active in various experimental designs.

The earlier and voluminous literature concerned with the thymus gland is beyond the scope of the present review and will not be considered here. It may be of value to the reader, however, to provide several references to literature surveys of the thymus which appeared prior to 1960 (Hammar, 1910, 1936; Park and McClure, 1919; Biedl, 1923; Perla and Marmorston, 1941). In 1961, a markedly increased rate of growth of experimental interest in the thymus gland was initiated as a consequence of the description of the deleterious consequences of the extirpation of the gland in the newborn of several species (Archer and Pierce, 1961; Fichtelius *et al.*, 1961; Good *et al.*, 1962; Miller, 1961; Jankovic *et al.*, 1962). A number of recent treatises and reviews (Good and Gabrielson, 1964; Metcalf, 1966; Miller and Osoba, 1967; Hess, 1968; White and Goldstein, 1968, 1970a,b; 1971; Goldstein and White, 1970, 1971; Goldstein *et al.* (1970b) have documented the major literature on the thymus subsequent to 1960. Publications that are pertinent to the present chapter will be referred to in the sections which follow.

II. Embryonic Development and Differentiation of the Thymus Gland

A. *Embryonic Development*

In most mammals, the thymus gland develops from proliferating endodermal cells evaginating from the region of the third pharyngeal pouch on each side of the midline (Maximow, 1909). In higher species these cells grow in cordlike fashion and migrate caudally out into the brachial mesenchyme from both sides and move down into the thorax, where both thymic anlage join and lose the connections with their points of origin although their parenchymas still remain separate. During the earliest stages of embryonic development, the thymus gland consists primarily of these cords of epithelial cells and bears a marked histological resemblance to a typical endocrine gland. It may be noted that the primordia of the thyroid, parathyroid, and ultimobranchial gland, whose humoral secretions have been well characterized, originate in close proximity to the thymic anlage in the same pharyngeal regions of the third and fourth pouch.

B. Origin of Thymic Lymphocytes

As the thymus develops, it becomes lobuled and the earliest lymphocytes, the lymphoblasts, begin to appear at a time before they are seen in the blood or other lymphoid organs. It has been a matter of some controversy whether the first lymphocytes develop autonomously within the thymus from epithelium or whether they enter the thymus primordium from surrounding mesenchyme (see Beard, 1899). Von Kolliken (1879), working with rabbit embryos, was the first to suggest the lymphoid transformation of thymic epithelial cells. These studies have been supported by histological studies in other animals (Ruth, 1961; Ackerman and Knoff, 1965) and by the observation of Sanel (1967) that lymphoid cells are seen within the embryonic thymus before its vascularization. In addition, Auerbach (1961) has demonstrated that the epitheliomesenchymal rudiments of 12-day-old embryonic mouse thymus differentiates *in vitro,* the epithelial fragments giving rise to lymphocytes and the mesenchymal rudiments giving rise to the stromal elements. In contrast to these studies, a number of other investigators (see Beard, 1899) have proposed that the first leukocytes (thymocytes) migrate into the thymic rudiment from surrounding mesenchyme. This hypothesis was supported by Maximow (1909), who described lymphoid-type cells, which he termed "Wanderzellen," that could presumably enter the thymic rudiment from the surrounding mesenchyme. Recent experiments in lethally X-irradiated mice given marrow cells with a chromosomal marker (T_6) indicate that lymphoid stem cell populations, in contrast to more mature lymphoid cells, migrate to the thymus, where they presumably can undergo further maturation (Ford and Micklem, 1963).

Burnet has proposed that a mutual inductive effect of epithelial primordium with primitive mesenchymal cells results in the differentiation of undifferentiated mesenchymal cells of the lymphocytic series (Burnet, 1969). This hypothesis would be in accord with evidence that adult bone marrow stem cells are the precursors of some classes of thymic lymphocytes in the thymus of X-irradiated animals (Ford, 1966).

C. Epithelial Secretory Cells

On the basis of histological studies, Sanel (1967) reported that during the final quarter before parturition and in the early neonatal period, many of the thymic epithelial cells contain secretory cells with pores or fenestrae which are similar to the cells found in typical endocrine organs. The presence of these epithelial secretory cells has also been confirmed by electron microscopy (Clark, 1966). The observations of Sanel and of Clark suggest that the thymus has a secretory role.

D. Postnatal Development

At birth, the thymus, in contrast to other lymphoid tissues, is well developed and has normal architecture (Blattner, 1963). In most species, it reaches its maximal size (ratio of thymus weight to body weight) during late fetal and early postnatal life (Ham, 1965). Shortly after birth, the thymus is metabolically very active. At this time the mitotic index of the thymic lymphocytes, for example, is five to ten times greater than that of peripheral lymphoid cell populations (Kindred, 1938). In the guinea pig, it has been estimated that the output of thymocytes to the general circulation is between approximately 12×10^6 (Kotani et al., 1966) and 74×10^6 cells per day (Ernström and Sandberg, 1970).

After a short period of progressive development and growth, involution of the thymus is initiated and becomes extensive. This occurs in man and most other mammals prior to puberty and involves primarily a depletion of the lymphoid elements (thymocytes) of the thymic cortex and also the medulla (Hammar, 1936). In other species such as the mouse (Metcalf, 1966) the same pattern of thymocyte depletion occurs with the result that the predominant cell type in the thymus of the older adult mouse is the reticuloepithelial stromal cell. This cell population includes the epithelial secretory cells described earlier.

III. Role of the Thymus in the Development, Maturation, and Function of the Lymphoid System

A. Early Experiences with Adult Thymectomy

Prior to 1961, the role of the thymus gland remained an enigma. Although this organ was the subject of extensive investigations for over 150 years, most investigators assigned a role of minor importance to the thymus. This was due mainly to the observation that removal of the thymus gland in a wide variety of animals (sheep, dogs, calves, rabbits, mice, hamsters, and man), was not associated with any immediately observable consequences. The only result reported frequently was death of the experimental animals due to infection. This outcome was thought to be due to inadequate nonsterile surgical techniques and poor housing facilities (cf. Park and McClure, 1919). Occasional reports appeared suggesting a relationship between the thymus and lymphoid cell-mediated host resistance. For example, Pappenheimer (1914) found that thymectomy of 10-day-old rats decreased the population of small lymphocytes in the blood. Also, Furth (1946) reported that thymectomized mice were more susceptible to the development of tumors under the influence of chemical carcinogens. Despite these suggestive data for a role of the thymus in regulating lymphoid tissue structure and function, no correlation was made between thymic function and host resistance.

B. Recent Experience with Thymectomy of the Newborn

Although it was long known that the thymus gland developed early in fetal life and reached a maximal size in relation to body weight shortly after birth (Friedleben, 1858), it is surprising that no apparent association between thymic development and the maturation of the lymphoid system was made until rather recently. This relationship was clearly recognized in 1961 when almost simultaneously J. F. A. P. Miller, then at the Chester Beatty Institute in London (Miller, 1961), and Archer and Pierce (1961) at the University of Minnesota reported that neonatal thymectomy resulted in acute and serious defects in the numbers and types of peripheral lymphoid cells and in host immunity. These initial observations were quickly extended and confirmed by a number of other investigators in a wide variety of species (cf. Miller and Osoba, 1967; Hess, 1968).

From the initial studies of thymectomized animals considered above, the important conclusion evident was that the thymus gland controls the development and expression of those aspects of the immunological system reflected in cell-mediated immunity and also has a role in certain aspects of the development of humoral immunity.

The defect in cell-mediated immunity following neonatal thymectomy is the basis for the development of a syndrome which has been termed a "wasting disease." This is characterized by an inability of the experimental animal to respond to a variety of viral, fungal, protozoan, and bacterial antigens and a consequent high degree of mortality due to generalized infection (cf. Good and Gabrielsen, 1964; Miller and Osoba, 1967; Hess, 1968). The operated animals lose the ability to reject foreign grafts (Dalmasso et al., 1962b; Miller, 1962), their lymphoid cells fail to elicit normal graft vs. host reactions (Dalmasso et al., 1962a; Miller et al., 1962), and most of the related delayed hypersensitivity responses, such as responses to tuberculin and to bovine serum albumin, are markedly deficient (Jankovic et al., 1962). The lymphoid cells from neonatally thymectomized animals fail to respond in vitro to mitogens such as phytohemagglutinin and do not exhibit the customarily seen blastogenesis of the mixed lymphocyte reaction (Dukor and Dietrich, 1967; Goldstein et al., unpublished observations). Recently, it has been shown by Bach and Dardenne (1971) that the spleen cell populations from neonatally thymectomized or genetically thymusless mice lack the specific rosette-forming cell types which are sensitive to azathioprine, antilymphocyte serum, and antitheta serum, and which have been designed as T-cells.

In addition to the resulting striking deficiencies in host immunity, thymectomy of the newborn results in a marked decrease in numbers of blood lymphocytes and a depletion of small lymphocytes from the peripheral lymphoid tissues, particularly in the "thymic dependent areas" (Parrott et al., 1966). Of the various lymphoid cells influenced by thymectomy, the small lymphocyte is the most susceptible. Recent studies have indicated that some of these cells are thymus dependent and these cells can be obtained in large numbers from the thoracic duct lymph (Gowans, 1965). This class of small lymphocyte has been proposed as being responsible for the surveillance role of lymphoid tissue (Burnet, 1959) in the body and also responsible for the typical cell-mediated responses (cf. Miller and Osoba, 1967). The small lymphocyte, or more specifically a class of small lymphocytes within this category, has been designated collectively by Medawar (1963) as "immunologically competent cells" or alternatively as "antigen-reactive cells" and has been demonstrated to have an extremely long life-span. Studies utilizing chromosomal markers have revealed that the immunologically competent cell in rats has a life-span of over 100 days (Little et al., 1962) and in man of several years (Buckton and Pike, 1964). This long life-span explains the lack of immediate immunological defects in adult animals following thymectomy. The number of immunologically competent cells in the circulation at the time of thymectomy would, under normal circumstances, be more than required to parry normal pathogenic challenges. Thus, the numerous older reports of the lack of effect of thymectomy in the adult animal can now be reconciled with present immunological understanding. Several studies in the literature indicate that a decrease in lymphocyte numbers and in immunological competence can be seen in adult thymectomized animals examined at a time significantly beyond operation (Metcalf, 1965; Miller, 1965; Taylor, 1965). This slow rate of decline in the numbers of immunologically competent cells in the adult, thymectomized animal can be accelerated by destruction of the existing lymphoid cell populations by use of lymphocytolytic agents such as X-irradiation (Miller *et al.*, 1963), antilymphocyte serum (Monaco *et al.*, 1965) or cyclophosphamide (Dukor and Dietrich, 1967). Adult, thymectomized animals treated in this manner cannot restore normal numbers of small lymphocytes and, histologically and immunologically, now resemble the neonatally thymectomized animal in their immunological incompetence.

IV. Thymic Malfunction; Clinical Disorders

A. *Recent Recognition of Thymic Involvement in Disease in Man*

It is now recognized that a large number of clinical disorders categorized as primary immunological deficiency diseases are directly related to an absence or malfunctioning of the thymus gland (Good, 1967). There are several excellent review articles and books which describe these diseases and correlate them with the growing number of newly reported immune disorders (Good, 1967; Miller, 1967; Rosen, 1968; Bergsma, 1968; Graf and Uhr, 1969; Alexander and Good, 1970).

The occurrence of these pathological states in the general population has only recently been established and is not, as yet, fully documented. Although these disorders differ outwardly in many of their clinical features, they share in common varying degrees of deficiency in cell-mediated immunological responses and in the ability of the individual to synthesize certain classes of immunoglobulins. More than 20 of these immune disorders have now been documented and this number is growing rapidly.

In some clinical disorders, such as the third and fourth pharyngeal pouch syndrome (DiGeorge syndrome), the thymus is either aplastic or fails to develop normally; absence of the parathyroid glands is often an accompanying feature. The DiGeorge syndrome is characterized immunologically by a marked failure to elicit typical delayed hypersensitivity and homograft reactions. Hence infants with this disorder are extremely susceptible to a wide range of infectious agents, particularly those which are viral or fungal. Although the antibody-producing mechanisms are intact and there is no significant deficiency in immunoglobulins, survival for more than one year is rare (DiGeorge, 1968).

Other types of immune diseases such as the Bruton sex-linked agammaglobulinemia are characterized by the cell-mediated response being normal in the presence of defects in humoral antibody production. Consequently, low levels of IgM, IgG, and IgA immunoglobulins are observed in the blood. Infants with this syndrome, although prone to recurrent pyrogenic pathogens, can live well into childhood and beyond if treated with γ-globulin and antibiotics (Bruton, 1952, 1968).

A third type of immunological disease, such as ataxia-telangiectasia, is characterized by defects in both cell-mediated and humoral antibody responses (Peterson and Good, 1968).

The majority of the primary immune disorders are congenital, but it is now recognized that a number of other disorders, such as autoimmune diseases (Burnet, 1962), certain lymphoid malignancies (Miller, 1962), as well as resistance to oncogenic viruses (Law, 1966) and many fungal and mycobacterial pathogens (Nahimias et al., 1967; Rees et al., 1967; August et al., 1968), are associated with thymic malfunction. For example, patients with cancer of lymphoid origin, particularly chronic lymphoid leukemia, exhibit deficient immunological responses and have increased susceptibility to debilitating infections (Shaw et al., 1960). Whether or not a preexisting immunological deficiency is related to the development of leukemia is still largely circumstantial, although leukemia has been observed to develop in patients with some preexisting immunological defects (Page et al., 1963). The rapid growth of tumors in some kidney transplant recipients receiving heavy immunosuppressive treatment is suggestive of a relationship between immunological competence and malignant growth (Russell, 1969). A considerable body of evidence is also available which suggests a causal relationship between immunological incompetence and the development of virus-induced (Law, 1966; Fefer et al., 1967), chemically induced (Stutman, 1969), and radiation-induced neoplasms (Kaplan, 1947).

The clinical study of Eilber and Morton (1970) also indicates that the state of cell-mediated resistance may influence the host's capacity to control malignant growth. These investigators found a positive correlation in cancer patients between the ability to manifest a delayed cutaneous hypersensitivity response to 2,4-dinitrochlorobenzene and the incidence of either inoperability, local recurrence, or distant metastases within 6 months postoperatively. Most recently, it has been reported (Johnson et al., 1971) that individuals refractive to the above aromatic nitro compound also do not exhibit an inflammatory response to croton oil. This last observation suggests that a basic defect may exist in patients with malignancy in their general capacity to respond to irritants.

The importance of the cell-mediated (thymus-dependent) segment of the immunological system in preventing many of the above-described clinical disorders has only recently been appreciated. Previously, humoral antibody-producing mechanisms were considered to be more important than cell-mediated mechanisms as a basis for general host resistance. This assumption no longer appears to be entirely correct. In fact, as indicated above from clinical and experimental studies, cell-mediated immunity appears to be responsible for a major degree of the body's immunological resistance in circumstances in which the classical immunoglobulin antibodies may not play a significant role.

V. Mechanism of Action of the Thymus

It is now well established that the thymus is the central organ in regulating the development and expression of cell-mediated immunity and general host resistance (cf. Miller and Osoba, 1967). Although the precise mechanisms by which the thymus exerts this influence on host resistance are still being defined, present evidence supports the concept that the thymus functions as both a donor of cells to the peripheral lymphoid system and by the production and secretion of one or more humoral factors (White and Goldstein, 1968, 1970a,b; 1971; Goldstein *et al.*, 1970b; Goldstein and White, 1970, 1971).

A. *Progenitor of Cells*

During fetal development, lymphoid-type cells appear in the thymus before they are detectable in other peripheral sites (Rowlands *et al.*, 1964; Miller, 1965). The thymus continues to produce large numbers of lymphocytes (thymocytes) during the last third of gestation and into the early postnatal period. This productive capacity of the thymus, based on measurements of mitotic indices, could account for 50–70% of all new lymphocytes (Metcalf, 1966). Although it was generally believed that the majority of the thymic lymphocytes are destroyed prior to departure from the thymus (Metcalf, 1966), recent studies in guinea pigs (Nossal, 1964) and rats (Weissman, 1967), using labeled thymocytes, suggest that thymocyte emigration from the thymus does occur. The extremely high rate of proliferation of thymic lymphocytes within the thymus is apparently independent of antigenic stimulation and is probably under the autonomous control of the epithelial elements within the thymic stromal network (Maximow, 1909). The basis for the extremely high rate of thymocyte proliferation within the thymus of the newborn animal, 5–10 times higher than that of any other lymphoid organ (Kindred, 1938), is not known. It has been proposed that this is a mechanism for the elimination of forbidden lymphoid clones (Burnet, 1969). An alternative explanation might be that the humoral secretion(s) of the thymic epithelial cells, with responsibility for the expansion of the lymphoid stem cell population throughout the body, will stimulate stem cells wherever they may exist. Obviously, the cells in closest proximity to the site of production of a secreted factor would be exposed to the highest concentration of this humoral agent and hence would manifest a marked degree of cell division.

B. Endocrine Function

There is a relatively recent but rapidly growing body of experimental evidence supporting the concept that the stimulatory influence of the thymic epithelial cells on thymic lymphocytes is humoral in nature. These data derive from experimental studies with thymectomized animals and involve replacement therapy with either thymic grafts, thymic tissue enclosed within cell-impermeable diffusion chambers, or cell-free thymic preparations.

1. Thymic Grafts

The first type of remedial experiments attempted in neonatally thymectomized animals consisted of transplanting one or more isogeneic thymic grafts in subcutaneous or intraperitoneal sites (Miller, 1962). These studies revealed that a single thymic graft was capable of preventing almost completely the "wasting syndrome," lymphocyte depletion, and immunological deficiencies usually seen in these experimental animals (Miller, 1962, 1964). It was further demonstrated that morphological and immunological restoration of lymphoid tissue structure and function could also be achieved with allogeneic (Dalmasso et al., 1963), but not heterologous, grafts (Yunis et al., 1964). Chromosomal marker studies (Miller, 1966) indicated that most of the immunologically competent cells appearing in the animals restored with allogeneic grafts were of host origin. In these studies with allogeneic thymus grafts, it was noted that such animals were tolerant also to skin grafts from animals of the same genotype of the donor of the transplanted thymus. Further studies revealed that lymphoid cell restoration could be achieved with thymoma grafts consisting of epithelial and reticular (mesenchymal) cells that were not lymphoid (Stutman et al., 1968).

In the clinical literature there have been at least two successful reports of implantation of thymic tissue in children with thymic aplasia. In one case, a 21-month-old male was implanted with fragments from a 16-week-old female fetus (August et al., 1968). Deficiencies of lymphocyte numbers and functions, such as failure to reject a foreign skin graft and lack of delayed hypersensitivity responses to *Monilia*, dinitrofluorobenzene, and phytohemagglutinin, were repaired within a dramatically short time. The rapid recovery of immune responses led the investigators to suggest that the clinical improvement was based on an endocrine or humoral mechanism.

In the second clinical case (Cleveland et al., 1968), a 7-month-old male received a transplant in the rectus abdominus muscle of three sections of thymic tissue from a 13-week-old female fetus. In this case also, there was a rapid restoration of blood lymphocyte numbers, as well as of the ability of the infant to resist infections. The rapidity with which recovery occurred of lymphoid and immunological responsiveness following implantation of the grafts again suggested an endocrine rather than a cellular mechanism as being involved in the clinical improvement.

August and his associates have published a subsequent report on the progress of their patient 18 months after thymic transplantation (August et al., 1970). Normal cell-mediated immunity was still present. The authors express the opinion that the transplantation approach promises to be of significant therapeutic value.

2. Thymic Grafts within Cell-Impermeable Diffusion Chambers

After the initial observations in experimental animals that the morphological and immunological deficiencies consequent to neonatal thymectomy could be reversed by thymic tissue transplantation, thymic grafts were placed within cell-impermeable Millipore diffusion chambers and transplanted into neonatally thymectomized mice to ascertain whether the recovery mechanisms required intact cells or humoral factors. In one of the first studies of this type, Levey and his colleagues (Levey et al., 1963a) found that neonatally thymectomized C_3Hf/Lw and C_3Hf/Bi mice implanted at 3–4 weeks of age with Millipore chambers (pore size, 0.45 μ) did not develop the characteristic depletion of blood lymphocytes or the typical wasting syndrome. At the same time, it was demonstrated independently by Osoba and Miller (1963) that neonatally thymectomized $(CBA \times T_6)F_1$ mice bearing thymic tissue in Millipore chambers (pore size, 0.3 μ) were similarly restored immunologically in that they could reject allografts, although they still showed depletion of lymphoid tissue. In the same year, Levey and his colleagues (Levey et al., 1963b) demonstrated that neonatally thymectomized Swiss mice, in contrast to normal mice, did not die when inoculated with lethal doses of lymphocytic choriomeningitis virus. Death from this virus is thought to be due to lymphocytic infiltration of the meninges and choroid plexus, possibly initiated by a hypersensitivity reaction which serves as a stimulus for lethal convulsions. The decrease in lethality of this virus in the neonatally thymectomized animal was apparently due to failure of development of host cell-mediated immunity as a consequence of early thymectomy. It was further shown by these investigators that restoration of cell-mediated immunity by isologous thymic tissue in Millipore diffusion chambers (pore size, 0.45 μ) resulted in the lethality of this virus again becoming manifested.

It thus appeared from these early experiments utilizing mice with thymic tissue transplants in Millipore diffusion chambers that the mechanisms of restoration of immunological parameters by thymic transplantation resided in a response elicited by a factor which could be released from the donor tissue enclosed in a cell-impermeable chamber.

These initial studies in mice with Millipore chambers did not provide answers to two basic questions: one, whether the humoral influence of the thymus was specific, that is, could other lymphoid tissues such as the spleen or lymph nodes also function in lieu of the thymus; and second, whether the humoral influence was species specific, that is, would allogeneic thymic grafts in diffusion chambers also be effective. These questions were both answered in the affirmative by the study of Osoba (1965). This investigator found that neonatally thymectomized CBA mice implanted at 9–12 days of age with Millipore diffusion chambers (pore size, 0.1 μ) containing either syngeneic (CBA) or allogeneic (C57Bl) thymic tissue restored the ability of the animals to reject foreign skin grafts (AKR), as well as to form hemagglutinins to sheep erythrocytes and to prevent wasting disease. However, under these experimental conditions there was no restoration of blood lymphocytes or of the normal histological appearance of the peripheral lymphoid tissues. Grafts of spleen or lymph node tissue within the same diffusion chambers failed to restore immunological competence of lymphocyte populations. Law and Ting (1965) have demonstrated that restoration of resistance to the polyoma virus in neonatally thymectomized mice could similarly be achieved by the implantation of thymic grafts within Millipore chambers. Similar restoration of resistance to syngeneic (Abdou and McKenna, 1969) and xenogeneic (Hallenbeck et al., 1969) transplanted tumors has been achieved by thymic grafts in Millipore chambers. Restoration of the allograft response in adult thymectomized, irradiated mice has been achieved with thymic tissue enclosed within Millipore chambers with pore sizes less than 0.1 μ (Barclay et al., 1964).

The effectiveness of thymic grafts within Millipore diffusion chambers in restoring immunological competence in mice has also been demonstrated in other species such as the rat (MacGillivray et al., 1964; Aisenberg and Wilkes, 1965; Biggart, 1966), the rabbit (Trench *et al.*, 1966), and the hamster (Wong *et al.*, 1966). However, most investigators have observed that, under the experimental conditions employed with Millipore chambers, reconstitution of normal lymphoid tissue morphology has been, at best, only partial.

Histological examination of the thymic tissue in Millipore chambers several weeks after implantation has revealed that the only viable structures present are reticuloepithelial cells (Levey *et al.*, 1963a; Osoba and Miller, 1963). This suggests that the humoral secretions of the thymus probably derive from this cell type. Light and electron microscopic studies of thymic tissue (Clark, 1966; Sanel, 1967) also suggest that some of the epithelial cells of the thymic stroma include what appear to be typical secretory cells. Recent studies by Stutman, Yunis, and Good (1968, 1969a,b) add support to the developing concept that the epithelial cells of the thymic stroma are secretory in nature. These investigators induced the formation of a nonlymphoid thymoma, consisting of reticuloepithelial cells, by instillation of 7,12-dimethylbenzanthracene directly into the thymus of mice. This thymoma was capable of fully restoring immunological responsiveness in neonatally thymectomized mice when it was implanted in Millipore diffusion chambers (pore size $<0.1 \mu$) into the operated animals.

3. Thymic Extracts

The influence of thymic extracts on physiological processes in normal and thymectomized animals has been studied for over 70 years (see White and Goldstein, 1968; Goldstein and White, 1970, for reviews of the older literature describing thymic extracts). The early studies with crude thymic extracts suggested that the thymus was involved in a multiplicity of regulatory mechanisms ranging from control of normal growth and development (Nowinski, 1930), to influences on calcium and phosphorus metabolism (Bracci, 1905; Potop *et al.*, 1966), fertility (Rowntree *et al.*, 1934), carbohydrate utilization (Bomskov and Sladovic, 1940), and the growth of tumors (Rohdenburg *et al.*, 1911). The enormous range of biological effects claimed, coupled with failure of confirmation of numerous reports, and the lack of chemical characterization of most of the extracts used, make it difficult to assess the significance of these earlier observations. In addition, the embryological development of the thymus gland occurs in such close proximity to the thyroid, parathyroid, and, in some species, the ultimobranchial body that, in many instances, tissue from one gland is enveloped in another, complicating the interpretation of reported biological effects of extracts of "thymic tissue." For example, the recent demonstration by Galante and his co-workers (1968) that calcitonin is present in the human thymus, although presenting a plausible explanation for the early observed influences of crude thymic extracts on calcium metabolism (Bracci, 1905), emphasizes the non-specific nature of the effect and may also provide a possible explanation for the reported failure by others to confirm a role for the thymus in calcium metabolism (cf. Park and McClure, 1919).

Evidence that the thymus gland produced a humoral factor capable of influencing the lymphoid system was first reported by Roberts and White (1949). Using ethanol-insoluble fractions of calf and rat thymic extracts, these investigators observed a stimulation of lymphocytopoiesis and an increase in lymphoid tissue size when these fractions were administered to normal rats. This initial observation was later confirmed by Gregoire and Duchateau (1956) in rats with extracts prepared from thymic tissue of irradiated pigs, by Metcalf (1956) in mice with extracts of mouse or human thymus, and by Nakamoto (1957) in rabbits with cow thymic extracts. From these early studies it was suggested that the thymus, a lymphoid organ, secreted a factor which could stimulate the growth and proliferation of peripheral lymphoid tissues. However, the relationship between lymphoid tissue proliferation under thymic influence and immunological competence was not suggested until 1961, when Miller (1961) and Archer and Pierce (1961) reported the results of their studies in neonatally thymectomized animals. In retrospect, suggestions did exist in the literature to the effect that thymectomized animals were very susceptible to infectious agents. By the early years of this century, numerous laboratories had reported that thymectomized animals frequently succumbed to infections (cf. Paton and Goodall, 1904; Park and McClure, 1919). At a more recent date, Furth (1946) showed that thymectomy in adult rats decreased host resistance to chemical carcinogens.

Subsequent to the experimental observations reported in 1961, a number of unsuccessful attempts were made in mice (Dalmasso et al., 1963; Miller, 1964) and in rats (Jankovic et al., 1962) to restore immunological and lymphocytic parameters in neonatally thymectomized animals with isologous, cell-free crude thymic fractions. These negative results may possibly have been due either to use of an inadequate dose of extracts or to inactivation of the active principles. In contrast, DeSomer and his associates (1963), using a cell-free extract prepared from incubated calf thymic slices *in vitro*, were able to restore peripheral lymphocyte counts, prevent the appearance of the wasting syndrome, and protect neonatally thymectomized animals against a fatal viral infection. Similarly, Jankovic and his colleagues (1965) reported that a crude "lipid rich" rat thymic fraction, when injected into neonatally thymectomized rats, induced a blood lymphocytosis and restored the ability of the experimental animals to elicit a delayed-type hypersensitivity reaction to bovine serum albumin.

The nature of a biologically active principle in crude thymic extracts was more precisely defined when the lymphocytopoietic factor present in the 105,000 g supernatant fraction of mouse, rat, and calf thymic tissue extracts (Klein et al., 1965, 1966) was partially purified (Goldstein et al., 1966). The biologically active component which induced a potent lymphocytopoietic response when injected in mice and guinea pigs and stimulated incorporation in vivo of precursors into the DNA, RNA, and proteins of mouse peripheral lymphoid tissue and spleen was termed *thymosin* (Goldstein et al., 1966).

Thymosin has been extracted and partially purified from calf thymic tissue by the following procedure. Fresh calf thymus is homogenized in 0.15 M NaCl and centrifuged at 1200 g to remove nuclei and cytoplasmic debris. The supernatant fluid is then centrifuged at 105,000 g for 60 minutes. The clear supernatant solution (fraction 1) contains the thymosin activity. This high speed supernatant is then subjected to a heat step ($>$80°C for 15 minutes). A large white voluminous precipitate which forms is removed by centrifugation at 20,000 g. The thymosin activity remains in the clear supernatant solution (fraction 2). The latter is then added slowly with constant stirring to 10 volumes of cold ($-$20°C) acetone. The acetone-insoluble precipitate (fraction 3), which contains the thymosin activity, is washed several times with cold acetone and dried *in vacuo*.

Fraction 3 can be stored at low temperatures ($< -$20°C) for periods of at least 6 months with little loss of activity (Goldstein and White, unpublished observations). In addition to its lymphocytopoietic activity *in vivo,* fraction 3 added to rat or rabbit mesenteric lymph node cells incubated in Eagle's minimal spinner culture media *in vitro,* was found to stimulate markedly the incorporation of tritiated thymidine into lymph node DNA (Goldstein et al., 1966).

Initially, it was believed that this activity of thymosin fractions *in vitro* could be the basis for a rapid assay in following further purification of thymosin. Examination of this *in vitro* activity indicated it to be associated with a low molecular weight component of fraction 3 (Goldstein et al., 1966). Subsequent purification, however, on P-10 polyacrylamide gel, DEAE-cellulose, CM Sephadex, and P-2 polyacrylamide gel revealed that this *in vitro* stimulatory activity was nonspecific and due to the presence in the acetone insoluble fraction of serine and, to a lesser extent, of glycine (Goldstein and White, unpublished observations). Both of these nonessential amino acids, which are not present in the Eagle spinner culture media (Eagle, 1959), are not active in our *in vivo* assay (Goldstein and White, unpublished observations).

The major portion of the thymosin lymphocytopoietic activity (Goldstein *et al.*, 1966), and the effects of thymosin on the enhancement of cell-mediated immunological competence (Law *et al.*, 1968a; Asanuma *et al.*, 1970; Goldstein *et al.*, 1970a, 1971a; White *et al.*, 1970b; Bach *et al.*, 1971) of fraction 3 have been found to reside in the protein fraction not retained on P-10 polyacrylamide gel (Goldstein *et al.*, 1966). Fraction 3 has been further purified by $(NH_4)_2SO_4$ fractionation. Activity is present in the fraction which is insoluble in 25–50% saturation with $(NH_4)_2SO_4$ (fraction 4). The latter is dialyzed free of salt and further purified by gel chromatography on Sephadex G-150 (fraction 5) and anion exchange chromatography on DEAE-cellulose or ECTEOLA (fraction 6) (Goldstein *et al.*, 1970b; unpublished observations).

The most highly purified lymphocytopoietic preparation available at this time (fraction 6) represents an approximately 500-fold purification in comparison with the activity, per milligram of protein, of the initial high speed supernatant fraction (fraction 1). The fraction obtained from the DEAE or ECTEOLA chromatography step (fraction 6) will induce the maturation *in vitro* of lymphoid stem cells to immunologically competent cells at concentrations of <0.01 µg of protein per 10^7 cells (Bach *et al.*, 1971). At concentrations of <25 µg protein per mouse per day for 3 days, thymosin also stimulates the incorporation of labeled precursors into the total DNA, RNA, and protein of the lymph nodes and spleens of normal (Goldstein *et al.*, 1966), irradiated (Goldstein *et al.*, 1970c), adrenalectomized (Goldstein *et al.*, unpublished observations), and germfree (Goldstein *et al.*, unpublished observations) mice, thus reflecting at a biological level the increase in lymph node weight seen following administration of thymosin.

Chemical studies of the purified thymosin fraction have yielded the following data (Goldstein *et al.*, unpublished observations). Polyacrylamide-gel electrophoresis in Tris–glycine buffer, pH 8.3 reveals one major and two minor components, all migrating toward the anode. On the basis of calibrated Sephadex-gel chromatography, the active component appears to have a molecular weight of less than 100,000 and exhibits some tendency to aggregate. The preparation has less than 1% of carbohydrate and a trace of lipid; the latter is not essential for biological activity. Thymosin activity is either identical to, or closely associated with, a protein. The most highly purified preparation available presently appears to have nothing unusual in its amino acid composition. The purified material, as described also for the early fractions, is relatively heat stable and does not contain nucleic acid. Lymphocytopoietic activity is unchanged after incubation with either RNase or DNase, but is destroyed by digestion with proteolytic enzymes.

Thymosin activity has also been found in the thymic tissue of a variety of animals including the rat, rabbit, guinea pig, hog, and the human. It may also be of interest to note that, although it has been generally accepted that the functional roles of the thymus are important primarily for the newborn and for younger animals prior to puberty, we have found that the quantity of thymosin lymphocytopoietic activity which can be isolated, per gram of thymus, is as great or greater in the thymus of older animals, for example, old cows and steers, as compared to young calves. These observations are in harmony with data suggesting that the thymic humoral factor is elaborated not by the mature thymocyte, but probably by the reticuloepithelial cells of the thymus (Clark, 1966; Sanel, 1967). In the thymus of the older animal, the relative proportion of epithelial cells to mature thymocytes is higher than in the thymus of the younger animal.

The administration of calf thymosin (fraction 3) to neonatally thymectomized CBA/Wh mice has been found to reduce the incidence of wasting disease, prolong survival, increase body weight gain and lymphoid tissue size, and elevate the number of absolute blood lymphocytes to a degree significantly greater than in operated animals given saline or other calf tissue extracts, such as calf spleen or liver; or protein antigens, such as bovine serum albumin; or lipopolysaccharide antigens, such as the endotoxin from *Salmonella enteritidis* (Asanuma et al., 1970; White and Goldstein (1970b). These studies extend the earlier observations of other investigators using less well-defined thymus cell-free fractions (DeSomer et al., 1963; Trainin et al., 1966).

The increase in life-span and the growth of lymphoid tissues following thymosin treatment in neonatally thymectomized CBA/Wh mice is reflected in a partial restoration of immunological capacities in the experimental animals (Goldstein et al., 1970a). Thymosin treated mice show completely normal cell-mediated immunological responses, such as the ability to reject a foreign skin allograft (Goldstein et al., 1970a), and their spleen cells can elect a graft vs. host reaction (White and Goldstein, 1970b; Goldstein et al., 1971a). In contrast, there is no significant influence of thymosin on humoral immunity in the operated animals as reflected by the lack of ability to make 19 S or 7 S antibody to sheep erythrocytes (Goldstein et al., 1970a).

In another experimental model, Law and his associates (1968a) have found that spleen cells from neonatally thymectomized C57Bl/KaLw mice treated with thymosin, in contrast to spleen cells from similar mice injected with a spleen fraction, were able to elicit a typical graft vs. host reaction, i.e., splenomegaly, when administered to newborn histoincompatible BALB/c mice. In the same study, it was noted that peripheral blood lymphocytes in the thymosin-treated mice were also significantly elevated.

The data presently available from these studies with neonatally thymectomized mice suggest that thymosin can restore cell-mediated immunological phenomena in the absence of an intact thymus but has little or no influence on humoral immunological responses to sheep erythrocytes under the experimental conditions used.

The influence of this endocrine function of the thymus has been explored also in adult thymectomized, lethally irradiated mice of the A/J strain given syngeneic bone marrow cells to maintain hemopoietic function. This animal is analogous to the neonatally thymectomized animal in that its lymphoid tissues remain depleted, it is very susceptible to infection, and its cell-mediated responses, as well as some of its humoral antibody-forming capacities, are markedly deficient. This exprimental animal, like the neonatally thymectomized animal, is unable to reject skin allografts (Miller *et al.*, 1963) or even xenografts (Davis *et al.*, 1964). Also, the ability to make antibody to some antigens, such as sheep erythrocytes, is depressed. Thymosin administration to these animals does not renew their capacity to make 19 S antibody after a challenge with sheep erythrocytes (Goldstein *et al.*, 1970a) but restores cellular immunity as measured by the ability to reject C57Bl/6 (histoincompatible) skin grafts (Goldstein *et al.*, unpublished observations).

The influence of thymosin on processes relating to cellular immunity are seen in normal mice as well as in the immunologically incompetent animal. Hardy and his colleagues (1968) have demonstrated that normal $B_{10}D_2/S_n$ mice, when treated with thymosin, reject first- and second-set C57Bl/6 skin grafts in an accelerated manner. In contrast, the ability to make hemagglutinating antibody titers to sheep erythrocytes in normal or irradiated mice is not increased by thymosin treatment (Goldstein *et al.*, 1970a). Wolf and Erb (1971), using lymph node explants from immunized rabbits, have made the interesting observation that the secondary response to diphtheria toxoid *in vitro* can be enhanced severalfold by the addition of low concentrations of thymosin (<1.0 μg). These observations suggest that thymosin may play some still undefined role in the manufacture and release of antibody during the secondary response to particular antigens.

Recent studies have demonstrated that the thymus gland is involved in host resistance to many types of viruses (Law, 1966; Miller, 1967). This resistance apparently resides, to a large extent, within the framework of the host cell-mediated segment of the immunological system (Law et al., 1966; Zisblatt et al., 1970). Any treatment which decreases cellular immunity, such as neonatal thymectomy, increases the susceptibility to oncogenic viruses. For example, Law and his associates (1966, 1968b) have shown that neonatal thymectomy in mice increases the incidence of progressive tumor growth in response to the Moloney sarcoma virus and the polyoma virus. Additional studies from the same laboratory demonstrated that resistance to these viruses can be achieved by grafting thymic tissue (Law et al., 1966, 1968b) or by implantation of thymic grafts within cell-impermeable Millipore chambers (Law et al., 1966).

Viruses such as the Moloney sarcoma virus (MSV) are excellent tools for studying the natural development of cell-mediated immunity since the lethality of this virus is directly related to the state of the host's cell-mediated immunological capacity (Zisblatt et al., 1970). In a normal immunologically competent animal, MSV inoculation in the proper concentration will induce the growth of a primary tumor in over 90% of the animals after a short latency period (4–8 days). This phase, i.e., growth of the primary tumor, is partly independent of the host's immunological competence. However, the regression of the tumor appears to depend upon the state of the host's cell-mediated immune system. For example, 85–100% of all CBA/Wh mice inoculated with a given dose of MSV from birth to 2 weeks of age succumb to progressive tumor growth. In contrast, only 40% of the mice inoculated at 3 weeks of age die as a result of the growth of the tumor. When mice have reached 5 weeks of age, none will succumb as a result of MSV inoculation. Thus, at some period between the second and third week of life the host's cell-mediated immunity is developed to a point at which it is partially capable of preventing progressive tumor growth and death, and the tumor regresses in a significant number of the mice. The acceleration of maturation of cell-mediated immunity would naturally be expected to accelerate the development of immunity to oncogenic viruses. That this can indeed occur, and that it depends upon an endocrine influence of the thymus, has recently been demonstrated by Zisblatt and his colleagues (1970). Calf thymosin administration from birth to 2 weeks of age in normal mice accelerated significantly the resistance to progressive tumor growth in animals inoculated with MSV at 2 weeks of age. The 2-week-old thymosin-treated mouse behaved, immunologically, similarly to a 3-week-old untreated mouse (Zisblatt et al., 1970). Other similarly prepared calf extracts from spleen or liver were without influence on the development of host resistance to the oncogenic MSV.

In adult immunosuppressed mice, as well, it has been shown that progressive growth of an MSV-induced tumor depends quantitatively upon the number of immunologically competent cells available to the host to challenge the tumor (Goldstein *et al.*, 1971b). Most recently it has been demonstrated by Hardy *et al.* (1971) that in adult mice which have been immunosuppressed with antilymphocyte serum or X-irradiation, and then inoculated with MSV, thymosin administration can restore the animal's capacity to resist progressive tumor growth.

Several recent studies concerned with the role of an antithymosin serum prepared in rabbits on host immunity and lymphoid tissue have been reported (Hardy *et al.*, 1968, 1969). In contrast to the accelerated skin graft rejection in normal mice treated with thymosin, treatment with antithymosin serum has been found to delay significantly first- and second-set allograft rejection in A/J mice (Hardy *et al.*, 1968). This antiserum appears to be unique in that it crosses species lines and is cytotoxic to and agglutinates thymocytes of several species *in vitro* but not lymphocytes or spleen cells (Hardy *et al.*, 1969). The potential uses of thymosin and antithymosin serum in conjunction with antilymphocyte serum to suppress the allograft response have been investigated by Quint and his colleagues (1969a,b). These investigators have observed that thymosin can either reduce or potentiate the immunosuppressive effects of mouse antilymphocyte serum (ALS) on cell-mediated immune processes depending upon the schedule of treatment. Thymosin, given 6 hours before ALS, prolongs allograft survival in A/J mice from 22 days, with ALS alone, to more than 50 days (Quint *et al.*, 1969a,b). In contrast, thymosin given following ALS, partially reverses the severe immunosuppressive action of ALS (Quint *et al.*, 1969a,b). Control calf tissue extracts prepared from brain, liver, and spleen were inactive under these experimental conditions (Quint, Hardy, and Monaco, private communication). The mechanism underlying the action of thymosin in this system with ALS is not completely understood. The hypothesis has been suggested (Quint *et al.*, 1969b) that thymosin administration increases the number and the rate of development and/or maturation of immunologically competent cells present in the circulation and, thus, enables ALS to come into contact with and inactivate a larger number of thymic dependent cells.

The capacity of purified thymosin fractions to restore the population of thymus dependent rosette forming cells in adult thymectomized mice has recently been examined (Bach *et al.*, 1971). The addition of thymosin *in vitro* to spleen cells from the operated animals restored normal numbers of thymus dependent rosette forming cells as measured by sensitivity to azathioprine, antilymphocyte serum, and antitheta serum.

In addition, it was demonstrated that thymosin can, *in vitro,* cause to appear on the surface of bone marrow cells immunologically functional receptor sites as reflected in the appearance of theta antigen.

VI. Concluding Comments

In this chapter we have described a number of the recently elucidated functions of the thymus in the development and maturation of lymphoid tissue and in the development of host immunity. While the complete role of the thymus gland in the homeostasis of the body is still being defined, it is apparent from the most recent experimental data in this area of research that part of the function of the thymus is based upon the production and secretion by the gland of one or more humoral factors. The mechanism by which the thymus exerts this apparent endocrine role and the number of hormones secreted by the thymus are in the early stages of exploration. The responses to partially purified thymic fractions of those functions of lymphoid tissue which are fundamental to host immunological competence and the similarity of these data to those of other reports using cell-free thymic extracts prepared in other laboratories, suggests that several of the diverse "crude" thymic fractions may contain a single biologically active substance similar to or identical with thymosin.

Although knowledge of the potential roles of the thymus gland and its functions is still incomplete, the recent experimental data indicate that these are dependent upon the secretion of one or more humoral factors. It is also established that the thymus is a major source of lymphocytes for the peripheral lymphoid tissues and circulation. Thus the thymus exerts a dual function, namely, as an endocrine gland and as a progenitor of lymphoid cells.

We have recently formulated a hypothesis which unifies the concepts of an endocrine and a cellular function of the thymus (White and Goldstein, 1970b; Goldstein and White, 1971). This hypothesis is based upon the newer experimental evidence that thymosin, probably secreted by the reticuloepithelial cells of the thymus, can act in lieu of the thymus to restore cell-mediated immunological competence in a number of experimental systems but is without action on humoral antibody synthesis (Goldstein *et al.,* 1970a; Goldstein and White, 1970, 1971; White and Goldstein, 1970a,b, 1971). The experimental data available suggest that there are at least two populations of thymus-dependent immunologically competent cells, in addition to at least a third large class of thymus-independent cells which are potential antibody-producing cells. The last class includes the cells that act in cooperation with a thymus-dependent

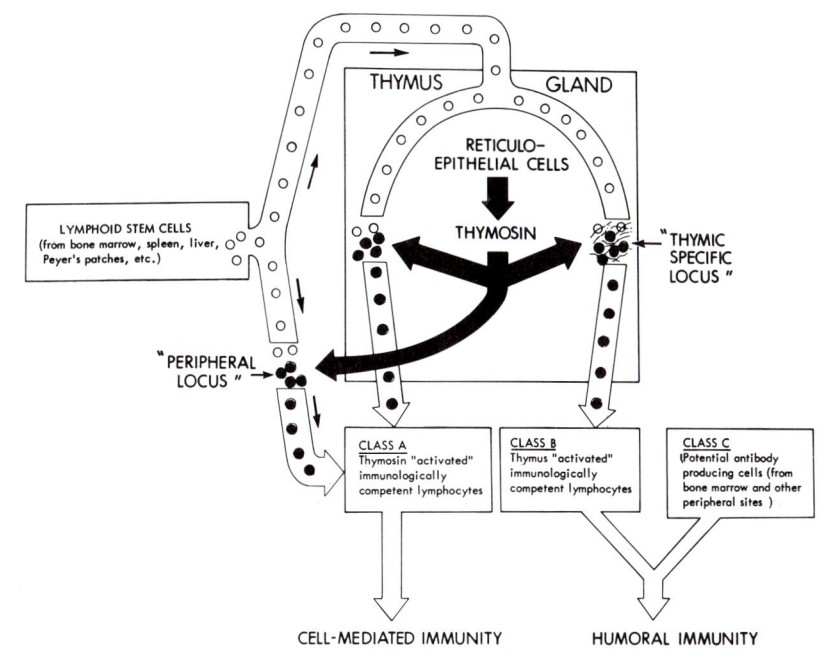

Fig. 1. Schematic representation of the role of thymosin in the development of immunologically competent cells. See text for details (from White and Goldstein, 1970b).

cell in the production of humoral antibody (Claman et al., 1966; Miller and Mitchell, 1968).

Figure 1 diagrams our suggested concept of the maturation of the two classes of thymus-dependent immunologically competent cells. One type, termed *Class A cells,* can mature solely under the influence of thymosin acting upon stem cell precursors (pre- or post-thymic cell populations) from bone marrow, spleen, liver, Peyer's patches or other peripheral sites; i.e., this maturation does not require an *in situ* thymic locus. The experimental data (Goldstein et al., 1970d, 1971a; White and Goldstein, 1970b, 1971) suggest that maturation of this type of immunologically competent cell occurs rapidly and may involve derepression or activation of an incompetent cell at a specific stage in its differentiation. The development of Class A cells may occur either within or outside of the thymic environment. The second type of lymphocyte, which we have termed *Class B cells,* are thymus-dependent cells involved in humoral immunity. This cell, once mature, can recognize either soluble antigens or antigens which have been solubilized by macrophages, and is capable of acting in cooperation with a population of thymus-independent cells (*Class C cells*) which contain the antibody-producing mechanism and thus are necessary to elicit a humoral response. Our experimental findings indicate that maturation of Class B lymphocytes requires specifically, in contrast to Class A lymphocytes, an intact thymic locus for proper development, as well as thymosin and/or other thymic factors. Thus, the stem cells from which Class B cells arise must, at some time in their development, reside within the thymus proper. The distinction between the two classes of thymus-dependent cells (*A and B*) is based upon whether or not maturation must occur within the thymic environment.

In a normal animal, the development of Class A cells can occur within the thymic environment, as well as peripherally. Our recent studies of the reconstitution of neonatally thymectomized mice by administration of thymosin (Law *et al.*, 1968a; Asanuma *et al.*, 1970; Goldstein *et al.*, 1970a) indicate that a thymic locus is not, however, an absolute requirement for the maturation of these cells. It is possible that the extremely high mitotic index within the thymus is a reflection of the influence of thymic humoral factors on the maturation and/or expansion of both Class A and Class B cells that are either indigenous to the thymus or have entered the gland from the periphery.

It appears that peripheral development of immunologically competent cells is influenced significantly by thymosin and possibly other thymic humoral factors which act upon stem cell populations at sites removed from the thymus. These stem cells may include cells that early in their development may have been in the thymus or have come under its influence, such as the post-thymic cells described by Stutman and his colleagues (Stutman *et al.*, 1969a). Our use of the term "stem cell" is to designate the progenitor of the cells involved in immunological reactions. Under the influence of thymosin, these stem cells can be activated to react immunologically. The term "activated" is used because we are not yet certain whether the process of maturation is based on an immediate derepression mechanism or represents a more prolonged process, perhaps occurring in stages. The suggestion that maturation of Class A cells occurs rapidly and may involve a derepression mechanism derives from evidence from several types of recently published investigations in our laboratory (Goldstein *et al.*, 1971a; Howe *et al.*, 1970a,b; White and Goldstein, 1970b). The findings point to the existence of a population of stem cells within which resides a number of latent cells which can be stimulated by thymosin to accelerate the maturation of their immunological competence.

It remains for future studies with completely defined thymic fractions to characterize precisely the nature and number of thymic factors secreted by the thymus and the mechanisms involved in the release and control of these hormones. An understanding of these processes will, it may be anticipated, aid in elucidation of the basis for the development and expression of host resistance and be of possible assistance in the diagnosis and treatment of diseases relating to a failure or defect of normal immunological processes.

References

Abdou, N. I., and McKenna, J. M. (1969). *Int. Arch. Allergy Appl. Immunol.* **35**, 20.
Ackerman, G. A., and Knouff, R. A. (1965). *Anat. Rec.* **152**, 35.
Aisenberg, A. C., and Wilkes, B. (1965). *Nature (London)* **205**, 716.
Alexander, J. W., and Good, R. A. (1970). "Immunobiology for Surgeons." Saunders, Philadelphia, Pennsylvania.
Archer, O. K., and Pierce, J. C. (1961). *Fed. Proc. Fed. Amer. Soc. Exp. Biol.* **20**, 26.
Asanuma, Y., Goldstein, A. L., and White, A. (1970). *Endocrinology* **86**, 601.
Auerbach, R. (1961). *Develop. Biol.* **3**, 336.
August, C. S., Berkel, A. I., Levey, R. H., Rosen, F. S., and Kay, H. E. M. (1970). *Lancet* **i**, 1080.
August, C. S., Rosen, F. S., Filler, R. M., Janeway, C. A., Markowsky, B., and Kay, H. E. (1968). *Lancet* **ii**, 1210.
Bach, J.-F., and Dardenne, M. (1971). *Cell. Immunol.* In press.
Bach, J.-F., Dardenne, M., Goldstein, A. L., Guha, A., and White, A. (1971). *Proc. Nat. Acad. Sci.* In press.
Barclay, T. J., Weissman, I. L., and Kaplan, H. S. (1964). *In* "The Thymus" (V. Defendi and D. Metcalf, eds.), Wistar Inst. Monogr. No. 2, pp. 117–119. Wistar Inst. Press, Philadelphia, Pennsylvania.
Beard, J. (1899). *Lancet* **i**, 144.
Bergsma, D. (1968). *In* "Immunologic Deficiency Diseases in Man." *Birth Defects, Orig. Artic. Ser.* **4**. National Foundation, New York.
Biedl, A. (1923). "The Internal Secretory Organs: Their Physiology and Pathology," pp. 110–124. William Wood, New York.
Biggart, J. D. (1966). *Brit. J. Exp. Pathol.* **47**, 586.
Blattner, R. (1963). *J. Pediat.* **62**, 445.
Bomskov, C., and Sladovic, L. (1940). *Deut. Med. Wochenschr.* **22**, 589.
Bracci, C. (1905). *Riv. Clin. Pediat.* **3**, 572.
Bruton, O. C. (1952). *Pediatrics* **9**, 722.
Bruton, O. C. (1968). *In* "Immunologic Deficiency Diseases in Man." *Birth Defects, Orig. Artic. Ser.* **4**. National Foundation, New York.
Buckton, K. E., and Pike, M. C. (1964). *Nature (London)* **202**, 714.
Burnet, F. M. (1959). *Brit. Med. J.* **ii**, 645.
Burnet, F. M. (1962). *Brit. Med. J.* **ii**, 807.
Burnet, F. M. (1969). "Cellular Immunity." Univ. of Melbourne Press, Carlton, Australia.
Claman, H. N., Chaperon, E. A., and Triplett, R. F. (1966). *Proc. Soc. Exp. Biol. Med.* **122**, 1167.

Clark, S. L., Jr. (1966). *Thymus Exp. Clin. Stud., Ciba Found. Symp.* 1966, Melbourne, pp. 3–38.
Cleveland, W. W., Fogel, B. J., Brown, W. T., and Kay, H. E. M. (1968). *Lancet* ii, 1211.
Dalmasso, A. P., Martinez, C., and Good, R. A. (1962a). *Proc. Soc. Exp. Biol. Med.* 111, 143.
Dalmasso, A. P., Martinez, C., and Good, R. A. (1962b). *Proc. Soc. Exp. Biol. Med.* 110, 205.
Dalmasso, A. P., Martinez, C., Sjodin, K., and Good, R. A. (1963). *J. Exp. Med.* 118, 1089.
Davis, W. E., Jr., Tyan, M. L., and Cole, L. J. (1964). *Science* 145, 394.
DeSomer, P., Denys, P., Jr., and Leyten, R. (1963). *Life Sci.* 11, 810.
DiGeorge, A. M. (1968). *In* "Immunologic Deficiency Diseases in Man." *Birth Defects, Orig. Artic. Ser.* 4, 116. National Foundation, New York.
Dukor, P., and Dietrich, F. M. (1967). *Int. Arch. Allergy Appl. Immunol.* 32, 131.
Eagle, H. (1959). *Science* 130, 432.
Eilber, F. R., and Morton, D. L. (1970). *Cancer* 25, 362.
Ernström, U., and Sandberg, G. (1970). *Acta Pathol. Microbiol. Scand.* 78, 362.
Fefer, A. G., McCoy, J. L., and Glynn, J. P. (1967). *Cancer Res.* 27, 1626.
Fichtelius, K. E., Laurell, G., and Phillipsson, L. (1961). *Acta Pathol. Microbiol. Scand.* 51, 81.
Ford, C. E. (1966). *Thymus: Exp. Clin. Stud., Ciba Found. Symp.,* 1966, Melbourne, pp. 131–152.
Ford, C. E., and Micklem,H. S. (1963). *Lancet* 1, 359.
Friedleben, A. (1858). "Die Physiologie der Thymusdrüse." Rütter, Frankfurt am Main.
Furth, J. J. (1946). *J. Gerontol.* 46, 1.
Galante, L., Gudmundsson, T. V., Matthews, E. W., Tse, A., Williams, E. D., Woodhouse, N. J. Y., and MacIntyre, I. (1968). *Lancet* ii, 537.
Goldstein, A. L., and White, A. (1970). *In* "Biochemical Actions of Hormones" (G. Litwack, ed.), Vol. 1, pp. 465–502. Academic Press, New York.
Goldstein, A. L., and White, A. (1971). *Adv. Metab. Disord.* 5, 149.
Goldstein, A. L., Slater, F. D., and White, A. (1966). *Proc. Nat. Acad. Sci. U.S.* 56, 1010.
Goldstein, A. L., Asanuma, Y., Battisto, J. R., Hardy, M. A., Quint, J., and White, A. (1970a). *J. Immunol.* 104, 359.
Goldstein, A. L., Asanuma, Y., and White, A. (1970b). *Recent Progr. Horm. Res.* 26, 505.
Goldstein, A. L., Banerjee, A., Schneebeli, G. L., Dougherty, T. F., and White, A. (1970c). *Radiat. Res.* 41, 579.
Goldstein, A. L., Guha, A., Zisblatt, M., Lilly, F., and White, A. (1970d). *Fed. Proc. Fed. Amer. Soc. Exp. Biol.* 7, 826.
Goldstein, A. L., Guha, A., Howe, M. L., and White, A. (1971a). *J. Immunol.* 106, 773.
Goldstein, A. L., Zisblatt, M., and Arvan, G. (1971b). *Fed. Proc. Fed. Amer. Soc. Exp. Biol.* 30, 241.
Good, R. A. (1967). *Hosp. Prac.* 7, 39.
Good, R. A., and Gabrielsen, A. E., eds. (1964). "The Thymus in Immunobiology, Structure, Function and Role in Disease." Hårper (Hoeber), New York.

Good, R. A., Dalmasso, A. P., Martinez, C., Archer, O. K., Pierce, J. C., and Papermaster, B. W. (1962). *J. Exp. Med.* **116**, 773.
Gowans, J. L. (1965). *Brit. Med. Bull.* **21**, 106.
Graf, M. W., and Uhr, J. W. (1969). *Advan. Intern. Med.* **15**, 397.
Gregoire, C., and Duchateau, G. (1956). *Arch. Biol.* **67**, 269.
Hallenbeck, G. A., Kubista, T. P., and Shorter, R. G. (1969). *Proc. Soc. Exp. Biol. Med.* **130**, 1142.
Ham, A. W. (1965). "Textbook of Histology," 5th Ed. Lippincott, Philadelphia, Pennsylvania.
Hammar, J. A. (1910). *Ergeb. Anat. Entwicklungsgesch.* **19**, 1.
Hammar, J. A. (1936). "Die Normal-morphologische Thymusforschung im Letzten Vierteljahrhundert." Barth, Leipzig.
Hardy, M. A., Quint, J., Goldstein, A. L., State, D., and White, A. (1968). *Proc. Nat. Acad. Sci. U.S.* **61**, 875.
Hardy, M. A., Quint, J., Goldstein, A. L., White, A., State, D., and Battisto, J. R. (1969). *Proc. Soc. Exp. Biol. Med.* **130**, 214.
Hardy, M. A., Zisblatt, M., Levine, N., Goldstein, A. L., Lilly, F., and White, A. (1971). *Transplant. Proc.* **3**, 926.
Hess, M. W. (1968). "Experimental Thymectomy, Possibilities and Limitations." Springer-Verlag, Berlin and New York.
Howe, M. L., Goldstein, A. L., and Battisto, J. R. (1970a). *Proc. Leukocyte Cult. Conf., 5th, 1970, Ottawa,* pp. 515–526.
Howe, M. L., Goldstein, A. L., and Battisto, J. R. (1970b). *Proc. Nat. Acad. Sci. U.S.* **67**, 613.
Jankovic, B. D., Waksman, B. H., and Arnason, B. G. (1962). *J. Exp. Med.* **116**, 159.
Jankovic, B. D., Isakovic, K., and Horvat, J. (1965). *Nature (London)* **208**, 356.
Johnson, M. W., Maibach, H. I., and Salmon, S. E. (1971). *New Engl. J. Med.* **284**, 1255.
Kaplan, H. S. (1947). *Cancer Res.* **7**, 141.
Kindred, J. E. A. (1938). *Amer. J. Anat.* **62**, 453.
Klein, J. J., Goldstein, A. L., and White, A. (1965). *Proc. Nat. Acad. Sci. U.S.* **53**, 812.
Klein, J. J., Goldstein, A. L., and White, A. (1966). *Ann. N.Y. Acad. Sci.* **135**, 485.
Kotani, M., Seiki, K., Yamashita, A., and Horit, I. (1966). *Blood* **27**, 511.
Krüger, J., Goldstein, A. L., and Waksman, B. H. (1970). *Cell. Immunol.* **1**, 51.
Law, L. W. (1966). *Cancer Res.* **26**, 551.
Law, L. W., and Ting, R. C. (1965). *Proc. Soc. Exp. Biol. Med.* **119**, 823.
Law, L. W., Ting, R. C., and Leckband, E. (1966). *Thymus: Exp. Clin. Stud., Ciba Found. Symp., 1966,* pp. 214–241.
Law, L. W., Goldstein, A. L., and White, A. (1968a). *Nature (London)* **219**, 1391.
Law, L. W., Ting, R. C., and Stanton, M. F. (1968b). *J. Nat. Cancer Inst.* **40**, 1101.
Levey, R. H., Trainin, N., and Law, L. W. (1963a). *J. Nat. Cancer Inst.* **31**, 199.
Levey, R. H., Trainin, N., Law, L. W., Black, P. H., and Rowe, W. P. (1963b). *Science* **142**, 483.

Little, J. R., Brecher, G., Bradley, T. R., and Rose, S. (1962). *Blood* **19**, 236.
MacGillivray, M. H., Jones, V. E., and Leskowitz, S. (1964). *Fed. Proc. Fed. Amer. Soc. Exp. Biol.* **23**, 189.
Maximow, A. A. (1909). *Arch. Mikrosk. Anat.* **74**, 525.
Medawar, P. B. (1963). *Ciba Found. Study Group* (*Pap.*) **16**, 1–15.
Metcalf, D. (1956). *Brit. J. Cancer* **10**, 442.
Metcalf, D. (1965). *Nature* (*London*) **208**, 1336.
Metcalf, D. (1966). "Recent Results in Cancer Research." Springer-Verlag, Berlin and New York.
Miller, J. F. A. P. (1961). *Lancet* **ii**, 748.
Miller, J. F. A. P (1962). *Ann. N.Y. Acad. Sci.* **99**, 340.
Miller, J. F. A. P. (1964). *In* "The Thymus in Immunobiology" (R. A. Good and A. E. Gabrielsen, eds.), pp. 436–464. Harper (Hoeber), New York.
Miller, J. F. A. P. (1965). *Nature* (*London*) **208**, 1337.
Miller, J. F. A. P. (1966). *Thymus: Exp. Clin. Stud., Ciba Found. Symp., 1966*, Melbourne, pp. 153–180.
Miller, J. F. A. P. (1967). *Modern Trends in Pathology* **2**, 140.
Miller, J. F. A. P., and Mitchell, G. F. (1968). *J. Exp. Med.* **128**, 801.
Miller, J. F. A. P., and Osoba, D. (1967). *Physiol. Rev.* **47**, 437.
Miller, J. F. A. P., Marshall, A. H. E., and White, R. G. (1962) *Advan. Immunol.* **2**, 111.
Miller, J. F. A. P., Doak, S. M. A., and Cross, A. M. (1963). *Proc. Soc. Exp. Biol. Med.* **112**, 785.
Monaco, A. P., Wood, M. L., and Russell, P. S. (1965). *Science* **149**, 432.
Nahimias, A. J., Griffith, D., Salsbury, C., and Yoshida, D. (1967). *J. Amer. Med. Ass.* **201**, 729.
Nakamoto, A. (1957). *Nippon Ketsueki Gakkai Zasshi* **20**, 187.
Nossal, G. J. V. (1964). *Ann. N.Y. Acad. Sci.* **120**, 171.
Nowinski, W. W. (1930). *Biochem. Z.* **226**, 415.
Osoba, D. (1965). *J. Exp. Med.* **122**, 633.
Osoba, D., and Miller, J. F. A. P. (1963). *Nature* (*London*) **199**, 653.
Page, A. R., Hansen, A. E., and Good, R. A. (1963). *Blood* **21**, 197.
Pappenheimer, A. M. (1914). *J. Exp. Med.* **19**, 319.
Park, E. A., and McClure, R. D. (1919). *Amer. J. Dis. Child.* **18**, 317.
Parrott, D. M. V., DeSousa, M. A. B., and East, J. (1966). *J. Exp. Med.* **123** 191.
Paton, D. N., and Goodall, A. (1904). *J. Physiol.* (*London*) **31**, 49.
Perla, D., and Marmorston, J. (1941). "Natural Resistance and Clinical Medicine." Little, Brown, Boston, Massachusetts.
Peterson, R. D. A., and Good, R. A. (1968). *In* "Immunologic Deficiency Diseases in Man." *Birth Defects, Orig. Artic. Ser.* **4**, 370. National Foundation, New York.
Potop, I., Boeru, V., and Mreană, G. (1966). *Biochem. J.* **101**, 454.
Quint, J., Hardy, M. A., and Monaco, A. P. (1969a). *Fed. Proc. Fed. Amer. Soc. Exp. Biol.* **28**, 694.
Quint, J., Hardy, M. A., and Monaco, A. P. (1969b). *Surg. Forum* **20**, 252.
Rees, R. J. W., Waters, M. F. R., Weddell, A. G. M., and Palmer, E. (1967). *Nature* (*London*) **215**, 599.
Roberts, S., and White, A. (1949). *J. Biol. Chem.* **178**, 151.

Rohdenburg, J., Bullock, F. D., and Johnston, P. J. (1911). *AMA Arch. Intern. Med.* **7**, 491.
Rosen, F. S. (1968). *New Engl. J. Med.* **279**, 643.
Rowlands, D. T., LaVia, M. F., and Block, M. H. (1964). *J. Immunol.* **93**, 157.
Rowntree, L. G., Clark, J. H., and Hansen, A. M. (1934). *J. Amer. Med. Ass.* **103**, 1425.
Russell, P. S. (1969). *Transplant. Proc.* **1**, 659.
Ruth, R. F. (1961). *Anat. Rec.* **139**, 270.
Sanel, F. T. (1967). *Z. Zellforsch. Mikrosk. Anat.* **83**, 8.
Shaw, R. K., Szed, C., Boggs, D. R., Fahey, J. L., Frei, E., Morrison, E., and Utz, J. P. (1960). *Arch. Intern. Med.* **106**, 467.
Stutman, O. (1969). *Science* **166**, 620.
Stutman, O., Yunis, E. J., and Good, R. A. (1968). *J. Nat. Cancer Inst.* **41**, 1431.
Stutman, O., Yunis, E. J., and Good, R. A. (1969a). *Transplant. Proc.* **1**, 614.
Stutman, O., Yunis, E. J., and Good, R. A. (1969b). *J. Nat. Cancer Inst.* **43**, 499.
Taylor, R. B. (1965). *Nature (London)* **208**, 1334.
Trainin, N., Bejerano, A., Strahilevitch, M., Goldring, D., and Small, M. (1966). *Isr. J. Med. Sci.* **2**, 549.
Trench, C. A. H., Watson, J. W., Walker, F. C., Gardner, P. S., and Green, C. A. (1966). *Immunology* **10**, 187.
Von Kolliken, R. A. (1879). "Entwicklungsgeschichte des Menschen und der höhren Thiere," pp. 815–880. Engelmann, Leipzig.
Weissman, I. L. (1967). *J. Exp. Med.* **126**, 291.
White, A., and Goldstein, A. L. (1968). *Perspect. Biol. Med.* **11**, 475.
White, A., and Goldstein, A. L. (1970a). *Contr. Processes Multicell. Organisms, Ciba Found. Symp., 1969*, pp. 210–237.
White, A., and Goldstein, A. L. (1970b). *Ciba Found. Study Group (Pap.)* **36**, 210–237.
White, A., and Goldstein, A. L. (1971). *In* "Immunogenecity" (F. Borek, ed.), North-Holland Publ., Amsterdam.
Wolf, B., and Erb, S. D. (1971). *Proc. Leukocyte Cult. Conf., 4th, 1971*, pp. 207–217.
Wong, F. M., Taub, R. N., Sherman, J. D., and Dameshek, W. (1966). *Blood* **28**, 40.
Yunis, E. J., Martinez, C., and Good, R. A. (1964). *Nature (London)* **204**, 664.
Zisblatt, M., Goldstein, A. L., Lilly, F., and White, A. (1970). *Proc. Nat. Acad. Sci. U.S.* **66**, 1170.

CALCITONIN

*J. T. Potts, Jr., H. D. Niall, and L. J. Deftos**

ENDOCRINE UNIT
MASSACHUSETTS GENERAL HOSPITAL
BOSTON, MASSACHUSETTS

I. Introduction 151
II. The Chemistry of Calcitonins 152
   A. Isolation 152
   B. Special Problems in Isolation 153
   C. Sequence Determination 154
   D. Synthesis 156
   E. Structure and Function in the Calcitonins 156
III. Control of Secretion of Calcitonin 161
   A. Control of Secretion 161
   B. Direct Estimation of Secretory Rate 163
   C. Effect of Gastrointestinal Factors 165
   D. Effect of Dietary Calcium 165
   E. Studies in Fish 167
   F. Studies in Humans 167
IV. Therapeutic Uses of Calcitonin 169
   References 172

I. Introduction

The study of the hypocalcemic peptide hormone calcitonin has progressed remarkably since the original experiments in which Copp,

* Cancer Research Scholar, American Cancer Society, Massachusetts division.

only a few years ago, demonstrated its existence (Copp et al., 1962). Independently, Hirsch, Gauthier, and Munson (1963) showed that the thyroid gland was the major source of the hormone in many mammalian species. The thyroid C-cell was found to secrete the hormone in mammals (Foster et al., 1964). In birds (Copp et al., 1967) and in other nonmammalian vertebrates calcitonin originates from a separate organ, the ultimobranchial body, which contains cells of a similar embryological origin to the C-cells of the thyroid (Pearse, 1970).

Even as recently as 1967, only porcine calcitonin had been obtained in highly purified form and there was no information whatever about its structure. Four years later, the complete covalent structures of seven different calcitonins from five different species have been elucidated, calcitonin produced by techniques of peptide synthesis is widely available, and detailed physiological, pharmacological, and clinical investigations are well advanced. The present review will summarize our current knowledge of the chemistry and comparative chemistry of calcitonin, factors affecting its secretion and metabolic degradation, and the results of its preliminary therapeutic application in the complex situation of disordered bone metabolism found in Paget's disease.

II. The Chemistry of Calcitonins

A. *Isolation*

Since the concentration of calcitonin in mammalian thyroid is low, the initial stages in its isolation depend upon large-scale handling and extraction techniques, first applied to hog thyroid. The development of these procedures with initial purification by column chromatography by the Armour Pharmaceutical Company made available comparatively large supplies of semipurified porcine calcitonin. This material has been used in many of the initial explorations of calcitonin physiology and pharmacology and after further purification by gel filtration and ion-exchange chromatography was also applied in the first structural analysis of a calcitonin (Potts et al., 1968). Subsequently similar techniques were found to be applicable to the isolation of bovine and ovine calcitonins.

Salmon calcitonin required the development of different approaches to isolation, as reported previously (Keutmann et al., 1970), since it differed in its tissue of origin (the ultimobranchial body) and in its chemical structure (Niall et al., 1969) when compared with the similar porcine, bovine, and ovine molecules. Human calcitonin also presented difficulties in purification due to its low levels in normal human thyroid obtained at autopsy, and to its lability to oxidation. So far it has not been purified from normal human tissues. However, the Ciba group were able to isolate a human calcitonin from several medullary carcinomata of the thyroid, which contain the hormone in high concentration. It is likely, though not yet definitely established, that this hormone has the same covalent structure as normal human calcitonin (Neher et al., 1968b).

B. Special Problems in Isolation

All calcitonins contain a disulfide bridge at the amino terminus linking half cystine residues at positions 1 and 7 (Fig. 1). This opens the possibility of oxidation or interchange reactions of the disulfide bonds during isolation. This can lead both to biological inactivation and to the formation of dimers or polymers of calcitonin not present in the original tissue extracts. Dimer formation seems to be particularly liable to occur with human calcitonin (Riniker et al., 1968), but there are also some indications of dimer formation during isolation of salmon and bovine calcitonins (Keutmann et al., 1970). The human dimer is probably not itself biologically active. Hypocalcemic effects obtained from dimer preparations are thought to be due to reconstitution of the active monomer under the conditions of the bioassay.

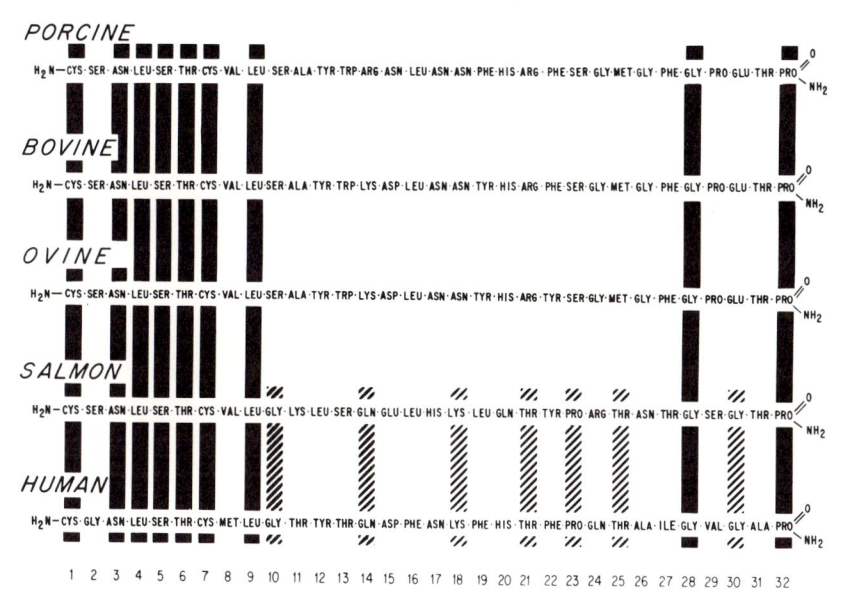

Fig. 1. Comparison of amino acid sequences of porcine, bovine, ovine, salmon, and human calcitonins. Solid bars indicate sequence positions homologous among all five molecules; cross-hatched bars indicate additional positions common to salmon and human calcitonin.

The presence of methionine in several calcitonins also provides opportunities for oxidation to the sulfoxide form during purification. Porcine calcitonin, for example, was isolated in two forms separable on ion-exchange chromatography and thin-layer chromatography (Brewer et al., 1968). These forms possessing equal biological potency differ only in the oxidation state of the single methionine at residue 25. Oxidation of the single methionine in human calcitonin, at residue 8, however, destroys biological activity (Riniker et al., 1968). Rat calcitonin also seems very liable to loss of potency during purification (Raulais and Milhaud, 1971), though the structural basis for this tendency is not yet known. Two other factors must be considered in the attempted isolation of a new calcitonin. Intraspecies microheterogeneity is well established for salmon calcitonin (Keutmann et al., 1970) and may occur also in other species. The presence of multiple, chemically differing, biologically active molecular species of calcitonin complicates interpretation of fractionation procedures. The variants may be totally or only partially resolved by the fractionation. They may differ in specific biological activity. Dimer formation, deamidation, and aggregation are further potential problems which may add to the complexity of the purification of any one component in homogeneous form.

The second problem results from the wide spectrum of biological potency of the calcitonins, ranging from 50 MRC Units per mg for bovine calcitonin to 2500 MRC Units per mg for salmon calcitonin. Since the specific activity of calcitonin from the species under investigation cannot be known in advance, a tissue extract containing, for example, 100 units of hypocalcemic activity might be contained in amounts of calcitonin varying from 2 mg down to 40 μg. In this situation estimates of the feasibility of isolation are little better than guesses. This has practical consequences for the study of comparative calcitonin chemistry since tissues from some of the species of potential interest (birds, fish, reptiles) are expensive and difficult to obtain.

C. Sequence Determination

The procedures used for the complete structural analysis of porcine, bovine, ovine, and salmon calcitonins as carried out in our laboratory have been described elsewhere (Potts et al., 1968, 1971a; Niall et al., 1969; Sauer et al., 1970). Independent completion of the porcine and bovine structures has been achieved in other laboratories (Brewer and Ronan, 1969; Bell et al., 1968; Neher et al., 1968a). The sequence of human calcitonin isolated from tumor tissue as discussed above was determined by the Ciba group (Neher et al., 1968b).

More recently, we have developed methods for sequence analysis of calcitonins at high sensitivity (Niall and Potts, 1970; Sauer *et al.*, 1970). These procedures involve the use of automated Edman degradation in the Beckman Model 890 Sequencer on submilligram quantities of peptide. The accelerated manual Edman degradation, and techniques of sequence analysis on unfractionated peptide mixtures have also been employed (Niall *et al.*, 1969).

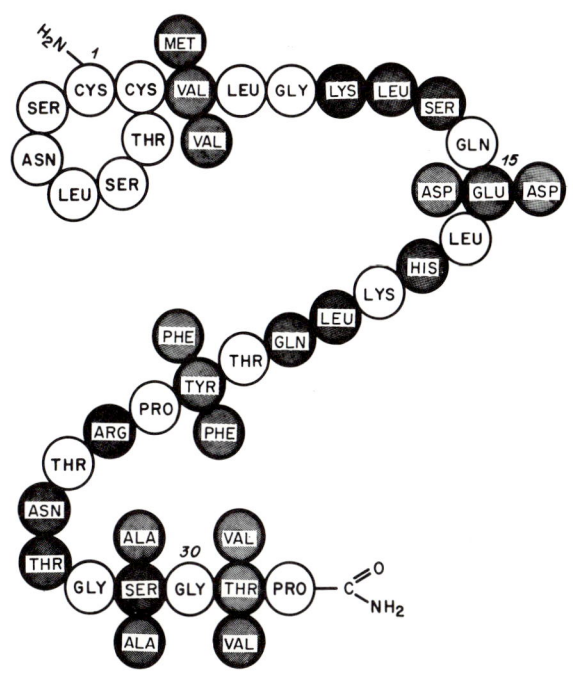

Fig. 2. The amino acid sequence of salmon calcitonins I, II, and III. The main peptide backbone represents the sequence of salmon calcitonin I, where darkened circles indicate those residues unique to this salmon molecule. The sequence positions in which calcitonins II and III differ from I are indicated by the darkened circles adjacent to the peptide backbone at positions 8, 15, 22, 29, and 31.

These approaches have now been used (Lequin *et al.*, 1971) in the sequence analysis of two variants of salmon calcitonin (II and III) which differ from the predominant form (I) in several sequence positions (Fig. 2). Total sequence analysis was achieved on only a few milligrams of material. Calcitonins from several other species are currently being sequenced using these procedures. The information regarding structure-function relationships in calcitonin based on the comparative chemical studies to date is discussed below.

D. Synthesis

Detailed synthetic studies on calcitonin have followed the elucidation of structure much more rapidly than with any other peptide hormone. This reflects the advances in the state of the art of peptide synthesis over the past few years and the degree of interest in the hormone itself. All syntheses published to date have been achieved using classical procedures with fragment condensation and purification of intermediates. This was due in part to the difficulties introduced by the presence of the C-terminal amide function when the solid phase method is used. However, recent advances in both the polymers themselves and the blocking groups used for solid phase synthesis have overcome some of these difficulties and several laboratories are currently developing solid phase procedures for calcitonin synthesis.

Synthesis for porcine and salmon calcitonin and their derivatives have been reported by Guttmann *et al.* (1968, 1970). Neher, Rittel, and colleagues at Ciba in Basel have synthesized porcine and human calcitonins and their derivatives (Rittel *et al.*, 1968; Sieber *et al.*, 1968). The information obtained from these syntheses relevant to structure-function studies in calcitonin is discussed below.

E. Structure and Function in the Calcitonins

1. THE CONSTANT AND VARIABLE REGIONS

Our current picture of the structural features in calcitonin important for biological activity is based on three lines of evidence. As outlined above, the amino acid sequences of 7 calcitonins from 5 different species have been determined (Figs. 1 and 2). A limited amount of information based on the study of derivatives of these naturally occurring calcitonins is also available. Finally a substantial number of synthetic calcitonins, calcitonin derivatives, and shorter fragments have been prepared and evaluated for biological activity.

Examination of the naturally occurring calcitonins reveals certain common structural features, together with a considerable amount of apparent variability. The common features include the 1,7 amino-terminal disulfide bridge and the carboxyl-terminal prolinamide residue. Seven of the amino-terminal 9 residues are identical in all calcitonins. Residues 28 (glycine) and 32 (prolinamide) are the only other sequence positions completely conserved. Between positions 10 and 27 there is considerable similarity between porcine, bovine, and ovine calcitonins, but both the human and salmon I molecule differ markedly from these three and from one another (Fig. 1).

Study of calcitonins from ultimobranchial glands isolated from four individual salmon species (Chum, Sockeye, Pink, and Cohoe) reveal that each species secretes two forms of calcitonin, I and either II or III. This intraspecies microheterogeneity is similar to that found for rat insulin. Salmon II differs from salmon I in positions 15, 22, 29, and 31. Salmon III is identical to salmon II in these positions, but differs from salmon I in an additional position (residue 8) where methionine replaces valine (Fig. 2).

On closer examination, the sequence variability of the middle region of calcitonin (residues 10–27 inclusive) is perhaps more apparent than real. Though no single amino acid in this region is constant in all 7 calcitonins, there is considerable similarity when the comparison is based on the chemical properties of the amino acid side chains. Acidic residues (aspartic or glutamic acid) are found only at position 15. (The only other acidic residue is found at position 30 in porcine, bovine, and ovine calcitonins.) Basic residues are also confined to a relatively few positions. Where substitutions are found for basic residues, asparagine or glutamine is the most common replacement. This is a conservative change since the amides are regarded as possessing weakly basic properties, and the basic amino acid-amide exchange is extremely common in other groups of related proteins and peptides. Hydrophobic residues (leucine, phenylalanine, or tyrosine) are distributed almost regularly along the peptide chain, occupying positions 4, 9, 12, 16, 19, and 22.

2. Importance of Specific Residues for Biological Activity

a. Acidic Residues. All calcitonins contain at least one acidic residue at positions 15 and/or 30. Biological activity of porcine calcitonin is retained when the single acidic residue (the glutamic acid at position 30) is present as the t-butyl ester derivative. Hence the presence of an acidic function is not an absolute requirement for hypocalcemic activity in calcitonins (Guttmann et al., 1970). In fact, substitution of asparagine for the aspartic acid found at position 15 in bovine calcitonin was actually found to result in a synthetic product possessing a 3-fold increase in biological potency (Guttmann et al., 1970).

b. Basic Residues. Moderate conservation regarding the distribution of basic residues has been observed, as discussed above. Positions 14, 17, 18, and 20 are occupied by either a basic residue (arginine, lysine, or histidine) or an amide. All calcitonins contain at least two basic residues.

c. Methionine. Methionine is found at 2 positions in the calcitonins, 8 and 25. Oxidation of the methionine at position 8 in human calcitonin to the sulfoxide form causes complete loss of biological activity (Riniker *et al.,* 1968). Oxidation or alkylation of the single methionine at position 25 in porcine calcitonin, however, is associated with either no change in biological activity or even a slight increase in the case of the polar carboxymethyl sulfonium derivative produced by alkylation with iodoacetic acid (Brewer, 1969). Methionine is not required, however, for biological activity since salmon calcitonins I and II lack methionine (Figs. 1 and 2).

d. Tryptophan. Tryptophan is present in porcine, bovine, and ovine calcitonins at position 13. Initial experiments suggested that the presence of this tryptophan might be essential for biological activity since its modification with Koshland's reagent (2-hydroxy-5-nitrobenzyl bromide) caused inactivation of the molecule (Brewer, 1969). This was not, however, the case since salmon and human calcitonins completely lack tryptophan.

e. Tyrosine. The number of tyrosines present in the calcitonins varies from zero (in salmon II and III) to 3 (in ovine calcitonin). When present, tyrosines occupy positions 12, 19, and/or 22. Though tyrosine is plainly not essential for biological activity, it is always replaced by a hydrophobic residue at these positions, as mentioned above.

3. Biological Activity of Synthetic Calcitonin Derivatives

A systematic study of the biological properties of synthetic calcitonin derivatives is just beginning. However, there is some preliminary information available from work already done. The most striking finding was that the entire 32 amino acid chain appears to be required for biological activity. Fragments of the molecule, whether derived from the amino-terminal, middle, or carboxyl-terminal region, are totally inactive (Fig. 3). Even the comparatively long fragments consisting of residues 10–32, or residues 1–10 joined to residues 20–32 with omission of the central nonapeptide, are inactive (Fig. 3). In fact, shortening the chain by omission of even a few amino acids causes almost complete loss of biological activity, even if the C-terminal prolinamide residue is retained (Fig. 3). There is some indication that a moderate increase in the size of the molecule may be associated with increased biological potency. For example, Guttmann *et al.* (1970) have observed that addition of the bulky tertiary butyloxycarbonyl group to the N-terminal α-amino group of porcine calcitonin is associated with retention or increase in biological potency. Guttmann has also found that substitutions of certain amino acid side chains by less bulky groups causes a decrease in biological activity (Fig. 4). For example, substitution of the tryptophan in position 13 of porcine calcitonin by glycine reduces the biological activity to one third of that of the native molecule. A logical extension of these

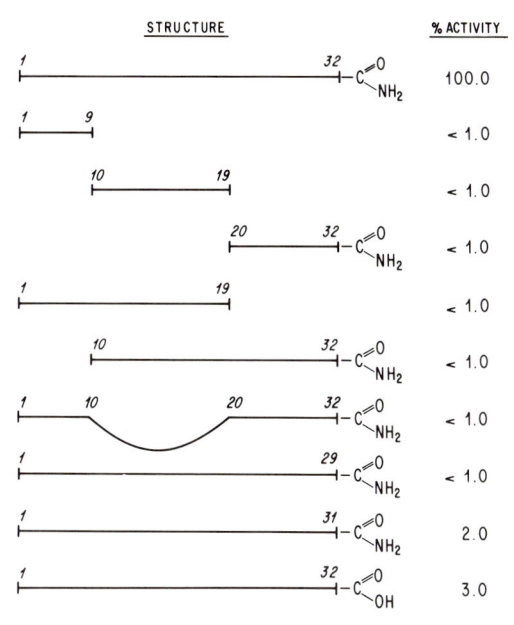

Fig. 3. Summary of biological potency studies of synthetic fragments of porcine calcitonin prepared by progressive shortening (Sieber et al., 1970; Guttmann et al., 1970).

observations would be to examine the effects of moderate lengthening of the chain, for example, to 33 or 34 amino acids.

In view of the loss of activity associated with omission of only one or two amino acids, while retaining constant the amino terminal sequence and the carboxyl terminal prolinamide, it is hardly surprising that the search for "active fragments" of calcitonin has not been rewarding. Fragments of calcitonin shortened at the amino terminus (e.g., residues 10–32) are almost totally inactive, as are fragments shortened at the carboxyl end (e.g., residues 1–28). The Ciba group (Sieber et al., 1970) observed a 20-fold increase in biological activity between 1 to 19 (0.04%) and 1 to 24 (0.8%) of porcine calcitonin. Further lengthening of the chain up to 1–31 made no further contribution to activity, however. They also found that the 1–32 peptide with the same covalent sequence as porcine calcitonin but lacking only the C-terminal amide group possessed only 3% biological activity. A similar loss of activity results in oxytocin when the carboxyl terminal amide is replaced by the free α-carboxyl group.

These limited observations suggest strongly that the whole peptide chain is involved in the biological activity of the hormone, the overall

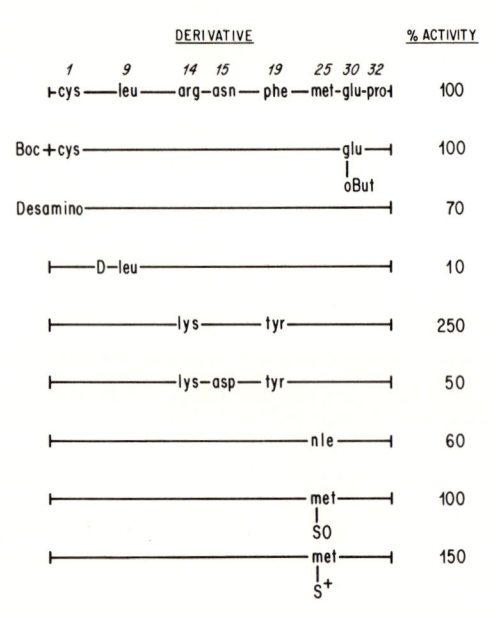

```
                DERIVATIVE                              % ACTIVITY

        1      9       14  15      19    25 30 32
        ⊢cys────leu────arg–asn────phe────met–glu–pro⊣      100

        Boc+cys───────────────────────glu─┤              100
                                      │
                                      oBut
        Desamino──────────────────────────┤              70

        ├────D–leu───────────────────────┤              10

        ├──────────lys────────tyr────────┤              250

        ├──────────lys–asp────tyr────────┤              50

        ├──────────────────────────nle───┤              60

        ├──────────────────────────met───┤              100
                                    │
                                    SO
        ├──────────────────────────met───┤              150
                                    │+
                                    S⁺
```

Fig. 4. Summary of biological potency studies of synthetic fragments of porcine calcitonin produced by substitution of functional groups of amino acid side chains (Sieber *et al.*, 1970; Guttmann *et al.*, 1970).

size and chain length and the chemical groupings at either end of the chain being particularly critical for binding to receptor sites.

4. Increased Potency of Salmon Calcitonin

The basis of the very great increase in biological potency of salmon calcitonin (O'Dor *et al.*, 1969; Keutmann *et al.*, 1970) compared to the calcitonins from other species is perhaps the most interesting unsolved problem in the study of structure and function in this group of related molecules. Because of its obvious relevance to the therapeutic use of calcitonin, it also has much practical importance.

The hypocalcemic activity of salmon calcitonin I in the rat bioassay varies from 2500 to 3000 U/mg, compared to the range of 50–200 U/mg for porcine, bovine, ovine, and human calcitonins. The exact biological potency of the salmon II and III variants has not been firmly established because of difficulties of isolation of these hormones in the native form. However, it seems that they also have high hypocalcemic activity, in the same range as the salmon I hormone.

This great potency of the salmon hormones must have a structural basis in one or more features of their covalent amino acid sequences (Fig. 2). There are two kinds of possible mechanism which could be operative, increased receptor site affinity or increased resistance to metabolic breakdown. These mechanisms are of course not mutually exclusive. However, there is now evidence, to be discussed elsewhere in this review, that the salmon molecule has a longer biological half-life than the other calcitonins. This would favor the second of the above alternatives.

Comparison of the amino acid sequence of the salmon hormones with the other 4 calcitonins does not reveal any obvious clues. All 7 calcitonins contain peptide bonds which would be expected to be cleaved both by trypsin-like and chymotrypsin-like enzymes in plasma or tissues. Since the amino-terminal 7 residues of the salmon calcitonin are identical to porcine, bovine, and ovine calcitonins one would not expect any greater resistance to aminopeptidases. The possible role of tertiary configuration of the calcitonins in altered resistance to metabolic breakdown is not known at present.

Two approaches currently under active investigation in our laboratory may help to elucidate the structural basis for the high potency of salmon calcitonin. Further comparative chemical studies on calcitonins both from other mammalian species and from other species of fish may reveal further sequence requirements for high potency. Synthesis of derivatives of salmon calcitonin and of "hybrid" molecules sharing some structural features of both mammalian and salmon hormones should also be informative. Finally, we are studying directly the patterns of metabolic degradation of salmon and of mammalian calcitonins *in vivo* and *in vitro* using region-specific antisera. This may allow the direct identification of the groups modified or the bonds cleaved during metabolic breakdown and thus provide a rational basis for the synthesis of derivatives which might be even more resistant to these degradative pathways.

III. Control of Secretion of Calcitonin

A. *Control of Secretion*

The development and application of sensitive and specific radioimmunoassays for the calcitonins has provided much detailed information about the control of secretion of this peptide (Deftos and Potts, 1969; Potts *et al.*, 1971a) (Fig. 5). The first immunoassay developed for this hormone was for porcine calcitonin (Deftos *et al.*, 1968; Lee *et al.*, 1969). This assay was sufficiently sensitive to detect peripheral concentrations of the peptide in both the rabbit and porcine species. These initial studies demonstrated that calcitonin is continuously secreted at physiological concentrations of blood calcium (Fig. 6). Measurements

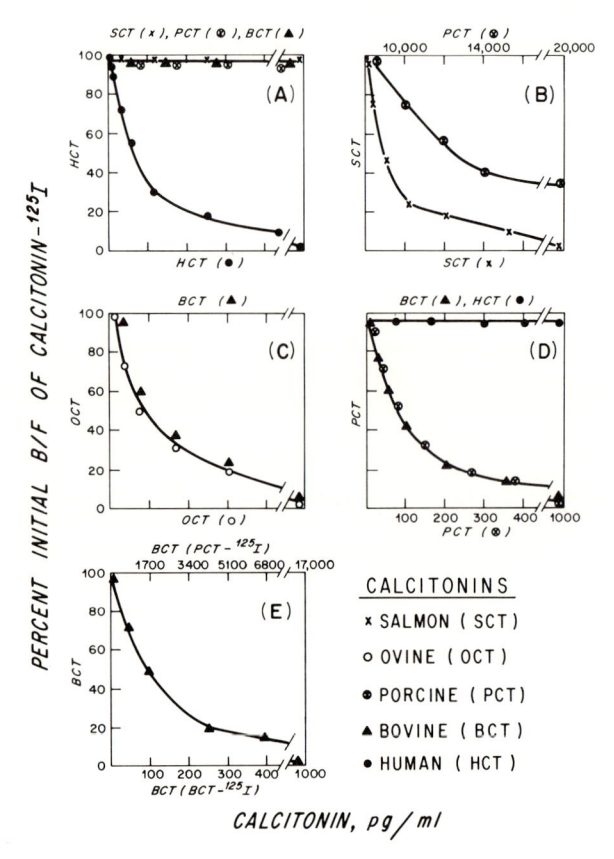

Fig. 5. Immunoassays for human (A), salmon (B), ovine (C), porcine (D), and bovine (E) calcitonin. In addition to each homologous immunoassay system, also illustrated are certain immunochemical relationships among the various calcitonins (see text for further discussion).

made during calcium infusion in these animals demonstrated that the concentration of the hormone rises within minutes of induced hypercalcemia. It was further shown that the secretion of the hormone is under the directly proportional control of blood calcium: an increase in calcium concentration causes an increase in the concentration of calcitonin, and a decrease in calcium concentration causes a decrease in the concentration of calcitonin. Calcitonin was shown to disappear rapidly from the circulation once secreted, with a half-life of 2–15 minutes. These aspects of the secretion and metabolism of calcitonin emphasize the dynamic turnover of the peptide in the blood and, in addition, are consistent with a hormonal role of calcitonin.

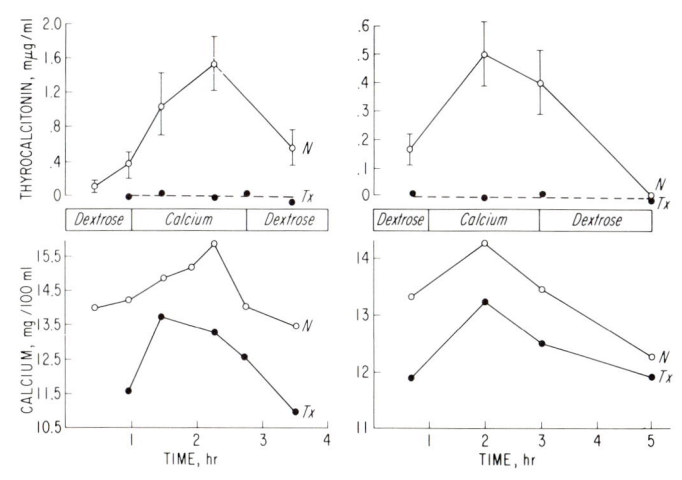

Fig. 6. Effect of calcium infusion on plasma calcium and calcitonin in two normal (N) and two thyroidectomized (TX) rabbits. Vertical bars indicate standard error. Since the parathyroids are intrathyroidal, thyroidectomized animals are also devoid of parathyroid hormone. This is the presumed cause of the initially lower calcium concentration in these animals.

B. Direct Estimation of Secretory Rate

In addition to studies of the peripheral concentration of calcitonin, the immunoassay for the porcine peptide was used for the detection of calcitonin in the effluent blood from the thyroid gland in the pig (Cooper et al., 1971) (Fig. 7). This enabled a direct estimation of the secretion of the hormone and permitted more accurate determinations of the magnitude of changes in hormone secretion that resulted from hypercalcemic challenge. Again, hormone was always detected under physiological conditions; its concentration was 30-fold over that found in peripheral blood. The concentration of the hormone rose several-hundred-fold during induced hypercalcemia and rapidly fell to undetectable levels when hypocalcemia was induced by EDTA. The thyroid gland was shown to respond rapidly with increased rates of hormone secretion during sequential episodes of hypercalcemia and hypocalcemia despite these alternate periods of stimulation and suppression. From these studies, it could be calculated that the basal secretory rate of calcitonin was 100 ng/min. Since the approximate calcitonin content of the thyroid gland is 100 μg, the stores of preformed calcitonin in the thyroid gland are large in relation to the basal secretion rates of hormone.

During hypercalcemic challenge, the secretory rate of calcitonin increased by at least 20-fold to 2000 ng/min. This relationship between

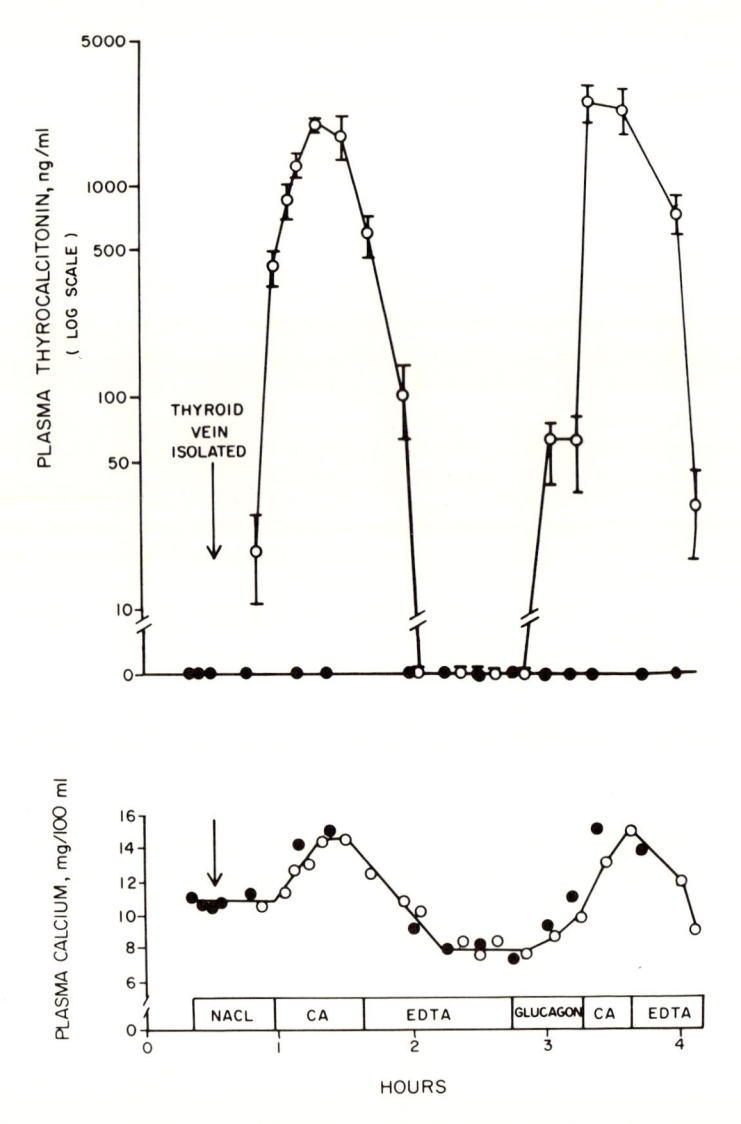

Fig. 7. Measurements of endogenous porcine calcitonin by radioimmunoassay in the thyroid effluent blood (open circles) and femoral blood (filled circles) of a pig during calcium, EDTA, and glucagon infusion. During calcium stimulation, there is a several-hundred-fold increase in the concentration of calcitonin. The lack of detectable hormone in the arterial blood (no thyroid effluent blood enters the general circulation) serves as a control for the specificity of the techniques. The slight rise in hormone concentration during glucagon infusion given during a period of hypocalcemia is significantly greater than the basal value.

calcitonin storage and secretion is in marked contrast to the small stores of preformed hormone in the parathyroid gland. During stimulation the maximum rise in parathyroid hormone secretion rate over basal is only of the order of 5- to 6-fold (Potts et al., 1971b).

C. Effect of Gastrointestinal Factors

Studies with the immunoassay for porcine calcitonin in this species confirmed (Cooper et al., 1971) that glucagon could also stimulate the secretion of calcitonin. This observation led to further evaluation of the role of gastrointestinal hormones in the control of secretion of calcitonin. It was demonstrated that oral ingestion of calcium in doses sufficient to cause an increase in blood calcium would also induce an increase in the secretion of calcitonin (Cooper and Deftos, 1970). Furthermore, doses of calcium could be given orally in amounts insufficient to cause an increase in the blood calcium concentration. Even under these circumstances, that is, oral calcium challenge without resulting hypercalcemia, there is an increase in the secretion of calcitonin. These findings strongly suggest that factors other than blood calcium concentration also modulate the secretion of calcitonin (Potts and Deftos, 1969). In relation to these observations, recent studies by Cooper et al. (1971) have demonstrated that gastrin when administered to the pig will cause a prompt and rapid increase in the secretion of calcitonin. The importance and physiological significance of gastrointestinal factors in the control of secretion of calcitonin await further investigation (Potts et al., 1971c).

D. Effect of Dietary Calcium

Development of an immunoassay for bovine calcitonin (Deftos et al., 1971a) permitted studies on the control of secretion of calcitonin in this species also. In the bovine species it was also found that calcitonin could be detected in the peripheral blood at physiological concentrations of blood calcium. Furthermore, induced hypercalcemia resulted in an increase in the secretion of calcitonin and induced hypocalcemia resulted in a decrease in the secretion of calcitonin (Fig. 8). Studies in this species also provided further evidence that diet, especially dietary calcium, influences the control of secretion of calcitonin. There is a marked difference in the basal concentration of calcitonin in cows and in bulls. The mean ($\pm$SE) in cows is 165 pg/ml ($\pm$12), significantly ($p < 0.01$) less than that seen in bulls, 303 pg/ml ($\pm$13). The entire reasons for this difference are not yet clear, but may be related to the high dietary intake of calcium by the bovine species. This high intake can be matched in the cow by losses which are incurred through lactation and pregnancy. Such means are, of course, not available to bulls. Accordingly, bulls

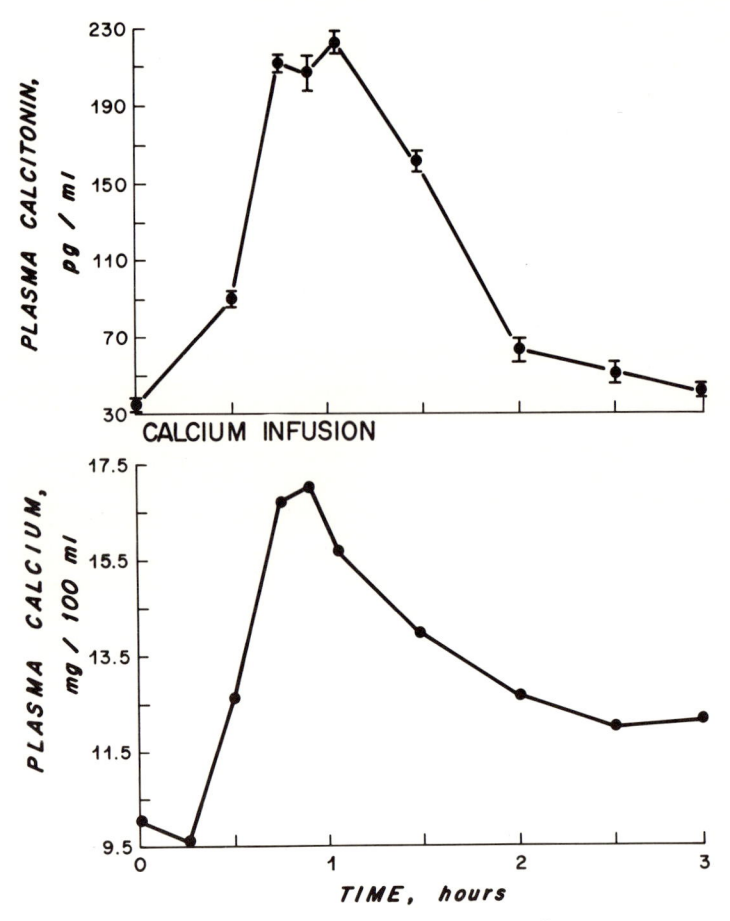

Fig. 8. The effect of calcium infusion on peripheral calcitonin concentration in a cow.

may secrete increased amounts of calcitonin to maintain a normal blood calcium concentration in the face of a great dietary calcium challenge well beyond their metabolic needs. Possibly related to this is the high incidence of tumors of the calcitonin-secreting cells (medullary thyroid carcinomas) in older bulls (Krook et al., 1969). The immunoassay has demonstrated that bulls with such tumors contain increased concentrations of calcitonin in their peripheral blood; furthermore, these thyroid tumors contain at least a 20-fold excess of calcitonin concentration when compared to normal bovine thyroid gland. It is of note that some of these bulls with medullary thyroid carcinoma also have coexistent pheochromocytomas and parathyroid neoplasias. This syndrome in bulls, therefore, bears a remarkable resemblance to one of the multiple endocrine adenomatoses (MEA Type II) seen in humans (Steiner *et al.*, 1968) (see further discussion below).

E. Studies in Fish

An immunoassay for salmon calcitonin has also been developed and applied to preliminary studies of the control of secretion of this peptide in the salmon species. It is noteworthy that the peripheral concentration of calcitonin in the salmon exhibits a much wider variation than that found in other species. Values ranging from 400 to 10,000 pg of calcitonin per milliliter of plasma have been detected in the salmon. Further studies are necessary to study the effect of such factors as migration, ambient salt and calcium concentration, and age on the secretion of calcitonin in fish.

F. Studies in Humans

Development of immunoassays for human calcitonin has permitted direct studies of the control of secretion of this peptide in the human (Deftos *et al.*, 1971a; Clark *et al*, 1969; Tashjian *et al.*, 1966; Deftos and Potts, 1970; Deftos *et al.*, 1971b). The immunoassay for human calcitonin was initially used to evaluate calcitonin secretion in patients with medullary thyroid carcinoma, a tumor which can occur sporadically or as part of a multiple endocrine syndrome. Excessive amounts of calcitonin are invariably found in the blood and in the tumor of involved subjects (Fig. 9). The immunoassay can therefore be used to establish the diagnosis of medullary thyroid carcinoma, even in patients in whom the tumor is not yet clinically apparent. The secretion of calcitonin by this malignant tumor is not autonomous (Fig. 10). As with normal calcitonin-secreting cells, calcium infusion causes a marked increase in the secretion of calcitonin by this tumor. Furthermore, the secretion of calcitonin by this malignancy can be suppressed by EDTA-induced hypocalcemia. Glucagon can have a variable effect on the secretion of calcitonin by medullary thyroid carcinoma, causing an increased secretion in some patients and a decreased secretion in other patients (Fig. 11). In addition to its usefulness in establishing the diagnosis of medullary thyroid carcinoma and in studying its secretion, the immunoassay can help to define the site and extent of this tumor. This can be accomplished by demonstrating a localized increase in the concentration of calcitonin in blood samples taken during catheterization from the venous drainage of the tumor and the major veins draining the neck, thorax, and abdomen.

The importance of calcitonin in normal human calcium and skeletal

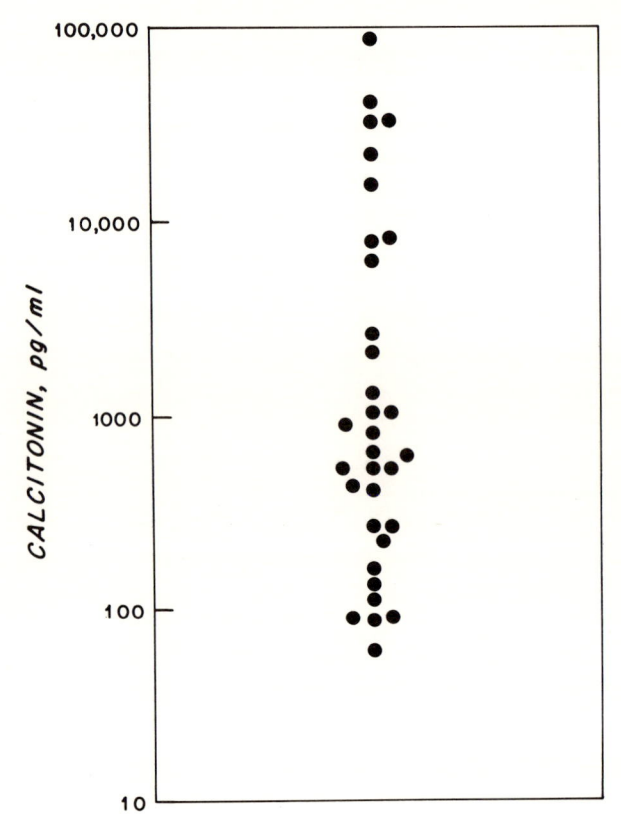

Fig. 9. Peripheral plasma concentration of calcitonin in patients with medullary thyroid carcinoma. Calcitonin concentration are plotted on a logarithmic scale. Note the wide range of variation in calcitonin concentration.

homeostasis has not been clearly established. In preliminary studies (Tashjian et al., 1970) the concentration of calcitonin in normal adults was reported as ranging from 20 to 400 pg/ml. However, the concentrations of hormone found were close to the detection limits of the assay, a situation in which nonspecific effects in immunoassay systems can be misleading. In addition, we have found that the concentration of calcitonin in the thyroid gland of normal human subjects is several orders of magnitude lower by both bioassay and immunoassay than that found in the thyroid gland of other mammals (Cooper et al., 1971; Deftos et al., 1971a). Furthermore, preliminary application of our immunoassay for human calcitonin (Deftos et al., 1971a,b,c) has shown the peptide to be undetectable (less than 100 pg/ml) not only in the peripheral plasma of many normal subjects, but also in thyroid venous blood taken

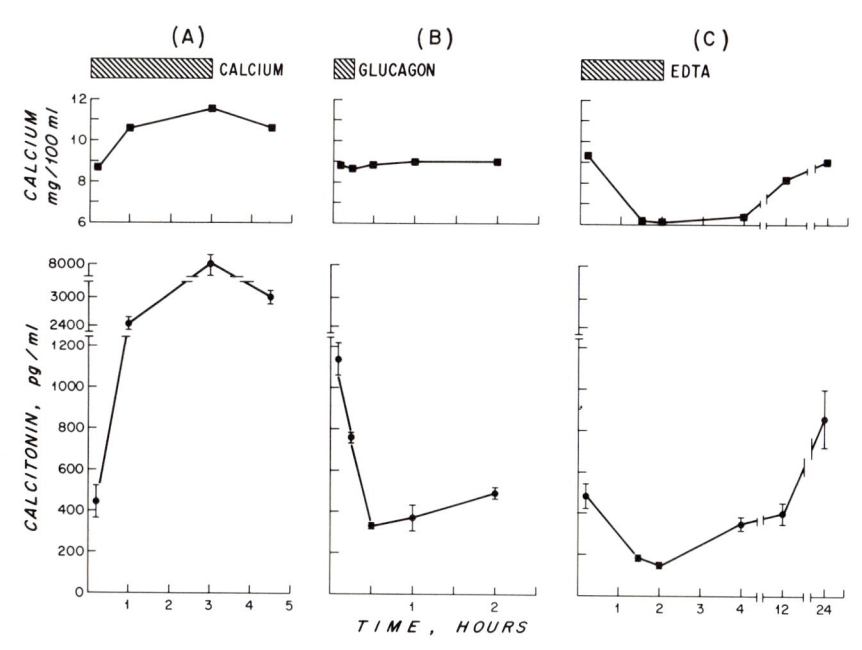

Fig. 10. Effect of calcium (A), glucagon (B), and EDTA (C) infusions on peripheral calcitonin concentration in a patient with medullary thyroid carcinoma. Calcium resulted in a marked increase in calcitonin. Glucagon led to an unexpected decrease in calcitonin. EDTA-induced hypocalcemia also resulted in a decreased plasma calcitonin concentration.

from patients, primarily with hypercalcemia, during selective venous catheterization or at surgery. These findings suggest that the concentration of calcitonin in the peripheral blood of humans is much lower than that found in other mammals. We would have to conclude that, at present, there is no convincing evidence that calcitonin has been detected in the peripheral circulation of normal man. Development of more sensitive assays will be required to decide whether calcitonin does circulate, but at very low concentrations, or whether the hormone is not secreted under normal physiological conditions.

IV. Therapeutic Uses of Calcitonin

Calcitonin because of its unique mode of action has recently been evaluated as a therapeutic agent in man in hypercalcemia states and in demineralizing bone disease. Most extensive use of calcitonin has been in patients with Paget's disease (Potts and Deftos, 1969). Although

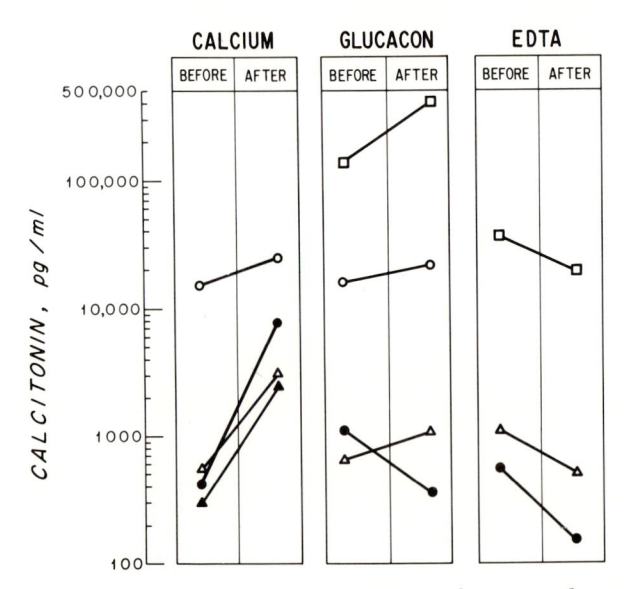

Fig. 11. Effect of calcium, glucagon, and EDTA infusion on the concentration of calcitonin in five patients with medullary thyroid carcinoma. In each case the postinfusion concentration is significantly different ($p < 0.01$) than the concentration of the preinfusion control.

the pathogenesis of Paget's disease is not well understood, the outstanding pathophysiological process is increased bone resorption, which is invariably matched by an increased bone formation. Since calcitonin strongly inhibits bone resorption, patients with Paget's disease were among the first to be treated with calcitonin (Singer et al., 1971). Acute trials confirmed that porcine and human calcitonin were effective in patients with Paget's disease; injections of the hormone resulted in a significant hypocalcemic effect, due to sudden inhibition of bone turnover. These acute trials have been followed by more prolonged administration of the drug in Paget's disease. Preliminary results of these clinical trials have been encouraging. Chronic administration of calcitonin resulted in a progressive decrease of the abnormally high bone resorption rate seen in Paget's disease. This has been documented by a decrease indices of bone turnover, urinary hydroxyproline excretion, and plasma alkaline phosphatase. Although more difficult to evaluate objectively, symptomatic response to calcitonin (relief of bone pain, etc.) has also been evident (Potts and Deftos, 1969).

Soon after the isolation and characterization of salmon calcitonin this hormonal peptide was found to be a more potent hypocalcemic agent by a factor of 25- to 200-fold (Potts and Deftos, 1969) in man, an observation in agreement with earlier findings that salmon calcitonin is more potent in all mammalian species tested. Because of its increased potency, salmon calcitonin has been recently introduced for the chronic treatment of patients with Paget's disease (Singer et al., 1971). Whereas milligram doses of porcine and human calcitonin were used in earlier treatment programs, we have found that microgram quantities of salmon calcitonin self-administered subcutaneously once daily are very effective and represent a practical approach to chronic treatment. Figure 12 shows

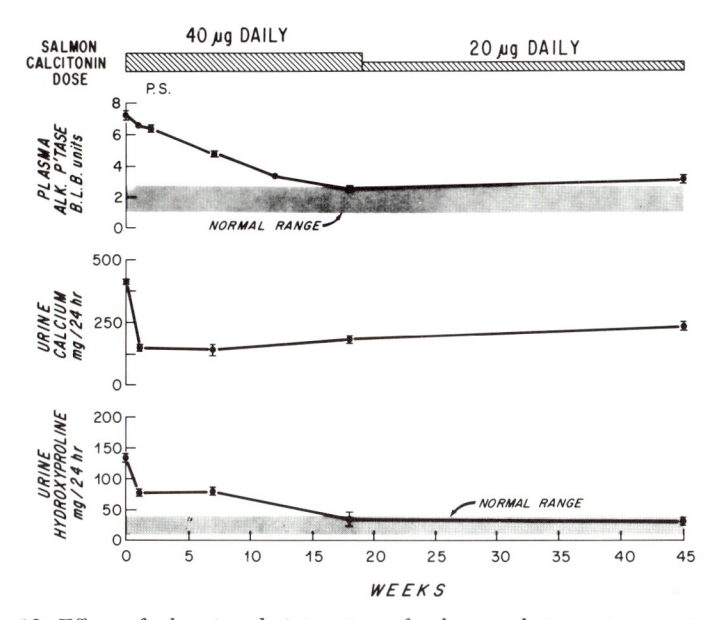

Fig. 12. Effect of chronic administration of salmon calcitonin in a patient with Paget's disease. The parameters of increased bone turnover, plasma alkaline phosphatase, and urine hydroxyproline show a progressive drop into the normal range.

the effects of long-term treatment with salmon calcitonin on Paget's disease in one patient. There is a progressive drop of the plasma alkaline phosphatase and urinary hydroxyproline into the normal range. There is also a decrease in 24-hour urinary calcium levels. Similar results have been seen in 18 other patients with Paget's disease on chronic salmon calcitonin therapy. Not all patients have shown a decrease to normal rates in skeletal turnover, perhaps because of inadequate dosage; other factors that may modify the course of long-term treatment are under investigation, as recently reviewed (Singer et al., 1971).

In summary, preliminary trials with calcitonin in the therapy of Paget's disease have been very promising. All the abnormal parameters of bone metabolism seen in this disease have reverted toward normal after chronic treatment with calcitonin. Further studies are, of course, needed to confirm these preliminary observations, to establish appropriate dose schedules, to examine in detail the clinical pharmacology of calcitonin action in man, and to determine the relative efficacy of porcine, human and salmon calcitonin for long-term treatment in man (Singer *et al.*, 1971).

References

Bell, P. H., Barg, W. R., Jr., Colucci, D. F., Davies, C. M., Dziobkowski, C., Englert, M. E., Heyder, E., Paul, R., and Snedeker, E. H. (1968). *J. Amer. Chem. Soc.* **90**, 2704.
Brewer, H. B., Jr. (1969). *Fed. Proc.* **28**, 383.
Brewer, H. B., Jr., and Ronan, R. (1969). *Proc. Nat. Acad. Sci. U.S.* **63**, 862.
Brewer, H. B., Jr., Keutmann, H. T., Potts, J. T., Jr., Reisfeld, R. A., Schlueter, R. J., and Munson, P. L. (1968). *J. Biol. Chem.* **243**, 5739.
Clark, M. B., Byfield, P. G. H., Boyd, G. W., and Foster, G. V. (1969). *Lancet* **ii**, 74.
Cooper, C. W., and Deftos, L. J. (1970). *Fed. Proc. Fed. Amer. Soc. Exp. Biol.* **29**, 253.
Cooper, C. W., Deftos, L. J., and Potts, J. T., Jr. (1971). *Endocrinology.* In press.
Copp, D. H., Cameron, E. C., Cheney, B. A., Davidson, A. G. F., and Henze, K. G. (1962). *Endocrinology* **70**, 638.
Copp, D. H., Cockcroft, D. W., and Kueh, Y. (1967). *J. Physiol. (London)* **45**, 1095.
Deftos, L. J., and Potts, J. T., Jr. (1969). *Brit. J. Hosp. Med.* (Nov.), p. 1813.
Deftos, L. J., and Potts, J. T., Jr. (1970). *Clin. Res.* **18**, 673.
Deftos, L. J., Lee, M. R., and Potts, J. T., Jr. (1968). *Proc. Nat. Acad. Sci. U.S.* **60**, 293.
Deftos, L. J., Murray, T. M., Powell, D., Habener, J. F., Singer, F. R., and Mayer, G. P. (1971a). *Int. Congr. Parathyroid Horm., 4th, Chapel Hill, 1971.* In press.
Deftos, L. J., Goodman, A. D., Engleman, K., Bury, A. E., and Potts, J. T., Jr. (1971b). *Metab. Clin. Exp.* **20**, 428.
Deftos, L. S., Burg, A. E., Habener, J. F., Singer, F. R., Potts, J. T., Jr. (1971c). *Metab. Clin. Exp.* In press.
Foster, G. V., MacIntyre, I., and Pearse, A. G. E. (1964). *Nature (London)* **203**, 1029.
Guttmann, St., Pless, J., Sandrin, E., Jaquenoud, P. A., Bossert, H., and Willems, H. (1968). *Helv. Chim. Acta* **51**, 1155.
Guttmann, St., Pless, J., Huguenin, R., Sandrin, E., and Zehnder, K. (1970). *Proc. Amer. Peptide Symp., 2nd, New York, 1970.* In press.
Hirsch, P. F., Gauthier, G. F., and Munson, P. L. (1963). *Endocrinology* **73**, 244.

Keutmann, H. T., Parsons, J. A., Potts, J. T., Jr., and Schlueter, R. J. (1970). *J. Biol. Chem.* **245**, 1491.
Keutmann, H. T., Dawson, B., and Potts, J. T., Jr. (1971). Unpublished observation.
Krook, L., Lutwak, L., and McEntee, E. (1969). *Amer. J. Clin. Nutr.* **22**, 115.
Lee, M. R., Deftos, L. J., and Potts, J. T., Jr. (1969). *Endocrinology* **84**, 36.
Lequin, R. M., Keutmann, H. T., Niall, H. D., and Potts, J. T., Jr. (1971). In preparation.
Neher, R., Riniker, B., Zuber, H., Rittel, W., and Kahnt, F. W. (1968a). *Helv. Chim. Acta* **51**, 917.
Neher, R., Riniker, B., Rittel, W., and Zuber, H. (1968b). *Helv. Chim. Acta* **51**, 1900.
Niall, H. D., and Potts, J. T., Jr. (1970). *In* "Peptides: Chemistry and Biochemistry" (S. Lande and B. Weinstein, eds.), p. 215. Dekker, New York.
Niall, H. D., Keutmann, H. T., Copp, D. H., and Potts, J. T., Jr. (1969). *Proc. Nat. Acad. Sci. U.S.* **64**, 771.
O'Dor, R. D., Parkes, C. O., and Copp, D. H. (1969). *Can. J. Biochem.* **47**, 823.
Pearse, A. G. E. (1970). *Proc. Int. Symp. Calcitonin, 2nd, London, 1969,* p. 125.
Potts, J. T., Jr., and Deftos, L. J. (1969). *In* "Duncan's Diseases of Metabolism" (P. K. Bondy, ed.), pp. 904–1069. Saunders, Philadelphia, Pennsylvania.
Potts, J. T., Jr., Niall, H. D., Keutmann, H. T., Brewer, H. B., Jr., and Deftos, L. J. (1968). *Proc. Nat. Acad. Sci. U.S.* **59**, 1321.
Potts, J. T., Jr., Keutmann, H. T., Deftos, L. J., and Niall, H. D. (1971a). *In* "Peptides: Chemistry and Biochemistry" (S. Lande and B. Weinstein, eds.). Gordon & Breach, New York. In press.
Potts, J. T., Murray, T. M., Peacock, M., Niall, H. D., Tregear, G. W., Keutmann, H. T., Powell, D., and Deftos, L. J. (1971b). *Amer. J. Med.* In press.
Potts, J. T., Jr., Niall, H. D., Keutmann, H. T., Tregear, G. W., Habener, J. F., Deftos, L. J., and Aurbach, G. D. (1971c). *Int. Congr. Parathyroid Horm., 4th, Chapel Hill, 1971.* In press.
Raulais, D., and Milhaud, G. (1971). Personal communication.
Riniker, B., Neher, R., Maier, R., Kahnt, F. W., Byfield, P. G. H., Gudmundsson, T. V., Galante, L., and MacIntyre, I. (1968). *Helv. Chim. Acta* **51**, 1738.
Rittel, W., Brugger, M., Kamber, B., Riniker, B., and Sieber, P. (1968). *Helv. Chim. Acta* **51**, 924.
Sauer, R., Niall, H. D., and Potts, J. T., Jr. (1970). *Fed. Proc. Fed. Amer. Soc. Exp. Biol.* **29**, 728.
Sieber, P., Brugger, M., Kamber, B., Riniker, B., and Rittel, W. (1968). *Helv. Chim. Acta* **51**, 2057.
Sieber, P., Brugger, M., Kamber, B., Riniker, B., Rittel, W., Maier, R., and Staehelin, M. (1970). *Proc. Int. Symp. Calcitonin, 2nd, London, 1969,* p. 28.
Singer, F. R., Keutmann, H. T., Neer, R. M., Potts, J. T., Jr., and Krane, S. M. (1971). *Int. Congr. Parathyroid Horm., 4th, Chapel Hill, 1971.* In press.
Steiner, A. G., Goodman, A. D., and Powers, R. S. (1968). *Medicine (Baltimore)* **47**, 371.
Tashjian, A. H. J., Frantz, A. G., and Lee, J. B. (1966). *Proc. Nat. Acad. Sci. U.S.* **56**, 1138.
Tashjian, A. H. J., Jr., Howland, B. G., Melvin, K. E. W., and Hill, C. S. (1970). *New Engl. J. Med.* **283**, 890.

THE LONG-ACTING THYROID STIMULATOR

D. S. Munro

DEPARTMENT OF PHARMACOLOGY AND THERAPEUTICS
THE UNIVERSITY OF SHEFFIELD, SHEFFIELD, ENGLAND

I. Introduction	176
A. The Discovery of Long-Acting Thyroid Stimulator (LATS)	177
B. Methods for Assay of LATS	177
C. Relationship to Earlier Theories of Thyrotoxicosis	179
D. Evidence That LATS Stimulates the Thyroid	181
E. Evidence That LATS Is Not of Pituitary Origin	182
II. Clinical Importance of LATS	183
A. Relationship Between LATS and Thyroid Function in Thyrotoxicosis	183
B. Clinical Markers of LATS	184
C. Relationship to Other Thyroid Autoantibodies	185
D. Relationship to Eye Signs	185
E. Relationship Between LATS, TSH, and Exophthalmos-Producing Substance (EPS)	186
III. Chemical Nature of LATS	186
A. Association of LATS with γG Immunoglobulins	186
B. The Proteolysis of LATS	187
C. Separation and Reaggregation of H and L Chain of LATS-γG	188
IV. Effects of LATS and Its Active Fragments in Relation to Actions of TSH	189
A. Altered Time Course of LATS *in Vitro* and *in Vivo*	189
B. Relationship Between Actions of LATS, TSH, and Cyclic AMP	190

V. Absorption of LATS by Thyroid Extracts 191
   A. Thyroid-Stimulating Effects of Antisera to Thyroid Extracts—Possibility of an Experimental Analog of Graves' Disease 191
   B. Partial Purification of LATS Absorbing Activity . . . 192
   C. Dissociation of LATS after Absorption 193
   D. Future Applications of LATS Absorption 193
   E. Importance of Better Assay for LATS 194
   References 195

I. Introduction

The long-acting thyroid stimulator (LATS) was discovered by Adams and Purves (1956) and owes its unusual name to the sustained stimulation of thyroid function which it causes in guinea pigs (Adams and Purves, 1953) or mice (McKenzie, 1958a).

Interest in LATS is related to its possible role in the pathogenesis of thyrotoxicosis. Although this remains a matter of dispute (Sellars et al., 1970), it is generally accepted that, with certain rare exceptions, LATS can be detected only in the circulating blood of patients with thyrotoxicosis or a past history of that disease. When purified from serum, LATS activity is associated with a protein fraction which has the characteristics of a member of the immunoglobulin G (γG) class of proteins. It has, therefore, been suggested that LATS may be a member of the group of circulating thyroid autoantibodies which are known to occur in patients with certain thyroid diseases, including thyrotoxicosis. Pursuing this hypothesis and hoping to identify the putative antigen to which LATS may be an antibody, several groups have studied the interaction between LATS and thyroid homogenates *in vitro*.

Thus, the concept of LATS as the ultimate cause of thyrotoxicosis also involves the acceptance of the idea of a thyroid-stimulating autoantibody. The evidence for the γG nature of LATS and in support of a pathogenetic role for LATS will be reviewed below. At this point it is only fair to stress some of the contrary arguments.

The major objection to accepting LATS as the cause of thyrotoxicosis is the acknowledged difficulty in detecting LATS in all patients. Assays of unconcentrated serum by the method of McKenzie (1958a) yield a variable proportion of "LATS positive" samples which at the most amounts to a little more than 50% of all cases. Even allowing for the lack of quantitative LATS assays in published serum surveys, there is in all series a substantial proportion of patients with undoubted thyrotoxicosis in whom LATS cannot be demonstrated.

Additional difficulties have arisen from the observation that among patients with Graves' disease there are two good "clinical markers" of a high serum LATS level: these are to have given birth to a baby suffering from neonatal thyrotoxicosis or to have the skin lesion known as localized or "pretibial" myxedema. This has tended to distract attention from study of the more general relationship between LATS and the severity of thyroid overactivity in thyrotoxicosis. There is evidence that such a relationship exists as a positive correlation between the serum level of LATS and the rate of radioiodine turnover in thyrotoxicosis has been demonstrated (Major and Munro, 1962; Carneiro *et al.*, 1966a); this correlation was shown only in patients in whom LATS could be detected in assays of unconcentrated serum. Other studies have failed to support this view (Chopra *et al.*, 1970; Sellars *et al.*, 1970). In common with many other problems concerning the significance of LATS, resolution of this conflict of evidence will come only when better methods for measuring LATS are available.

The evidence for the statements in these introductory comments may now be examined in detail.

A. *The Discovery of Long-Acting Thyroid Stimulator (LATS)*

Adams and Purves (1956) discovered LATS when they observed a prolonged and sustained discharge of radioiodine from the thyroid glands of thyroxine-treated guinea pigs following the intravenous injection of serum from a patient with thyrotoxicosis. This effect contrasted with the much briefer stimulation which resulted when extracts of pituitary thyroid-stimulating hormone (TSH) or serum from a patient with untreated myxedema was injected under comparable conditions. It is, of course, because of this characteristic time course of action in this type of assay that the long-acting stimulator has received its name. The term LATS persists in spite of the objections to its use—for example, observations which show that this difference in the contrasting time course of action between TSH and LATS does not always persist when they are studied *in vitro* (Brown and Munro, 1967). A plea has been made to rename LATS as thyroid-stimulating globulin, but this has not found general favor (Adams, 1965).

B. *Methods for Assay of LATS*

Ever since McKenzie transferred the principles of Adams and Purves' guinea pig assay to mice, the McKenzie (1958a) bioassay method has been preferred. Mice are easier to handle and much cheaper, and there may be an improvement in sensitivity when mice are compared with guinea pigs although no direct comparisons have been published. Another advantage is the ease of intravenous injection in mice, although many workers are now using the intraperitoneal route for LATS assays (Kriss et al., 1964). So far, none of the in vitro systems which detect LATS has proved to be more sensitive, although precision may be slightly superior (Brown et al., 1968), and the McKenzie assay is likely to continue in favor unless some entirely new approach, such as a LATS assay based on competitive binding, overtakes it (see Section V, D).

There are many variants on McKenzie's original assay (Ason, 1967; Furth et al., 1969; Levy et al., 1965; McKenzie and Williamson, 1966; Major and Munro, 1962; Shishiba and Solomon, 1969), but all use basically the same type of preparation, in which mice are partially depleted of iodine, then injected with radioiodine and treated with thyroid hormones to suppress endogenous TSH release. Schedules of preparation vary mostly in the type of thyroid hormone used to achieve endogenous TSH suppression. This can be achieved by oral thyroid powder feeding, the addition of thyroid hydrolyzate to the drinking water, or the injection of thyroxine or triiodothyronine. The radioactive isotope used is either ^{131}I or ^{125}I. The latter has the distinct advantage of achieving an increased counting rate in the peripheral blood samples without a comparable increase in radiation dose to the thyroid which, in McKenzie's original design, was pushed to the limit set by radiation damage to the gland. There are also a number of ways in which the results of a response in the McKenzie assay may be expressed. Leaving on one side (see Section I, B, 1) the question of nonspecific responses in the assay system, the differences between the laboratories depend partly on the way in which the results are expressed and partly on the relationship between assay responses due to the injection of active sera and the effects of an inert control solution. No doubt there are also other factors which also contribute to variability in assay performance. The constitution of the inert control solution used varies but most groups now prefer to use a protein-containing solution which is approximately isotonic with normal serum and to express their assay responses in terms of a laboratory standard for LATS or in terms of the MRC reference standard for LATS (Dorrington and Munro, 1964). In earlier papers, responses were usually expressed as the percentage increase in blood radioactivity in venous samples withdrawn at intervals after the injection of various solutions—practice regarding the deduction of responses to inert control solutions varied. Now that a standard for LATS is available, it is desirable that all laboratories working in this field of study should make some attempt to relate the sensitivity of their assays by its use. It must be accepted that the nature of LATS is such that a standard made, as the available standard is, from a single serum may not always be appropriate for comparing responses with activity from other individuals (see Section III, A, 1). Nevertheless, it would be a great advantage to all workers in this field to establish that their assay system was of comparable sensitivity to other centers.

1. Nonspecific Effects

A separate section is required to discuss nonspecific effects in the McKenzie type of assay. Although the precise nature of these nonspecific effects cannot be defined there can be little doubt that, after the injection of some sera, a spurious response does occur. This point is of importance in interpretation as nonspecific effects may be either short- or long-acting and thus mimic either TSH or LATS. In some experimental situations the interpretation of results may be quite different according to whether the existence of the possibility of a nonspecific effect is acknowledged or not. The author believes that assay responses less than a doubling of the baseline radioactivity in control blood samples should always be interpreted extremely cautiously. It is clearly impossible to say merely from inspection of the level of response whether it is due to a nonspecific effect or to a low level of LATS or TSH. Both could produce similar effects on the circulating radioiodine, but it cannot be assumed that low assay responses are necessarily due to TSH or LATS. The use of specific antisera may help to resolve difficulties of this type.

C. Relationship to Earlier Theories of Thyrotoxicosis

1. Psychosomatic Theory

The most commonly advanced hypothesis concerning the nature of thyrotoxicosis has been that it must be a disorder precipitated by a period or an episode of exceptional mental strain. Many physicians are impressed by the convincing histories that many patients give in which they attribute the onset of their symptoms of thyroid overactivity, and sometimes the appearance of eye signs, to some abrupt shock or period of mental distress due to a variety of factors and, in individual cases the sequence of events, corroborated by relatives, is certainly authentic. The existence of a link between the brain and the pituitary release of TSH offers an appropriate mechanism. Nevertheless, most objective studies which have attempted to define whether the incidence of mental shock or strain was more frequent among patients with thyrotoxicosis than among the general population have failed to establish that the patients with thyrotoxicosis suffer such strains with any greater frequency than the general population (Wittkower and Mandelbrote, 1955;

Dewhurst *et al.*, 1968). It has been objected that this does not necessarily overthrow the psychosomatic hypothesis for thyrotoxicosis because this group of patients may also have a genetic predisposition to develop thyrotoxicosis after this type of experience (McKenzie, 1968a). To the author, it seems probable that the increased nervousness, tremor, and irritability of thyrotoxicosis could easily suggest to the patient that the whole illness, sharing these features with the effects of anxiety, has arisen as a result of mental distress.

Many patients with other diseases will similarly relate specific incidents to clearly quite unrelated pathological results. For example, patients with painful conditions of the skeleton such as Paget's disease or myelomatosis, will recount how their symptoms began with an injury which is obviously not related to the underlying cause of their discomfort. However, until it was established that LATS was fully effective in stimulating the thyroid of assay animals after hypophysectomy (Munro, 1959; Adams *et al.*, 1961), the possibility did exist that the whole phenomenon of delay in onset of response and the sustained action of LATS might be due to an excess of thyroid-stimulating hormone-releasing hormone (TRH) in the circulating blood. This evidence has now been reinforced by the activity of LATS on many *in vitro* thyroid preparations (Section IV).

2. Genetic Factors

The well-known studies of Bartels (1941) and Martin and Fisher (1945, 1951) revealed an increased prevalence of thyrotoxicosis among the relatives of patients. An unexpectedly high incidence of goiter was found by both groups, and of myxedema by Bartels (1941), suggesting a familial predisposition to thyroid disturbances of several types. Another clue, which is at any rate compatible with a genetic basis for thyrotoxicosis, is the abnormally low proportion of nontasters of phenylthiocarbamide (PTC), which has been used as a "genetic marker" (Kitchin *et al.*, 1959). Ingbar and Freinkel (1958) found an abnormally rapid turnover of iodine in euthyroid relatives of patients with toxic diffuse goiter. Recently Wall *et al.* (1969) have detected LATS in the same group.

There is, therefore, evidence from family studies that genetic influences are of importance in thyrotoxicosis and in the distribution of LATS activity. It is known that the relatives of patients with thyroid disturbances have an increased incidence of circulating autoantibodies to thyroid proteins (Hall *et al.*, 1960), and the evidence that LATS may be a member of this group of antibodies is discussed later (Section III).

Thus, the genetic evidence is entirely compatible with the immunoglobulin G nature of LATS.

3. "Jod-Basedow" Phenomenon

Another type of sequence which has been believed to have been of pathogenetic significance in thyrotoxicosis deserves discussion at this point. It is the phenomenon known for many years as the "Jod-Basedow" phenomenon. This is the precipitation of thyroid overactivity in patients suffering from long-standing iodine deficiency by the administration of an iodide dietary supplement. The original descriptions were on purely clinical grounds, but there has been at least one well-documented example in which radioiodine studies in an area of iodine deficiency preceded the apparent induction of thyrotoxicosis by the administration of dietary iodide (Stanbury *et al.*, 1954). Recently, work on the influence of a small iodide supplement on the tendency of drug-treated patients with thyrotoxicosis to relapse after the cessation of therapy has been examined. The results suggest that relapse may be at least accelerated, if not actually precipitated, by the administration of as little as 100 μg of excess dietary iodide per day. If, indeed, dietary iodide intake is a critical factor in determining the onset of thyrotoxicosis, then it may be that two factors operate in these cases. Certainly, it is possible theoretically to envisage a severe iodide restriction protecting a patient from the development of thyrotoxicosis; if iodinated thyronines cannot be synthesized, then thyroid overactivity could not become manifest. A further example of the tendency of iodide supplementation to accelerate the onset of thyrotoxicosis may exist in the recent reports from Tasmania where iodide supplements in bread appear to have precipitated an outbreak of thyrotoxicosis (Clements *et al.*, 1970; Connolly *et al.*, 1970).

4. Toxic Adenoma

Rarely, excessive thyroid activity may be confined to a solitary hyperfunctioning adenoma of the thyroid, and in this group LATS has not been incriminated as an etiological factor; it has been suggested that sometimes overactive adenomata may be multiple so that there may be some patients with more than one adenoma which become overactive without the intervention of LATS (McKenzie, 1966); further detailed documentation of this is needed.

D. *Evidence That LATS Stimulates the Thyroid*

It is clear that in the McKenzie (1958a) type of bioassay any influence which disturbed the integrity of thyroid cell membrane might release radioiodine from the gland into the peripheral blood and thus appear to cause thyroid stimulation. Such effect may underly some of the nonspecific responses already mentioned as a difficulty in this field. It was, therefore, necessary in the early stages of studying LATS to examine whether this stimulator was capable of affecting other parameters of thyroid function other than increasing radioiodine discharge. In several different types of experiment involving other parameters it has been shown that LATS exerts a stimulatory effect on thyroid function. Thus, radioiodine uptake is stimulated by the injection of LATS into thyroxine-treated mice, the histological advances of thyroid activation are also evident after similar LATS treatment (Major and Munro, 1960, 1962; McKenzie, 1960). It has also been shown that the uptake of tritiated thymidine is stimulated showing that the rate of cell division is increased by LATS (Garry and Hall, 1970). The various *in vitro* experiments showing a stimulatory response to LATS are discussed in detail below.

E. Evidence That LATS Is Not of Pituitary Origin

The first step in studying LATS was to examine whether it could be extracted from 'the pituitary of patients suffering from thyrotoxicosis. Clearly, studies were possible only in patients who had been known to suffer from the disease earlier in life, and most of the autopsy examinations were made on pituitary glands removed after death from other causes. Nevertheless, it was soon clear that in such pituitaries the thyroid-stimulating activity resembled conventional TSH in all respects (Major and Munro, 1962; McKenzie, 1962a). The time course of action of human TSH was identical with bovine pituitary TSH, and the effects of pituitary extracts could be annulled with specific antisera (Dorrington and Munro, 1965). This type of evidence is supported by the considerable number of reported cases in which thyrotoxicosis has been observed to develop in patients known to have pituitary failure following postpartum necrosis (Fajans, 1958), after stalk section (McCullagh *et al.*, 1960), or after surgical pituitary ablation (Christensen and Binder, 1962). There is also additional evidence that in patients with thyrotoxicosis pituitary TSH can be detected in the circulating blood when the disease is overtreated with antithyroid drugs. Under these circumstances, as soon as the circulating thyroid hormone falls below the normal range, the anticipated normal response of the pituitary, namely to release excess TSH, ensures that the peripheral blood can be shown to contain both TSH and LATS (Adams and Kennedy, 1965). This evidence is now reinforced by measurements in similar patients by immunoassay (Kriss *et al.*, 1967). It is generally agreed that immunoreactive TSH is low in untreated thyrotoxicosis (Utiger, 1965; Odell *et al.*, 1965; Lemarchand-Béraud and Vanotti, 1965; D'Angelo, 1963). Recently patients with overt thyrotoxicosis have been shown not to respond to the administration of thyrotropin-releasing hormone (TRH) with the anticipated rise in serum TSH which is seen most vigorously in hypothyroid subjects but can be detected with ease in normals (Ormston *et al.*, 1971a,b; Hershman and Pittman, 1970). Preliminary observations suggest that this may also be a feature of euthyroid Graves' disease (Lawton *et al.*, 1971).

II. Clinical Importance of LATS

A. *Relationship Between LATS and Thyroid Function in Thyrotoxicosis*

A major difficulty to accepting that LATS is the cause of the excessive thyroid activity of Graves' disease is the failure to detect LATS in the serum of a large proportion of patients who have undoubtedly severe thyrotoxicosis. This experience has been widespread (Major and Munro, 1962; Pinchera *et al.*, 1965a; Adams, 1965; Kriss *et al.*, 1967; Carneiro *et al.*, 1966a), and the proportion of positive LATS assays in unconcentrated serum when measured by the McKenzie bioassay has been as low as 30% in some series. Clearly, there could be several explanations for this situation. It may be that there are two types of thyrotoxicosis [leaving aside autonomous toxic adenomata in which LATS cannot be implicated (Pinchera *et al.*, 1965a; McKenzie, 1966)] and that LATS is of importance in only one of these. It seems to the author more probable, however, that the failure to detect LATS in Graves' disease results from the relative insensitivity of the bioassay procedure. In support of this, when concentration procedures for LATS have been applied to sera which were negative when assayed, the proportion of positive LATS responses increased (Carneiro *et al.*, 1966b). In concentrating LATS it is important to remember that the distribution of LATS activity in γG molecules is such that recovery of the first peak (unabsorbed) protein from chromatography on DEAE-cellulose is not invariably adequate for concentrating LATS from all sera. The report of Smith *et al.* (1969a) showed clearly that unless all protein with γG molecules was included in any concentration procedure, it was possible, inadvertently, to discard highly active electrophoretic subfractions. Thus, when Bonnyns and Vanhaelst (1969) used a method for IgG separation which concentrated only protein which was not absorbed by DEAE-Sephadex A-50, they failed to recover LATS activity from some samples. Another important line of evidence has been the study of correlations between the serum LATS levels and thyroid function. Positive correlations have been obtained only in patients in whom LATS could be demonstrated in assays of unconcentrated serum. Two reports from the same laboratory have established that in this group there is a strong positive correlation between the rate of radioiodine turnover in the patients' thyroid and the serum LATS response (Major and Munro, 1962; Carneiro et al., 1966a). Others have failed to confirm this, but the methods of study applied have not been identical and the number of patients in other series has usually been small (Hoffmann and Hetzel, 1966; Lipman et al., 1967; Chopra et al., 1970). It is difficult to escape the conclusion that, in those patients with whom a positive correlation has been demonstrated between serum LATS and radioiodine turnover, LATS is the ultimate cause of their thyroid overactivity.

B. Clinical Markers of LATS

1. Pretibial Myxedema

It was Kriss and his associates (1964) who first established that there is a strong association between the presence of localized myxedema of the skin, usually in the pretibial region, and a high LATS response on serum assay. This observation, confirmed by several groups (Pimstone et al., 1964; Pinchera et al., 1965a; Carneiro et al., 1966a; Bonnyns et al., 1968), has led Kriss to suggest that LATS cannot be the cause, but is one of the consequences, of Graves' disease (Kriss, 1968a). Nevertheless, those patients in whom localized myxedema is present are not infrequently suffering from severe thyrotoxicosis with an exceptionally rapid turnover of radioiodine in their thyroids, and it is in such patients that Carneiro et al. (1966a) found that the correlation between LATS and thyroid function was clearly demonstrable.

2. Neonatal Thyrotoxicosis

The second interesting clinical correlation which is generally agreed between different groups of workers is that mothers who bear babies suffering from the rare syndrome of neonatal thyrotoxicosis have very high serum LATS levels (Major and Munro, 1960; Rosenberg et al., 1963; McKenzie, 1964; Sunshine et al., 1965; Holmes et al., 1965). Most such mothers have, in fact, been successfully treated for Graves' disease at an early age usually by partial thyroidectomy, and are usually euthyroid at the time of their pregnancy and delivery. It is accepted that, in such circumstances, serum LATS may remain very high and the patient is presumably protected from recurrent thyrotoxicosis by lack of an adequate thyroid mass. In view of the evidence (see Section III) that LATS is a member of the γG class of immunoglobulins there is no difficulty in accepting on theoretical grounds that such a protein could be transferred from mother to fetus and may, therefore, cause the congenital syndrome. Indeed, this is only one of a group of diseases caused in this way (Scott, 1966). The evidence, however, goes further than this because serum LATS has been demonstrated in the cord blood of babies suffering from congenital thyrotoxicosis and, in a few instances, has been known to disappear from the neonatal circulation with a half-life compatible with the γG nature of LATS. There is no widespread objection to the hypothesis that LATS can cause this rare form of thyrotoxicosis, yet the controversy concerning the role of LATS in adult Graves' disease still continues.

C. Relationship to Other Thyroid Autoantibodies

Because LATS has so many chemical characteristics suggesting that it is a member of the γG class of immunoglobulins and, therefore, may well be an autoantibody to a thyroidal component, there has been a search in different laboratories for positive correlations between serum LATS and the titer of known thyroid autoantibodies (Major and Munro, 1962; Hoffmann and Hetzel, 1966; Bonnyns and Vanhaelst, 1969). On balance, the results suggest that such a correlation cannot be demonstrated. This does not constitute a serious impediment to the hypothesis that LATS may be an unusual thyroid autoantibody, because the relative sensitivity of the procedures being applied to this type of investigation clearly varies greatly for the different antibodies being studied. Inasmuch as LATS is, to all intents and purposes, confined to the serum of patients with a history of Graves' disease, a correlation can, indeed, be claimed. Recently, an interesting study by Volpé *et al.* (1969) reported that LATS persisted after total thyroid ablation with radioiodine whereas thyroid autoantibodies declined, suggesting that LATS may not depend on a thyroid antigenic stimulus.

D. Relationship to Eye Signs

It was only to be anticipated that the well known, but unexplained, association between eye involvement and thyroid overactivity in Graves' disease should provoke speculation concerning the possible etiological role of LATS in the eye signs. Surveys of serum LATS activity in patients with and without a severe eye involvement have yielded conflicting results (Major and Munro, 1962; Pinchera *et al.*, 1965a; Noguchi *et al.*, 1964; Hoffmann and Hetzel, 1966). The balance of opinion is against any association and, certainly, from any large series it is possible to select illustrative examples which confirm that serum LATS levels vary widely in patients with equally severe eye involvement. Kriss *et al.* (1967) have studied the progress of the eye signs associated with hyperthyroidism in patients treated with radioiodine. Serial LATS assays and measurement of antibodies to thyroglobulin were made, and they observed a tendency for serum LATS to rise after treatment in those patients in whom the eye signs deteriorated. This was interpreted as indicating that LATS might cause the eye signs. However, there are also serial LATS measurements in patients with a rapidly deteriorating eye involvement which failed to show any consistent rise in serum LATS levels as the eye signs got worse (Major, 1961).

E. Relationship Between LATS, TSH, and Exophthalmos-Producing Substance (EPS)

It is evident that whereas LATS is not of pituitary origin, both TSH and EPS activity probably are. EPS activity is usually assayed by its effect on the intercorneal distance of fish after the intraperitoneal injection of pituitary extracts rich in this activity. Morris (1962) has shown that TSH activity and LATS activity are closely related, and in TSH rich fractions varying in potency by a factor of 2000-fold or more he finds close correlation between TSH and EPS levels using a modification of the sensitive Shubunkin goldfish assay (McGill, 1960). Unfortunately, this assay cannot be applied effectively to the measurement of serum EPS activity because, after single intraperitoneal injection of serum, adhesions prevent any further use of the assay fish in crossover experiments which are essential for precision. This type of assay may well also be prone to nonspecific effects due to toxic factors which affect the general condition of the fish adversely, and the maximum range of response is severely limited by the anatomical circumstances. McGill (1960) detected EPS activity in two patients with severe malignant exophthalmos in whom eye signs were deteriorating rapidly, but otherwise his serum studies with this assay method were largely negative. It must be concluded that it is extremely unlikely that LATS and EPS activity are related in any way, and at the present time there is no clear evidence linking EPS activity in pituitary extracts with the eye signs of Graves' disease.

III. Chemical Nature of LATS

A. Association of LATS with γG Immunoglobulins

1. Distribution of LATS in γG Molecules

It was quickly established that LATS activity was associated with serum proteins, but the tendency for LATS activity to be found in protein fractions of differing electrophoretic mobility in early experiments failed to reveal the specific association with γG immunoglobulins, using chromatography on DEAE-cellulose (Munro, 1959; McKenzie, 1961b). Other workers showed a clear relationship between the serum LATS and γG protein (Adams and Kennedy, 1962; McKenzie, 1962b; Meek et al., 1964; Kriss et al., 1964). The explanation for the early conflicting results emerged in the detailed study of Smith et al. (1969a). From some sera, LATS activity can be recovered solely with the first peak of unabsorbed protein on chromatography on DEAE-cellulose or DEAE-Sephadex. Indeed, immunoelectrophoretically "pure" γG protein of high specific LATS activity has been commonly used in studies on the chemical nature of LATS described below.

The more common pattern of distribution of LATS activity is to show an irregular distribution among γG immunoglobulins of differing electrophoretic mobility, as has been shown for antibody activity (Sela and Mozes, 1966).

2. Methods for Concentrating LATS

This potentially widespread distribution of LATS in differing γG subfractions imposes limitations on serum concentration procedures for LATS. These are discussed in Section II, A. It is unlikely that any of the commonly available methods for serum protein fractionation would allow greater than 5-fold concentration if all γG protein is included. It is probable that a globulin precipitate produced by adding ammonium sulfate to a final concentration of 1.8 M will ensure the total recovery of LATS activity from serum. Care must be taken in preparing this precipitate for assay that no activity is discarded with euglobulins which tend to remain insoluble after dialysis, as in one potent serum described by Munro et al. (1967) in which all the LATS activity was confined to this particular small γG subfraction. Additional confirmatory evidence for the γG nature of LATS has come from the application of techniques originally developed for the study of antibodies (Cohen and Porter, 1964).

B. The Proteolysis of LATS

Proteolytic digestion of γG molecules of LATS activity has shown that the active groupings in the molecule are associated with the Fab or the Fab' fragments. This result has been achieved consistently in different centers (Meek et al., 1964; Kriss et al., 1965; Dorrington et al., 1965, 1966a; Burke, 1969), and the evidence from both peptic and papain digestion in the presence of cysteine is consistent.

1. Relation Between the Time Course of Action of LATS and Active Fragments Derived from γG

From these early proteolytic studies small active fragments of LATS-γG were shown to have a short-acting time course in the McKenzie bioassay. Even those fragments whose molecular size may be of the same order as purified human TSH remain immunologically quite distinct from pituitary TSH and show no cross-reaction with specific antisera. There is reason to presume from *in vitro* studies that these active fragments have a short time course of action because, in the intact animal, they have a shorter half-life compared with the parent molecules from which they are derived. Certainly, the converse fact is established in both rats (Adams, 1960) and mice, (McKenzie, 1961b), namely that the circulating half-time of γG molecules of LATS activity is very much longer than that of pituitary TSH fractions and, when assayed *in vitro*, the short-acting (*in vivo*) fragments of LATS-γG have an enhanced potency and identical course of action compared with either TSH or the parent molecule (Brown *et al.*, 1968).

C. *Separation and Reaggregation of H and L Chain from LATS-γG*

An alternative approach to the subfractionation of γG molecules is, of course, separation of H and L chain (Meek *et al.*, 1964; Dorrington *et al.*, 1964; McKenzie, 1965). The techniques originally described for antibody structure analysis destroyed most of the LATS activity, but Smith *et al.* (1969b) have developed modifications of the original method which greatly diminish the severity of the chemical conditions to which the protein was exposed. The principal changes were to reduce greatly the molarity of the mercaptoethanol used in the reduction and to collect the fractions from the gel filtration on Sephadex G-75 directly into cooled buffer. Even with these precautions, there was a substantial loss of LATS activity, but it was possible to establish quite clearly that with sufficiently potent LATS-γG preparations the thyroid-stimulating activity was confined to the heavy chain. Of the greatest importance is the observation made by Smith *et al.* (1969b) that, when heavy chain with thyroid-stimulating activity was allowed to reaggregate under appropriate chemical conditions with light chain, the 7 S molecules which were re-formed then reacquired long-acting thyroid-stimulating activity, in the McKenzie bioassay, of the parent LATS-γG molecules from which the chains were prepared. The potency of the reaggregated complexes was substantially enhanced in terms of the size of the maximum response when compared with that of the equivalent amount of H chain alone, but the clear reversion to the long-acting time course is the most striking evidence that the activity of LATS-γG is located in the Fd fragment, which is the site for antigen binding by γG-immunoglobulins. It remains possible that, in spite of the chemical evidence from these widely differing approaches to the analysis of LATS-γG, that the association of the thyroid-stimulating groupings in the LATS-γG molecule with the fractions which contain antigen binding activity in known antibodies is fortuitous. However, it seems much more probable that LATS is indeed an unusual autoantibody which possesses thyroid-stimulating activity. This is a hypothesis capable of examination by further experiment (see Sections IV and V) and, so far, the accumulated evidence remains consistent with this view.

IV. Effects of LATS and Its Active Fragments in Relation to Actions of TSH

Once LATS was accepted as a true stimulator of thyroid function (Section I, D), it was of great interest to determine whether its mode of action differed in any way from the effects of pituitary thyroid-stimulating hormone (TSH). This was clearly of great importance in assessing the significance of LATS in Graves' disease, particularly in relation to the possibility that LATS might produce an excess of the relatively more potent triiodothyronine. There was also considerable interest to observe whether, in different types of assay systems, the differences in time course of action between TSH and LATS persisted (see Section IV, A. On the whole, the early results have tended to show a remarkable similarity between the effects of TSH and LATS; no matter whether their actions were compared by the handling of radioactive iodine (McKenzie, 1960; Shishiba et al., 1967) or by histology (McKenzie, 1967) or whether some aspect of intermediary metabolism in the thyroid, such as glucose oxidation (Scott et al., 1966; Shishiba et al., 1970), the incorporation of ^{32}P into phospholipid or RNA synthesis (Field, 1968; Ochi and DeGroot, 1968), both stimulators were inhibited in mice treated with actinomycin D (McKenzie and Williamson, 1966).

A. Altered Time Course of LATS in Vitro and in Vivo

It has also been a feature of such studies that, in general, when tested in vitro, the time courses of action of these two different thyroid-stimulating materials were found to be very similar (Brown and Munro, 1967; Brown et al., 1968) although a slight latency in the in vitro actions has been observed in some circumstances (Shishiba et al., 1970; Kaneko et al., 1970). Strangely, this does not apply to in vitro studies on adenyl cyclase activation by TSH and LATS (Levey and Pastan, 1970; Kendall-Taylor, unpublished observations). There can be little doubt that the outstanding discrepancy in time course of action which exists in the McKenzie type of bioassay, using an intact animal, does not persist when the materials are being tested in in vitro experiments in which extrathyroidal degradation and excretion factors no longer operate. So far as can be tested at the present time, TSH and LATS appear to act through similar mechanisms in stimulating the thyroid, and no clear qualitative difference in their effects has been defined. The change in the time course of action of molecular fragments derived from LATS-γG when compared with the original γG molecule has already been stressed (Section III, B, 1). The evidence from the use of specific antisera shows quite definitely that there is no possibility that the fragmentation of the LATS-γG molecule resulted in the release of pituitary thyroid-stimulating hormone which had been hitherto associated with it (Dorrington *et al.*, 1966a). Thus, even with active Fab or Fab' fragments derived from γG with LATS activity, in which the size of the active fragments approximate to the current estimates of the molecular size of pituitary thyroid-stimulating hormone, there remains a clear antigenic distinctness between the two types of thyroid-stimulating activity. The result of reaggregation of active H with inactive L chain also tends to confirm the view that the biological potency of LATS cannot be attributed to the association of pituitary TSH with a protein molecule. Finally, Kriss (1968b) has shown that LATS, but not TSH, is inactivated by anti-kappa and anti-lambda antisera.

B. Relationship Between Actions of LATS, TSH, and Cyclic AMP

The widespread interest in the role of cyclic adenosine 3',5'-monophosphate (c-AMP) as a "second messenger" in the mediation of the effects of many different hormones has led to several comparisons of the thyroidal effects of TSH and LATS with c-AMP (Ensor and Munro, 1969; McKenzie, 1967) or with dibutyryl c-AMP (Kendall-Taylor and Munro, 1970). Experiments have also been performed in which the effects of thyroid stimulation on intrinsic thyroidal adenylcyclase activity has been assayed (Kaneko *et al.*, 1970). Direct measurement of thyroidal c-AMP content has been made after thyroidal stimulation by TSH in sheep thyroid homogenates (Klainer *et al.*, 1962) bovine thyroid slices (Gilman and Rall, 1966) and in canine and bovine homogenates (Levey *et al.*, 1969). Another line of study in this field has been to examine the effects of theophylline, a known inhibitor of phosphodiesterase, the enzyme responsible for the degradation of c-AMP. All these approaches have provided supporting evidence for the view that both TSH and LATS activate adenylcyclase and may well owe the greater part of their intrathyroidal effects to the mediation of c-AMP. A wide variety of different techniques has been applied. Many of the studies, in common with other work in this field, have been by *in vitro* methods. There can, however, be little doubt that the overall picture is one which again supports the view that LATS and TSH must in many respects have very similar intrathyroidal effects. This is an aspect of the study of LATS which will undoubtedly be examined in greater detail as knowledge concerning the mode of action of TSH grows.

V. Absorption of LATS by Thyroid Extracts

Pursuing the concept that LATS might be a member of the γG class of proteins and, therefore, a thyroidal autoantibody, there is now great interest and activity in the field of studying the effects of absorption of LATS by thyroid homogenates. The original phenomena were reported by Kriss *et al.* (1964), who observed that when serum potent in LATS activity was incubated *in vitro* with homogenates of whole thyroidal tissue or, subsequently, of partially purified preparations of thyroidal microsomes, there was a loss of the thyroid-stimulating activity from the potent serum (Beall and Solomon, 1966; Dorrington *et al.*, 1966b). Evidence that LATS absorption by tissue extracts was not specifically a property of the thyroid has been presented by Benhamou-Glynn *et al.* (1967), but other tissues were much less effective and did not completely remove LATS activity. It has been presumed that *in vitro* absorption of LATS is, in fact, analogous to an antigen–antibody interaction. Clearly, such experiments open up several new approaches to the study of the nature of LATS. If the basic presumption that the *in vitro* absorption of LATS is the result of antigen–antibody combination is valid, then the purification and identification of the intrathyroidal activity which is capable of combining with LATS would reveal the nature of the antigen to which LATS is an antibody. Such a preparation would clearly be of great use in experiments in which an experimental analog in Graves' disease might be created in animals by the deliberate raising of antisera to such a purified material; these are discussed below.

A. *Thyroid-Stimulating Effects of Antisera to Thyroid Extracts— Possibility of an Experimental Analog of Graves' Disease*

There are now many different experiments in the literature in which attempts have been made to raise a thyroid-stimulating antibody. Most workers have used rabbits and immunized them by a variety of routes, with or without Freund's adjuvants; the commonest antigenic materials injected have been whole thyroidal homogenates or thyroid microsomes (Pinchera *et al.*, 1965b; McKenzie, 1968b; Beall and Solomon, 1968; Solomon and Beall, 1968; Burke, 1968). The results, on the whole, have been disappointing. There is some evidence that, in some rabbits, a weak form of thyroid-stimulating activity can be created by such immunization procedures, and it has also been shown that this thyroid-stimulating activity is concentrated with γG protein. Nevertheless, no clear analog to Graves' disease has resulted, and studies of thyroidal function in the affected animals has not tended to reveal a state analogous to the human Graves' disease. Because of the relative remoteness of rabbits as a species from man, several groups have been tempted to immunize monkeys or apes. One extremely interesting experiment reported by Beall *et al.* (1970) has shown that the injection of human thyroidal homogenates into baboons does result in the excess thyroid-stimulating activity in the serum of immunized animals, but this thyroidal stimulating activity has been shown to be due to excess endogenous TSH, and the thyroids of the injected animals have shown a form of thyroiditis very analogous to the autoimmune thyroiditis so widely studied by Rose and his associates (Kite *et al.*, 1966; Andrada *et al.*, 1968). It is clear, therefore, that in this species the administration of human thyroid extracts induces thyroidal damage with an excess of pituitary thyroid-stimulating hormone resulting, no doubt, from a diminution in circulating thyroid hormone levels. It is to be anticipated that further work on this line will be pursued when LATS absorbing activity is available in more purified form.

B. Partial Purification of LATS Absorbing Activity

Although most workers have continued to study particulate fractions in purifying LATS absorbing activity, it was Berumen *et al.* (1967) who first observed that the majority of the absorbing activity from thyroidal homogenates could, in fact, be recovered from the soluble supernatant protein left after centrifugation at 105,000 g for 2 hours. Centrifugation at this speed is usually accepted as being capable of precipitating particulate fractions from thyroidal homogenates, although it is clearly difficult to be absolutely certain on this point. Nevertheless, the availability of LATS-absorbing activity in a soluble form or, at worst, associated with very small particles, has allowed the purification of LATS-absorbing activity by fractionation methods for protein solutions. For example, Smith (1970) has shown that, when subjected to gel filtration on Sephadex G-200 in molar sodium chloride, LATS-absorbing activity may be recovered in a fraction quite separate from 19 S thyroglobulin with 4 S thyroid protein. This does not agree with the results of Berumen *et al.* (1967), who concluded that 19 S thyroglobulin was responsible for LATS absorption, nor with Beall *et al.* (1969), who also found LATS-absorbing activity to be completely excluded by Sephadex G-200. Smith and Munro (1970) have also shown that the LATS-absorbing activity may be separated from serum albumin, a point of importance because of the claim that a factor associated with serum albumin inhibits the effects of LATS (Burke, 1967). There is, at present, a good reason to hope that, with modern techniques for protein purification, LATS-absorbing activity may be recovered in purified form.

C. Dissociation of LATS after Absorption

Recent work on the effects of chaotropic ions on the antigen–antibody complex (Hatefi and Hanstein, 1969) prompted the study of the exposure of the complex formed when LATS has been absorbed by LATS-absorbing activity to sodium thiocyanate. It was found that the response to this treatment was, in fact, closely analogous to the described dissociation of antigen and antibody. Optimal yields of LATS activity from the inactive complex were obtained when 2 M sodium thiocyanate was employed.

D. Future Applications of LATS Absorption

The use of dissociation of LATS after absorption has already been exploited to locate the complex formed between LATS and thyroid proteins in fractions prepared by gel filtration on Sephadex G-200 (Smith and Munro, 1970). This has shown that LATS-absorbing activity (LAA) must be a molecule of relatively low molecular weight (around 30,000) compared with LATS-γG. Until this maneuver was applied to the problem, it was possible to observe the loss of LATS activity only after absorption, but now many features of the interaction and the nature of the reaction product can be elucidated.

Another application has been in the purification of LATS-γG. It has been possible to allow γG immunoglobulins possessing LATS activity to react with 4 S thyroid protein and subsequently to separate the LATS–LAA complex. Subsequently, exposure to sodium thiocyanate allowed a 70-fold purification of LATS-γG (Smith, unpublished observations).

Exposure to 2 M sodium thiocyanate inactivates LAA (Smith, 1970), which is also unstable to heating at 56°C for 1 hour (Sharard and Adams, 1965; Smith, 1970). However, the complex between LATS and LAA does not release any LATS activity when heated at 56°C for 1 hour (Smith, 1970). This last observation is of considerable importance, as it confirms that the interaction between LATS and LAA occurs *in vitro* and is not due to an inhibitory action of LAA on the capacity of the thyroid of the mice used for assay to respond. The importance of this observation is enhanced by the demonstration by Floresheim (1970) that the responses of the McKenzie assay can be influenced by the treatment of the mice with thyroxine or thyroidal proteins.

E. Importance of Better Assay for LATS

In addition to revealing fundamental information concerning the nature of the interaction of LATS and thyroid homogenates *in vitro*, such a reaction also, of course, opens up the possibility of a radioimmune type of assay for LATS. There is now a clear need for better LATS assay procedures. At present, bioassay detects LATS activity in approximately one half of all patients with Graves' disease (Section I), and it is not known to what extent LATS may be present in other patients. Concentration procedures suggest that some patients have LATS in lower concentrations than can be detected in assays of unconcentrated serum. They could not readily be applied to the serial study of LATS levels in large groups of patients.

Furthermore, better precision in assay would assist in assessing the effects of different forms of treatment on LATS activity about which there is only fragmentary information at present (Snyder et al., 1964). Kriss and his group (Mori et al., 1970) have been in the forefront of this type of development and have made preliminary reports of the use of thyroidal microsomes as an immunoabsorbent for LATS-γG which has been absorbed after being labeled with radioactive iodine. The results, as at present reported, have not yet established a new assay for LATS, but other work also suggests that this field is still worthy of continued study. One great difficulty arises from the need to purify LATS-absorbing activity before exposing LATS-γG labeled with radioactive iodine. Clearly, in a disease in which several different autoantibodies are known to circulate and in the present state of purification of LATS-γG from sera, it will be difficult to interpret the results of absorption of γG serum proteins by thyroidal protein preparations which may not be absolutely specific for LATS. The greatest care will be required to establish that there is no cross reaction between the binding protein used in this type of assay from LATS and any of the known thyroid autoantibodies.

In spite of these difficulties it is clear that progress is being made (Wong and Litman, 1969), although it is the author's belief that the use of particulate thyroid fraction to absorb LATS will always be difficult because of contamination with thyroglobulin and other thyroid antigens.

When such an assay is available, the controversial issues concerning the nature and significance of LATS may all be speedily resolved. The study of the problems concerning the mechanism of LATS production will no doubt be equally fascinating.

References

Adams, D. D. (1960). *Endocrinology* 66, 658.
Adams, D. D. (1965). *Brit. Med. J.* i, 1015.
Adams, D. D., and Kennedy, T. H. (1962). *Proc. Univ. Otago Med. Sch.* 40, 6.
Adams, D. D., and Kennedy, T. H. (1965). *J. Clin. Endocrinol. Metab.* 25, 571.
Adams, D. D., and Purves, H. D. (1953). *Proc. Univ. Otago Med. Sch.* 31, 38.
Adams, D. D., and Purves, H. D. (1956). *Proc. Univ. Otago Med. Sch.* 34, 11.
Adams, D. D., Purves, H. D., and Sirett, N. E. (1961). *Endocrinology* 68, 154.
Andrada, J. A., Rose, N. R., and Kite, J. H., Jr. (1968). *Clin. Exp. Immunol.* 3, 133.
Ason, E. K. (1967). *J. Clin. Endocrinol Metab.* 27, 1529.
Bartels, E. D. (1941). "Heredity in Graves Disease." Munksgard, Copenhagen.
Beall, G. N., and Solomon, D. H. (1966). *J. Clin. Invest.* 45, 552.
Beall, G. N., and Solomon, D. H. (1968). *J. Clin. Endocrinol. Metab.* 28, 503.
Beall, G. N., Doniach, D., Roitt, I. M., and El Kabir, D. J. (1969). *J. Lab. Clin. Med.* 73, 988.
Beall, G. N., Daniel, P. M., Pratt, O. E., and Solomon, D. H. (1970). *J. Clin. Endocrinol. Metab.* 29, 1460.
Benhamou-Glynn, N., El Kabir, D. J., Doniach, D., and Roitt, I. M. (1967). *In* "Thyrotoxicosis" (W. J. Irvine, ed.), pp. 29–39. Livingstone, Edinburgh.
Berumen, F. O., Lobsenz, I. L., and Utiger, R. D. (1967). *J. Lab. Clin. Med.* 70, 640.
Bonnyns, M., and Vanhaelst, L. (1969). *Clin. Exp. Immunol.* 4, 597.
Bonnyns, M., Demeester-Mirkine, N., Calay, R., and Bastenie, P. A. (1968). *Acta Endocrinol. (Copenhagen)* 58, 581.
Brown, J., and Munro, D. S. (1967). *J. Endocrinol.* 38, 439.
Brown, J., Ensor, J., and Munro, D. S. (1968). *Proc. Roy. Soc. Med.* 61, 652.
Burke, G. (1967). *J. Lab. Clin. Med.* 69, 713.
Burke, G. (1968). *J. Lab. Clin. Med.* 72, 17.
Burke, G. (1969). *Endocrinology* 84, 1063.
Carneiro, L., Dorrington, K. J., and Munro, D. S. (1966a). *Lancet* ii, 878.
Carneiro, L., Dorrington, K. J., and Munro, D. S. (1966b). *Clin. Sci.* 31, 215.
Chopra, I. J., Solomon, D. H., Johnson, D. E., Chopra, U., and Fisher, D. A. (1970). *J. Clin. Endocrinol. Metab.* 30, 524.
Christensen, L. K., and Binder, V. (1962). *Acta Med. Scand.* 172, 285.
Clements, F. W., Gibson, H. B., and Howeler-Coy, J. F. (1970). *Lancet* i, 489.
Cohen, S., and Porter, R. R. (1964). *Advan. Immunol.* 4, 287.
Connolly, R. J., Vidor, G. I., and Stewart, J. C. (1970). *Lancet* i, 500.
D'Angelo, S. A. (1963). *J. Clin. Endocrinol. Metab.* 23, 229.
Dewhurst, K. E., El Kabir, D. J., Harris, G. W., and Mandelbrote, B. M. (1968). *Confin. Neurol.* 30, 161.
Dorrington, K. J., and Munro, D. S. (1964). *J. Endocrinol.* 31, 21.
Dorrington, K. J., and Munro, D. S. (1965). *Clin. Sci.* 28, 165.
Dorrington, K. J., Munro, D. S., and Carneiro, L. (1964). *Lancet* ii, 889.
Dorrington, K. J., Carneiro, L., and Munro, D. S. (1965). *Curr. Top. Thyroid Res., Proc. Int. Thyroid Conf., 5th, Rome, 1965,* pp. 455–463.

Dorrington, K. J., Carneiro, L., and Munro, D. S. (1966a). *Biochem. J.* **98**, 858.
Dorrington, K. J., Carneiro, L., and Munro, D. S. (1966b). *J. Endocrinol.* **34**, 133.
Ensor, J. M., and Munro, D. S. (1969). *J. Endocrinol.* **43**, 477.
Fajans, S. S. (1958). *J. Clin. Endocrinol. Metab.* **18**, 271.
Field, J. B. (1968). *J. Clin. Invest.* **47**, 1553.
Florsheim, W. H. (1970). *Proc. Int. Thyroid Conf., 6th, Vienna.* (Abstr.)
Furth, E. D., Rathbun, M., and Posillico, J. (1969). *Endocrinology* **85**, 592.
Garry, R., and Hall, R. (1970). *Lancet* **i**, 693.
Gilman, A. G., and Rall, T. W. (1966). *Fed. Proc. Fed. Amer. Soc. Exp. Biol.* **25**, 617.
Hall, R., Owen, S. G., and Smart, G. A. (1960). *Lancet* **ii**, 187.
Hatefi, Y., and Hanstein, W. G. (1969). *Proc. Nat. Acad. Sci. U.S.* **62**, 1129.
Hershman, J. M., and Pittman, J. A. (1970). *J. Clin. Endocrinol. Metab.* **31**, 457.
Hoffmann, M. J., and Hetzel, B. S. (1966). *Australas. Ann. Med.* **15**, 204.
Holmes, R. A., Engring, N. H., and Enestrom, W. W. (1965). *Ann. Intern. Med.* **62**, 1008.
Ingbar, S. H., and Freinkel, N. (1958). *J. Clin. Invest.* **37**, 1603.
Kaneko, T., Zor, U., and Field, J. B. (1970). *Metab. Clin. Exp.* **19**, 430.
Kendall-Taylor, P. (1971). Unpublished observations.
Kendall-Taylor, P., and Munro, D. S. (1970). *J. Endocrinol.* **47**, 333.
Kitchin, F. D., Howel-Evans, W., Clarke, C. A., McConnell, R. B., and Sheppard, P. M. (1959). *Brit. Med. J.* **i**, 1069.
Kite, J. H., Jr., Argue, H., and Rose, N. R. (1966). *Clin. Exp. Immunol.* **1**, 139.
Klainer, L. M., Chi, Y. M., Freidberg, S. L., Rall, T. W., and Sutherland, E. W. (1962). *J. Biol. Chem.* **237**, 1239.
Kriss, J. P. (1968a). *Advan. Metab. Disord.* **3**, 209.
Kriss, J. P. (1968b). *J. Clin. Endocrinol. Metab.* **28**, 1440.
Kriss, J. P., Pleshakov, V., and Chien, J. R. (1964). *J. Clin. Endocrinol. Metab.* **24**, 1005.
Kriss, J. P., Pleshakov, V., Rosenblum, A., and Chien, J. R. (1965). *Curr. Top. Thyroid Res., Proc. Int. Thyroid Conf., 5th, Rome, 1965*, pp. 432–444.
Kriss, J. P., Pleschakov, V., Rosenblum, A. L., Holderness, M., Sharp, G., and Utiger, R. (1967). *J. Clin. Endocrinol. Metab.* **27**, 582.
Lawton, N. F., Ekins, R. P., and Nabarro, J. D. N. (1971). *Lancet* **ii**, 14.
Lemarchand-Béraud, T., and Vanotti, A. (1965). *Curr. Top. Thyroid Res., Proc. Int. Thyroid Conf., 5th, Rome, 1965*, p. 527.
Levey, G. S., and Pastan, I. (1970). *Life Sci.* **9**, 67.
Levey, G. S., Roth, J., and Pastan, I. (1969). *Endocrinology* **84**, 1009.
Levy, R. P., McGuire, W. L., Shaw, R. K., and Bartsh, G. E. (1965). *Endocrinology* **76**, 890.
Lipman, L. M., Green, D. E., Snyder, N. J., Nelson, J. C., and Solomon, D. H. (1967). *Amer. J. Med.* **43**, 486.
McCullagh, E. P., Reynolds, C. W., and McKenzie, J. M. (1960). *J. Clin. Endocrinol. Metab.* **20**, 1029.
McGill, D. A. (1960). *Quart. J. Med.* **29**, 423.
McKenzie, J. M. (1958a). *Endocrinology* **63**, 372.
McKenzie, J. M. (1958b). *Endocrinology* **62**, 865.
McKenzie, J. M. (1960). *J. Clin. Endocrinol. Metab.* **20**, 380.

McKenzie, J. M. (1961a). *Advan. Thyroid Res., Trans. Int. Goitre Conf., 4th, London, 1960,* pp. 210–214.
McKenzie, J. M. (1961b). *J. Clin. Endocrinol. Metab.* **21**, 635.
McKenzie, J. M. (1962a). *Proc. Roy. Soc. Med.* **55**, 539.
McKenzie, J. M. (1962b). *J. Biol. Chem.* **237**, 3571.
McKenzie, J. M. (1964). *J. Clin. Endocrinol. Metab.* **24**, 660.
McKenzie, J. M. (1965). *Trans. Ass. Amer. Physicians* **78**, 174.
McKenzie, J. M. (1966). *J. Clin. Endocrinol. Metab.* **26**, 779.
McKenzie, J. M. (1967). *Recent Progr. Horm. Res.* **23**, 1.
McKenzie, J. M. (1968a). *Physiol. Rev.* **43**, 252.
McKenzie, J. M. (1968b). *J. Clin. Endocrinol. Metab.* **28**, 596.
McKenzie, J. M., and Williamson, A. (1966). *J. Clin. Endocrinol. Metab.* **26**, 578.
Major, P. W. (1961). Ph.D. Thesis, Univ. of Sheffield, Sheffield, England.
Major, P. W., and Munro, D. S. (1960). *J. Endocrinol.* **20**, xix.
Major, P. W., and Munro, D. S. (1962). *Clin. Sci.* **23**, 463.
Martin, L. C., and Fisher, R. A. (1945). *Quart. J. Med.* **14**, 207.
Martin, L. C., and Fisher, R. A. (1951). *Quart. J. Med.* **20**, 293.
Meek, J. C., Jones, A. E., Lewis, U. J., and VanderLaan, W. P. (1964). *Proc. Nat. Acad. Sci. U.S.* **52**, 342.
Mori, T., Fisher, J., and Kriss, J. P. (1970). *J. Clin. Endocrinol. Metab.* **31**, 119.
Morris, C. J. O. R. (1962). *Proc. Roy. Soc. Med.* **55**, 540.
Munro, D. S. (1959). *J. Endocrinol.* **19**, 64.
Munro, D. S., Brown, J., Dorrington, K. J., Smith, B. R., and Ensor, J. (1967). *In* "Thyrotoxicosis" (W. J. Irvine, ed.), p. 1. Livingstone, Edinburgh.
Munro, D. S., Brown, J., Dorrington, K. J., Ensor, J., Smith, B. R., and Kendall-Taylor, P. (1968). *In* "Progress in Endocrinology" (C. Gual, ed.), pp. 1192–1199. Excerpta Med. Found., Amsterdam.
Noguchi, A., Kurihara, H., and Sato, S. (1964). *J. Clin. Endocrinol. Metab.* **24**, 160.
Ochi, Y., and DeGroot, L. J. (1968). *Biochim. Biophys. Acta* **170**, 198.
Odell, W. D., Wilber, J. F., and Paul, W. E. (1965). *J. Clin. Endocrinol. Metab.* **25**, 1179.
Ormston, B. J., Cryer, R. J., Garry, R., Besser, G. M., and Hall, R. (1971a). *Lancet* ii, 10.
Ormston, B. J., Kilborn, J. R., Garry, R., Amos, J., and Hall, R. (1971b). *Brit. Med. J.* ii, 199.
Pimstone, B. L., Hoffenberg, R., and Black, E. (1964). *J. Clin. Endocrinol. Metab.* **24**, 976.
Pinchera, A., Pinchera, M. G., and Stanbury, J. B. (1965a). *J. Clin. Endocrinol. Metab.* **25**, 189.
Pinchera, A. Liberti, P., and Badalamenti, G. (1965b). *Folia Endocrinol.* **18**, 523.
Rosenberg, D., Grand, M. J. H., and Silbert, D. (1963). *New Engl. J. Med.* **268**, 292.
Scott, J. S. (1966). *Brit. Med. J.* i, 1559.
Scott, T. W., Good, B. F., and Ferguson, K. A. (1966). *Endocrinology* **79**, 929.
Sela, M., and Mozes, E. (1966). *Proc. Nat. Acad. Sci. U.S.* **55**, 445.
Sellars, E. A., Awad, A. G., and Schönbaum, E. (1970). *Lancet* ii, 335.
Sharard, A., and Adams, D. D. (1965). *Proc. Univ. Otago Med. Sch.* **43**, 25.
Shishiba, Y., and Solomon, D. H. (1969). *J. Clin. Endocrinol. Metab.* **29**, 405.

Shishiba, Y., Solomon, D. H., and Beall, G. N. (1967). *Endocrinology* **80**, 957.
Shishiba, Y., Solomon, D. H., and Davidson, W. D. (1970). *Endocrinology* **86**, 183.
Smith, B. R. (1970). *J. Endocrinol.* **46**, 45.
Smith, B. R., and Munro, D. S. (1970). *Biochim. Biophys. Acta* **208**, 285.
Smith, B. R., Munro, D. S., and Dorrington, K. J. (1969a). *Biochim. Biophys. Acta* **188**, 89.
Smith, B. R., Dorrington, K. J., and Munro, D. S. (1969b). *Biochim. Biophys. Acta* **192**, 277.
Snyder, N. J., Green, D. E., and Solomon, D. H. (1964). *J. Clin. Endocrinol. Metab.* **24**, 1129.
Solomon, D. H., and Beall, G. N. (1968). *J. Clin. Endocrinol. Metab.* **28**, 1496.
Stanbury, J. B., Brownell, G. L., Riggs, D. S., Perinetti, H., Itoiz, J., and Del Castillo, E. B. (1954). "Endemic Goitre: The Adaptation of Man to Iodine Deficiency." Harvard Univ. Press, Cambridge, Massachusetts.
Sunshine, P., Kusomoto, H., and Kriss, J. P. (1965). *Pediatrics* **36**, 869.
Utiger, R. D. (1965). *J. Clin. Invest.* **44**, 1277.
Volpé, R., Desbarats-Schönbaum, M., Schönbaum, E., Row, V. V., and Egrin, C. (1969). *Amer. J. Med.* **46**, 217.
Wall, J. R., Good, B. F., and Hetzel, B. S. (1969). *Lancet* **ii**, 1024.
Wittkower, E. D., and Mandelbrote, B. M. (1955). "Modern Trends in Psychosomatic Medicine." Butterworth, London.
Wong, E. T., and Litman, G. W. (1969). *J. Clin. Endocrinol. Metab.* **29**, 72.

ENDOCRINOLOGICAL IMPLICATIONS OF PROSTAGLANDINS*

John D. Flack, Peter W. Ramwell, and Jane E. Shaw

WORCESTER FOUNDATION FOR EXPERIMENTAL BIOLOGY
SHREWSBURY, MASSACHUSETTS
AND
ALZA CORPORATION
PALO ALTO, CALIFORNIA

I.	Introduction	200
II.	Tropic Hormone Effects	202
	A. Growth Hormone	202
	B. ACTH—Adrenals	203
	C. TSH—Thyroid	206
	D. Gonadotropin—Ovaries	207
	E. Gonadotropin—Testes	209
III.	Neuroendocrinological Considerations	210
IV.	Posterior Pituitary	212
	A. Uterus	212
	B. Fallopian Tubes	214
	C. Kidney	215
V.	Exocrine Hormone Interaction	218
	A. Pancreas	218
	B. Stomach	218
VI.	Actions on Lipid and Carbohydrate Metabolism	220
VII.	Conclusions	222
	References	223

* Supported in part by Office of Naval Research Contract N00014-67-C-0351; NR 101-695; National Institute of Mental Health Grant MH-10624 and National Institutes of Health Grant NB-06444.

I. Introduction

Recent identification of a whole series of highly active substances called prostaglandins (Fig. 1) is currently having a dramatic impact on conventional endocrinology, for these compounds have now been shown to mimic or inhibit the action of nearly all hormones. The prostaglandins are biosynthesized in most tissues from essential fatty acids; however, no specific source or target tissue has yet been located. At present, no disease has been convincingly identified with under- or overproduction of prostaglandins, although prostaglandin release has been tentatively associated with peptide amine-secreting tumors (Sandler et al., 1969), hypertension (Edwards et al., 1969), and renal ischemia (McGiff et al., 1969a). Prostaglandins have remarkably low toxicity (Bergström et al., 1968), but their side effects are such as to suggest that some of the symptomatology of shock may be due in part to hypersecretion of prostaglandins. Their ready release on neuronal or hormonal stimulation of tissues (Ramwell and Shaw, 1970) reflects biosynthesis, not release from a bound form, since no cellular storage sites have been

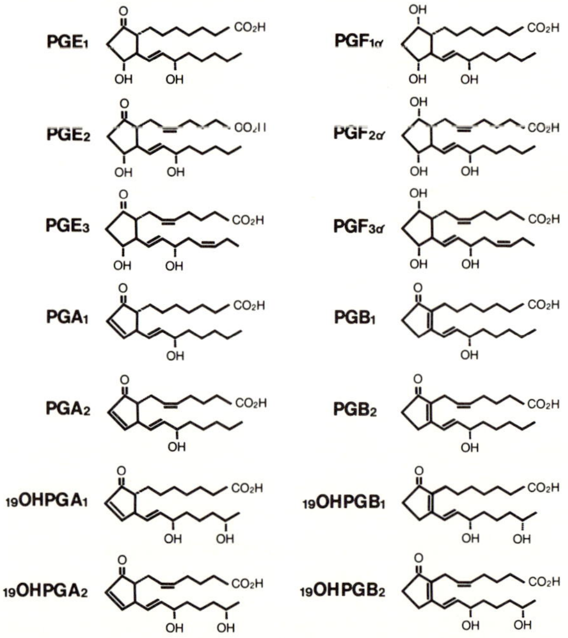

Fig. 1. Structural formulas of some naturally occurring prostaglandins.

identified and more prostaglandin is released from tissues on stimulation than can be extracted. Formation appears to be governed by availability of precursors, which are polyenoic ω6 C_{20} fatty acids, including homo-γ-linolenic and arachidonic acids. These fatty acids are endogenous constituents of tissue phospholipids and are thought to be released from the esterified form following activation of phospholipase on hormonal stimulation (Vogt et al., 1969). The liberated fatty acid then undergoes microsomal cyclization by a complex reaction to form prostaglandins, a process that has not been completely defined but is known to involve the introduction of molecular oxygen (Samuelsson, 1965). Dihydroxy (PGE) and trihydroxy (PGF) compounds are formed from the same precursor, and the degree of unsaturation within the compounds depends upon the particular precursor employed; thus the tri-, tetra-, and pentanoic precursors yield mono-, di-, and trienoic E and F prostaglandins, respectively. The direction of the synthesis may be modified by altering the conditions of incubation, and there is evidence that the composition of prostaglandins released following stimulation may be qualitatively different from the basal composition (Shaw and Ramwell, 1968a). The prostaglandins exhibit a wide range of pharmacological effects *in vivo*, which are of short duration (Bergström et al., 1968). Autoradiographic studies have indicated that 1 hour after administration, radioactivity initially associated with prostaglandin E_1 (PGE_1) is generally distributed throughout the body, with exclusion of the central nervous system; most radioactivity was concentrated in the lungs, liver, and kidneys. Metabolism studies have indicated rapid removal of circulating prostaglandins by the lungs and liver, and urinary analysis indicates that the prostaglandin molecule undergoes rapid modification, including oxidation of the 15-hydroxyl group, β-oxidation, and reduction of the Δ^5, Δ^{13}, and Δ^{17} bonds where present, prior to excretion.

These observations concerning the metabolism of prostaglandins, which leads to formation of less active products, possibly explain the short duration of effect of prostaglandins on systemic injection. This evidence, together with the failure to detect significant amounts of circulating prostaglandins except in special circumstances, would suggest that the biological effect of endogenous prostaglandins will be localized to their tissue of origin, and argues against a classical humoral role for these compounds. There is considerable speculation that prostaglandins are local humoral substances associated with regulation of tissue perfusion (Ramwell and Shaw, 1967). Thus, it has been suggested that the vasodilator prostaglandins are responsible for functional hyperemia seen on activation of adipose tissue (Lewis and Matthews, 1969), adrenals (Maier and Staehelin, 1968), or skeletal muscle (Beck et al., 1968). Conversely, the luteolytic effect obtained with $PGF_{2\alpha}$ has been ascribed to a vasoconstrictor action; it is proposed that the prostaglandin causes constriction of the ovarian vein, which produces ischemia of the corpus luteum sufficient to induce luteal regression (Pharriss et al., 1970). Finally, there is the possibility that the prostaglandins exert their pharmacological effects through modification of intracellular cyclic AMP. The concept of Sutherland that cyclic AMP is the intracellular mediator of hormone action has received wide confirmation (see Breckenridge, 1970). The evidence to be reviewed here indicates that the prostaglandins modify cyclic AMP formation in all tissues so far examined, but once cyclic AMP is formed in response to a hormone, prostaglandins are thought to have little effect on the action of this nucleotide in mediating its intracellular effects. The knowledge that increased biosynthesis of prostaglandins also occurs on hormonal stimulation of a tissue has led to the suggestion that the endogenous prostaglandins may serve some function in regulating hormone action at the tissue level.

II. Tropic Hormone Effects

Examination of the effects of prostaglandins on the release of tropic hormones from the anterior pituitary began with *in vitro* studies. Zor et al. (1969a) showed that prostaglandins and extracts of ovine hypothalamus stimulate adenyl cyclase activity and cyclic AMP formation in rat pituitary glands, while in the same test system epinephrine (adrenaline), norepinephrine (noradrenaline), histamine, 5-HT, dopamine, and vasopressin were all ineffective. The change in adenyl cyclase activity and cyclic AMP with a hypothalamic extract, but not prostaglandin, was accompanied by increased release of luteinizing hormone. There is no information on the interactions of prostagandins with release of prolactin or FSH.

A. Growth Hormone

Growth hormone (GH) is released from rat pituitaries by epinephrine, norepinephrine, theophylline, or cyclic AMP (Garay and Martin, 1970). These results have been confirmed in part by Cehovic et al. (1970), who also obtained release with porcine MSH. MacLeod and Lehmeyer (1970) found that PGE_1 (10^{-6} to 10^{-8} M) increased both synthesis and release of GH in a dose-dependent manner. PGA_2 (10^{-6} M) increased synthesis only, while $PGF_{2\alpha}$ was totally ineffective; adenyl cyclase activity in pituitary extracts was increased by both PGE_1 and PGA_1 (10^{-4} M). Further, interactions between prostaglandins and growth hormone have been reported by Fain (1968), who showed that growth hormone (plus dexamethasone) induced lipolysis of white fat cells and that the effect was inhibited by PGE_1. This inhibitory effect of PGE_1 was overcome in a dose dependent manner by norepinephrine (see also Fain, 1970).

B. ACTH—Adrenals

In vivo studies have indicated that PGE_1 (0.125–4.0 μg/i.v.), but not PGA_1 or $PGF_{2\alpha}$ (5 μg i.v.), increased ACTH release as determined by increase in plasma corticosterone concentration and depletion of adrenal ascorbic acid and cholesterol in the rat. The log-dose relationship between PGE_1 and adrenal ascorbic acid was found to be linear between 0.5 and 2.0 μg. Since this effect of the prostaglandins was not observed in hypophysectomized rats or those treated with morphine-pentobarbitone, Peng *et al.* (1970) concluded that PGE_1 was effective, possibly via an action on higher centers in the brain, in stimulating ACTH release from the pituitary and that PGE_1 did not act directly on the pituitary or adrenal glands.

In contrast, de Wied *et al.* (1969) tested PGE_1, PGE_2, $PGF_{1\alpha}$, and $PGF_{2\alpha}$ (10μg/rat i.v.) in several systems for corticotropic activity and found that, in the sodium pentobarbital and chlorpromazine treated rat, PGE_1 and PGE_2 stimulated ACTH release. Angiotensin II, arginine vasopressin, carbachol, and a crude corticotropin-releasing factor (CRF) also activated the pituitary–adrenal system. The crude CRF preparation was the only agent to cause release of ACTH in all tests, but solvent extraction and analysis did not reveal prostaglandin-like activity in these preparations. These results and those of Flack *et al.* (1969), who obtained a corticosteroidogenic response to prostaglandins only in acutely hypophysectomized rats, indicated that PGE_1 and PGE_2 were unlikely to be direct ACTH-releasing factors. The mechanism of release of ACTH by prostaglandins may be due to peripheral effects resulting from a direct action on vascular or alimentary smooth muscle, since the doses used modify blood pressure and cause diarrhea.

However, evidence to indicate a direct stimulatory effect of prostaglandins on the adrenal gland has also been obtained, for when adrenal glands from acutely hypophysectomized rats (3–4 hours) were superfused *in vitro* with PGE_2 (2.8×10^{-5} M), corticosterone secretion was doubled (Flack *et al.*, 1969). All prostaglandins tested under these conditions were effective, the order of potency being $PGE_2 > PGF_{2\alpha} > PGA_2 > PGE_1$. As stated above, this stimulation was not observed with adrenals from intact rats, and furthermore, the response to PGE_2 was insignificant 12 hours after hypophysectomy. Injection of PGE_2 into acutely hypophysectomized rats also caused a significant increase of plasma and adrenal concentrations of corticosterone; however, PGE_1 in vivo did not increase plasma corticosterone levels 24 hours after hypophysectomy.

The steroidogenic response to PGE_2 in the superfused decapsulated adrenal has been compared with the response to ACTH, cyclic AMP, and dibutyryl cyclic AMP (Flack and Ramwell, unpublished observations). PGE_2 caused a transient stimulation of corticosteroidogenesis (about 60 minutes) whereas ACTH and cyclic AMP maintained steroid secretion for several hours. The transient nature of the response to PGE_2 suggested that the prostaglandin may be releasing preformed corticosterone, but further experiments indicated that PGE_2 increased both the concentration of corticosterone in the adrenal gland and in the medium, and furthermore, increase was inhibited by cycloheximide, a protein synthesis inhibitor. Doses of ACTH and PGE_2 which gave submaximal stimulation of steroidogenesis were additive, and there was no potentiation or additive effect when PGE_2 was added to adrenal glands maximally stimulated with ACTH. These results indicate that ACTH and PGE_2 may stimulate steroidogenesis via similar mechanisms. In no case, either in vitro or in vivo, has prostaglandin inhibition of basal or ACTH induced corticosterone secretion been detected when intact or hypophysectomized rats have been used. In the autotransplanted adrenal gland of the sodium-depleted sheep, PGE_1 increased adrenal blood flow, but in some animals corticosterone, cortisol, and aldosterone secretion was inhibited, while in others there was an increase in cortisol and corticosterone with no effect on aldosterone (Funder et al., 1969).

There are currently two theories as to the mechanism by which prostaglandins may directly activate the adrenal gland and modulate corticosteroid secretion. One is by regulation of intracellular cyclic AMP levels, and the second is by controlling the flow of blood through the adrenal vasculature (Flack et al., 1969). However, PGE_2 neither increased nor decreased cyclic AMP in adrenal glands from hypophysectomized rats (Zor et al., 1970), although a significant decrease in corticosterone content was detected. Thus the increase in corticosterone production by PGE_2 may be independent of cyclic AMP formation.

Many of the pharmacological effects of the prostaglandins are known to be associated with alteration of cellular calcium movements (Ramwell and Shaw, 1970), and since ACTH has also been shown to have effects on cation transport and calcium uptake in the adrenal gland (Leier and Jungmann, 1970; Margoulies et al., 1969), prostaglandin may possibly induce corticosteroid production through such a mechanism. Thus other actions of ACTH, including effects on steroid precursors and production of cyclic AMP which are not mimicked by prostaglandins, may be responsible for the sustained action of the tropic hormone, when compared with the transient effect of the prostaglandins.

It has been shown that adrenal hyperemia observed after ACTH stimulation is not a consequence of increased corticosterone secretion, but apparently results from an increase in some other factor, perhaps a prostaglandin. Grant (1968) and Maier and Staehelin (1968) suggested that, on stimulating the adrenal with ACTH, cleavage of cholesterol esters may liberate prostaglandin precursors which would undergo cyclization and form vasodilator prostaglandins. However, it is unlikely that the steroidogenic effect of PGE_1 is a consequence of vasodilatation, for Funder *et al.* (1969) have shown that PGE_1 may increase blood flow independently of steroid secretion. If prostaglandins do mediate the hyperemia observed after ACTH, it should be possible to demonstrate an increase in prostaglandin content of the adrenal, or release from the gland. However, after *in vivo* or *in vitro* stimulation of corticosterone production with ACTH, no increase in PGE or PGF compounds was observed, but rather a consistent decrease in the release and content of these prostaglandins was detected (Flack and Ramwell, unpublished observations); no measurement of PGA compounds was performed. One possible explanation for the decrease in prostaglandin content of the adrenal on stimulation was that ACTH increased the metabolism of prostaglandins; however, no stimulation of 15-dehydrogenation or β-oxidation of 1-^{14}C-labeled PGE_1 by adrenal slices or homogenates was detected in the presence of ACTH. Furthermore, neither PGE_2 nor $PGF_{2\alpha}$ caused swelling in adrenal mitochondria, or altered the conversion of 11-deoxycorticosterone (DOC) to corticosterone effected by isocitrate or succinate. Another possibility to explain the decrease in prostaglandin content on ACTH stimulation was that corticosterone may be inhibiting prostaglandin synthetase, but addition of corticosterone to microsomal fractions of beef seminal vesicles failed to alter the rate of formation of prostaglandin from labeled arachidonic acid (Flack *et al.*, unpublished observations).

Unlike the adrenal cortex, the adrenal medulla responds to acetylcholine stimulation with increased release of prostaglandins (mainly $PGF_{1\alpha}$) as well as catecholamines and free fatty acids (Ramwell *et al.*, 1966a). Both acetylcholine and ACTH increased prostaglandin formation in rat adrenal homogenates (Shaw and Ramwell, 1967). However, in adrenal slices no release of free fatty acids or prostaglandins was detected on stimulation with ACTH, although an ACTH-sensitive lipase has been reported (Macho and Palkovic, 1965).

C. TSH—Thyroid

Prostaglandins have been isolated from the thyroid of different species (Karim et al., 1968a), from medullary carcinoma of the human thyroid (Williams et al., 1968), and from tissue culture fluid of medullary carcinoma (Grimley et al., 1969). No studies as to the effect of TSH stimulation on endogenous prostaglandin concentration have been reported, but there are several studies concerning the effects of exogenous prostaglandins on thyroid function.

Rodesch et al. (1969) compared the actions of TSH, PGE_1 (5.6×10^{-5} M) and cyclic AMP on dog thyroid function in vitro. PGE_1 was found to mimic the actions of TSH and cyclic AMP in stimulating glucose oxidation at C-1 and iodide binding to proteins, but PGE_1 did not stimulate intracellular colloid droplet formation as did TSH or cyclic AMP. Onaya and Solomon (1969, 1970) reported that in slices of dog thyroid, PGE_1 (3.6–36 μg) stimulated the oxidation of glucose-1-^{14}C to $^{14}CO_2$ and colloid droplet formation. PGE_1 (10–75 μg i.v.) also stimulated colloid droplet formation in vivo and ^{131}I release in thyroxine-suppressed mice; the time course was similar to that obtained with TSH in that peak ^{131}I blood levels were attained 2 hours after injection. The actions of PGE_1 on glucose oxidation and colloid droplet formation were inhibited by the lysosome stabilizer chlorpromazine and were additive, with submaximal doses of TSH. Field et al. (1969) also found that PGE_1 increased glucose oxidation and cyclic AMP in dog thyroid homogenates but did not augment ^{32}P incorporation into phospholipids. In thyroid slices it has been confirmed that PGE_1 (0.95×10^{-6} M to 2.8×10^{-5} M) increases glucose oxidation, but again no effect on phospholipogenesis has been evident (Zor et al., 1969b). PGE_1 (0.57×10^{-5} M) neither inhibited nor potentiated the effects of TSH on $^{14}CO_2$ production. PGE_2 reproduced the effects of TSH on glucose-1-^{14}C oxidation and cyclic AMP concentration; however, $PGF_{1\alpha}$ (2.8×10^{-5} M) stimulated glucose oxidation without any effect on cyclic AMP levels; PGE_1 (2.8×10^{-5} M) had no effect on either parameter. If cyclic AMP does mediate the effect of TSH on glucose oxidation, ^{32}P incorporation into phospholipid and colloid droplet formation in the thyroid, then the differential effects of PGE_1 and $PGF_{1\alpha}$ on these parameters are difficult to explain. There is evidence, however, that cyclic AMP may not mediate the glucose oxidation effects of TSH. Cyclic AMP levels are increased by TSH within 1 minute in canine slices and homogenates (Zor et al., 1969b), but this was not well correlated with glucose oxidation since the stimulation of adenyl cyclase was transient and that of glucose oxidation sustained. However, the transient increase in cyclic AMP may be sufficient to initiate the requisite biochemical and morphological changes. Conversely, neither cyclic AMP nor its dibutyryl analog were effective in stimulating glucose oxidation, although dibutyryl cyclic AMP did induce colloid droplet formation (Onaya and Solomon, 1969). PGE_1 (0.01 mM) also increased the proteolysis of labeled iodoprotein in dog thyroid slices (Ahn and Rosenberg, 1970). Cyclic AMP, TSH, and PGE_1 effects were not additive at maximal doses, indicating that on this parameter of thyroid function, a common pathway may be operating. More recently Burke (1970) using sheep thyroid slices has confirmed that PGE_1 (5×10^{-5} M) stimulated adenyl cyclase, endocytosis, and glucose oxidation, but did not effect phospholipogenesis. Somewhat disconcertingly, in none of these parameters was a dose-response relationship established.

The situation regarding the prostaglandins and the thyroid is obviously complex, especially since there are discrepancies in the literature on the metabolic actions of TSH and cyclic AMP. Nevertheless, prostaglandins should prove to be useful tools in elucidating the mechanism of action of TSH.

D. Gonadotropin—Ovaries

Over the past two years there has been tremendous interest in the potential for prostaglandins in the field of reproductive physiology. A recent review has covered this field in more detail than will be attempted here (Speroff and Ramwell, 1970a).

The recent surge of interest stems from the studies of Pharriss et al. (1968), who demonstrated that $PGF_{2\alpha}$ caused regression of rat corpora lutea; these studies have since been extended to primates (Kirton et al., 1970a), guinea pigs (Blatchley and Donovan, 1969), hamsters (Hansel, unpublished observations; Weeks, 1969), and sheep ovarian transplants (McCracken et al., 1970); in all species $PGF_{2\alpha}$ was found to be luteolytic. $PGF_{2\alpha}$ infusion (1 mg/kg per day) into the uterus of the rat for 2 days decreased progesterone and increased 20α-dihydroprogesterone content of the ovarian tissue; a similar observation was made when $PGF_{2\alpha}$ was infused into the right heart. Furthermore, pseudopregnant rats treated with $PGF_{2\alpha}$ (0.8 mg per 12 hours) returned to vaginal estrus after 8 days compared with 17 days for saline-treated controls (Pharriss and Wyngarden, 1969). It was considered that $PGF_{2\alpha}$ may cause venoconstriction of the utero-ovarian vein, which would then lead to regression of the corpus luteum. In support of this hypothesis was the finding that pituitary LH content remained unchanged during treatment with $PGF_{2\alpha}$ and that $PGF_{2\alpha}$ was not luteolytic in vitro (Pharriss et al., 1968). Subsequently, $PGF_{2\alpha}$ was indeed shown to constrict the utero-ovarian vein in rabbits and thereby reduce the ovarian drainage (Weeks, 1969). However, when Blatchley and Donovan (1969) treated hysterectomized guinea pigs with PGF$_{2\alpha}$ (0.5 μg/day for 7 days) and then examined the ovaries on the eighth day, all the corpora lutea had regressed, but the follicles were normal, indicating a near normal blood supply to the ovary. McCracken et al. (1970) demonstrated a decrease in progesterone secretion after infusion of PGF$_{2\alpha}$ (50 and 100 μg per hour for 6 hours) directly into the artery of the autotransplanted ovary of the ewe. There was subsequent regression of the corpus luteum as indicated by an increase in peripheral LH values and a return to behavioral estrus. In these studies, however, infusion of PGF$_{2\alpha}$ (50 μg per hour) was not accompanied by a decrease in blood flow through the transplanted ovary; at higher infusion rates (100 μg per hour) a decrease in venous flow was evident (62%). Aldridge et al. (1970) using a similar preparation have observed that PGF$_{2\alpha}$ decreased progesterone secretion without changing blood flow.

In women, where a luteolysin has not been demonstrated, PGF$_{2\alpha}$ is present in the endometrium in higher concentrations in the secretory phase than in the proliferative stage, and this correlates with the activity of the corpus luteum (Pickles et al., 1965). However, PGF$_{2\alpha}$ was shown to be luteolytic (as determined by plasma progestin levels) in rhesus monkeys (30 μg s.c., twice a day for 5 days) if administration began on day 11, 12, or 13, but not if the injections were given earlier in the luteal phase. If the monkeys were mated and pregnancy ensued (as indicated by increasing progestin levels), the injections of PGF$_{2\alpha}$ caused an immediate decline in progestin levels, and 24–48 hours after injections, menstruation occurred (Kirton et al., 1970b).

Sheep endometrial extracts which were luteolytic in two assay systems were nondialyzable, and did not contain significant concentrations of PGF$_{2\alpha}$; unlike PGF$_{2\alpha}$, these extracts caused significant lysis of granulosa cells in tissue culture (Caldwell et al., unpublished observations). The hamster luteolytic factor is thermolabile and also nondialyzable (Mazer and Wright, 1968). These results indicate that the uterine factor controlling the life-span of the corpus luteum may not be an F prostaglandin.

Although it has been well established that PGF$_{2\alpha}$ is luteolytic *in vivo*, at a concentration of 2.8×10^{-5} M, this prostaglandin increased the production of progesterone in incubated rat ovaries (Pharriss et al., 1968) indicating a luteotropic action. PGE$_2$ (2.8 to 5.6×10^{-6} M) increased 20α-hydroxypregn-4-en-3-one concentration in chopped rabbit ovaries (Bedwani and Horton, 1968). Speroff and Ramwell (1970b) extended these observations to the bovine corpus luteum, where the ascending order of potency on progesterone formation was PGA$_1$ < PGF$_{2\alpha}$ < PGE$_1$ < PGE$_2$ at 2.8×10^{-5} M. The mechanism of prostaglandin action appeared to be similar to that of HCG and LH since the specific activity of the newly formed progesterone after incubation with prostaglandins and acetate-1-^{14}C was of the same order of magnitude as the progesterone formed on gonadotropin stimulation. Moreover, prostaglandins added to luteal slices that were maximally stimulated with LH did not elicit further increases in progesterone production. Cycloheximide inhibited the stimulatory effects of both prostaglandins and gonadotropin. This evidence lent strong support for the contention that prostaglandins were utilizing the same steroid precursor pool as the gonadotropins. Cyclic AMP has been shown to mediate progesterone secretion in the corpus luteum (Dorrington and Baggett, 1969; Marsh and Savard, 1966). Recently it has been shown that PGE$_2$ also increases adenyl cyclase activity and cyclic AMP formation in bovine corpus luteum slices (Marsh, 1970).

All prostaglandins so far tested are luteotropic, whereas *in vivo* the luteolytic effect appears to be specific for PGF$_{2\alpha}$. PGE$_1$ perfused into the transplanted ovary of the sheep had no effect on luteal maintenance (Kaltenbach *et al.*, 1969), and in the rat PGA$_1$, PGE$_1$, and PGF$_{2\beta}$ were also without effect (Pharriss *et al.*, 1968).

The luteolytic effect of PGF$_{2\alpha}$ is unlikely to be due to inhibition of LH release since Pharriss *et al.* (1968) failed to find changes in pituitary LH in rats where pseudopregnancy was terminated by PGF$_{2\alpha}$ (5 mg/day for 5 days). Similarly, Gutknecht *et al.* (1969) found that PGF$_{2\alpha}$ did not inhibit lactation, which also implies that the pituitary is not involved.

Clearly, definitive experiments are required using sensitive specific assay for tropic hormones since PGF$_{2\alpha}$ definitely has vasoconstrictor properties not possessed by the PGE and PGA series (DuCharme *et al.*, 1968). The hypophysial portal system is a susceptible locus for such interfering substances.

E. *Gonadotropin—Testes*

In contrast to work on the ovaries, little has been done on the testes in spite of the large amounts of prostaglandin present in the semen of some species. However, the prostaglandin in the case of the human probably comes from the seminal vesicles since it is present with alkaline phosphatase in the split ejaculate. However, prostaglandins are present in testicular tissue (Carpenter and Wiseman, 1970), and moreover, the hormone secretion of the testes is responsive to exogenous prostaglandins. Eik-Nes (1969), using the dog perfused testes, has shown that the PGE compounds stimulate secretion of testosterone.

III. Neuroendocrinological Considerations

The prostaglandins are widely distributed in mammalian tissues, including the central nervous system (CNS) of various species (Bergström et al., 1968; Holmes and Horton, 1968). To date, no specific concentration of prostaglandins has been identified as characteristic of any particular part of the brain, but the concentration in gray matter does appear to be the highest (Holmes and Horton, 1968). Biosynthesis from the C_{20} ω6 polyenoic precursors readily occurs in a microsomal preparation (Kataoka et al., 1967; Wolfe et al., 1967).

Following systemic injection of radiolabeled PGE_1, or $PGF_{1\alpha}$ very little radioactivity was detected in the CNS, indicating the presence of a blood–brain barrier to circulating prostaglandins (Hansson and Samuelsson, 1965; Holmes and Horton, 1968). This finding implies that the prostaglandins within the CNS are formed *in situ*, and indeed increased biosynthesis of prostaglandins on electrical or hormonal stimulation of nervous tissue has been detected (Ramwell and Shaw, 1966). By use of sensitive bioassay procedures, release of prostaglandins from cerebral ventricles (Holmes, 1970), cerebellar cortex (Coceani and Wolfe, 1965), parietal and somatosensory cortex (Ramwell and Shaw, 1966), and spinal cord (Ramwell et al., 1966b) has been demonstrated. Release of prostaglandins from the somatosensory cortex of the cat was increased on direct or indirect electrical stimulation or after peripheral administration of central stimulants such as leptazol or picrotoxin (Ramwell and Shaw, 1966). Furthermore, prostaglandin release from the somatosensory cortex of an *encéphale isolé* preparation of the cat was found to be directly related to electrocortical arousal. In these studies, stimulation of the reticular formation (300 c/s, 2–5 V) produced both electrocortical arousal and prostaglandin release. Chlorpromazine (1.0–8.0 mg/kg i.v.) not only depressed the spontaneous release of prostaglandins, but blocked the increase evoked by stimulation concomitantly with blocking electrocortical arousal. By increasing the stimulating voltage to restore the arousal response, the evoked release of prostaglandins was also restored (Bradley et al., 1969). Further studies have shown that the discharge rate of brain stem neurons is modified following iontophoretic application of PGE or PGF compounds (Avanzino et al., 1966).

All these observations, together with detection of prostaglandins in nerve ending fractions prepared from rat cerebral cortex (Kataoka et al., 1967), have strongly implicated the prostaglandins in CNS function.

The CNS contains extremely high levels of adenyl cyclase activity (Sutherland et al., 1962) and cyclic AMP (Weiss and Costa, 1968), particularly in the cerebellum (Kakiuchi and Rall, 1968), but despite the knowledge that prostaglandin formation and action are closely associated with changes in intracellular cyclic AMP, there are to date no reports concerning the effects of prostaglandins on cyclic AMP levels in the cerebral or cerebellar cortex. However, indirect evidence implicating a possible interaction between prostaglandins and cyclic AMP in modifying CNS activity has evolved from the work of Bloom and his associates. During a study of the responsiveness of rat and rabbit cerebellar Purkinje cells to the electrophoretic administration of various chemical agents, it was found that almost all cells exhibited reproducible reductions in spontaneous discharge rate in response to norepinephrine (Hoffer et al., 1969). The administration of cyclic AMP from a second barrel of the micropipette also reduced mean discharge rates of Purkinje cells. Theophylline (i.v.) or aminophylline (electrophoretic application) increased the magnitude and duration of the response to both norepinephrine and cyclic AMP. PGE_1 and PGE_2 administered electrophoretically had the reverse effect and increased the mean firing rate of Purkinje cells; in addition, the PGE compounds antagonized the inhibitory effect of simultaneously applied norepinephrine, but had no effect on the inhibition induced by cyclic AMP or γ-aminobutyric acid (GABA). These well controlled studies indicate that norepinephrine-induced depression of Purkinje cells may be mediated via cyclic AMP formation and are consistent with the possibility that PGE_1 and PGE_2 may antagonize norepinephrine-induced cyclic AMP formation in these cells; an analogous situation prevails in isolated fat cells (Butcher and Baird, 1968).

Other studies with prostaglandins have indicated that PGE_1 will protect rats from death due to maximal electroshock convulsions (Holmes and Horton, 1968). Injection of PGE_1 into the third ventricle of cats modified body temperature in a dose-dependent manner (Milton and Wendlandt, 1970). Horton (1964) observed that injection of PGE_1 into cat cerebral ventricles resulted in behavioral effects which could still be detected 48 hours after injection. Similarly, PGE_1, $PGF_{1\alpha}$, and $PGF_{2\alpha}$ have been found to produce long-lasting depolarization (up to 20 minutes) of the dorsal and ventral roots of the toad spinal cord, in contrast to the depolarization elicited by glutamate which returned to control levels within 1 minute (Phillis and Tebecis, 1968). In the chick spinal cord preparation, PGF compounds have a strychnine-like action (Horton and Main, 1967), and after intra-arterial injection close to the spinal cord, Duda et al. (1968) noted a reduction in the monosynaptic reflex which was slow in onset and lasted for as long as 3 hours. The possibility that prostaglandins modify the cell membrane to induce a long lasting depolarization has been considered to explain these diverse effects, but no confirmatory evidence is yet available. While it seems unlikely that the endogenous prostaglandins themselves function as synaptic transmitters in the CNS, the evidence suggests that they may modify the action of other transmitters, possibly via modification of cyclic AMP as seen in peripheral tissues.

IV. Posterior Pituitary

A. Uterus

The actions of prostaglandins on the uterus and fallopian tubes both *in vivo* and *in vitro* have been studied extensively, and for more detailed information on the earlier work, the reader is referred to recent reviews (Pickles, 1969; von Euler and Eliasson, 1967; Speroff and Ramwell, 1970a).

$PGF_{2\alpha}$ contracts the human uterus, and since this prostaglandin was found in greatest concentrations during the secretory phase, the suggestion was made that $PGF_{2\alpha}$ was responsible for uterine movements and expulsion of the menses (Pickles, 1957). This was supported by the findings that patients with dysmenorrhea had higher $PGF_{2\alpha}$ concentrations than in controls (Pickles et al., 1965), and that the menses from a girl of 14–16 had higher concentrations of $PGF_{2\alpha}$ in ovulatory than in anovulatory cycles (Pickles, 1967).

Karim (1966), following up the work of Pickles, found that there was a large proportion of PGF compounds (mainly $PGF_{2\alpha}$) in human amniotic fluid during labor. No detectable amounts of prostaglandin in the amniotic fluid were found in those patients who were not in labor (Karim and Devlin, 1967) or in plasma of patients prior to cesarean section (Karim, 1968). $PGF_{2\alpha}$ was also detected in the peripheral venous blood of patients in labor. $PGF_{2\alpha}$ was highest 1 minute prior to and during the initial phase of contraction; between contractions no prostaglandin was detected. This observation implies that the uterine contraction is initiated by a surge of circulating $PGF_{2\alpha}$ at this time, and suggests a possible hormonal role for $PGF_{2\alpha}$ in induction of labor (Karim, 1968).

Kirton et al. (1970b) terminated pregnancy in rhesus monkeys with both PGE_2 and $PGF_{2\alpha}$. In women, infusion of $PGF_{2\alpha}$ at term has been used successfully to induce labor and delivery (Karim et al., 1968b). Uterine contractions started 15–20 minutes after the onset of infusion, and the average induction to delivery interval was 6 hours 46 minutes. Amniotic fluid pressure during the $PGF_{2\alpha}$ infusion (25–50 µg/kg per minute) was similar to that of normal labor, and neither mother nor fetus suffered cardiovascular irregularities. The infusion was stopped when labor was initiated (one contraction per minute with cervical dilatation of 5–6 cm).

Induction of labor has also been successful with PGE_1 or PGE_2 (0.5–2.0 µg/minute) in 23 of 25 patients. The pattern of uterine motility produced resembled that of normal labor; hypertonus was not observed nor were there any undesirable side effects (Embrey, 1970). Karim has also successfully induced labor with an infusion of PGE_2 (7.5–10 ng/kg per minute) and found that there was a normal pattern of uterine contractions. It is perhaps of significance that PGE_2 is also present in maternal blood during labor, with a ratio of $PGE_2:PGF_{2\alpha}$ of 1:5, and PGE_2 was five times more potent than $PGF_{2\alpha}$ in inducing human labor. In earlier work PGE_1 and PGE_2 had been used in patients with threatened abortion in the second and third trimester of pregnancy (Wiqvist et al., 1968; Bygdeman et al., 1968). PGE_1 (i.v. infusion) during mid-pregnancy did cause an increase in uterine tone with some small contractions, and there was a gradual increase in response with increasing doses. Above a dose level of 50 µg PGE_1 side effects of nausea and increased pulse rate were apparent, but large doses of 75 µg or more i.v. caused a uterine contraction which lasted 30 minutes with a tone of 40–50 mm Hg. In patients at term, or near term, it was observed that the difference in dose which increased the amplitude and frequency of contractions and that which increased tone alone was very small, thus offering no advantages over the oxytocic drugs. PGE_2 had similar properties to PGE_1, and the two were approximately equiactive.

More recently Karim and Filshie (1970) have used $PGF_{2\alpha}$ for therapeutic abortion in fifteen patients with gestational age between 9 and 22 weeks. $PGF_{2\alpha}$ (50 µg i.v. per minute) stimulated uterine activity in all women after a latent period of only 1–3 minutes. An increase in tone (20–50 mm Hg) which lasted for 10–15 minutes was accompanied by small and irregular contractions. After disappearance of the hypertonus, the uterus began to contract regularly and rhythmically with an increase in frequency and amplitude of contractions. With continuing infusion the contractions became stronger, frequency increased, and complete abortion ensued in 13 out of 15 women. The minimum induction–abortion interval was 4 hours 20 minutes, and the maximum 27 hours 15 minutes. There were quantitative and qualitative differences between the action of $PGF_{2\alpha}$ on the uterus at term and on the uterus in the first and second trimester of pregnancy; at term there is no increase in resting tone, and the dose of $PGF_{2\alpha}$ required for induction of labor at term was 10 times less than that required to induce early abortion. In seven cases the infusion was accompanied by diarrhea or vomiting or both;

in contrast, PGE_2 (5 μg per minute) was successfully used in 12 women without producing diarrhea.

Roth-Brandel et al. (1970) infused two patients with $PGF_{2\alpha}$ for short durations (10–50 μg per minute for 6 hours) and confirmed the increase in uterine hypertonus with the subsequent strong uterine contractions which were observed by Karim and Filshie (1970). However, neither case aborted, but this was to be expected since in only 1 in 13 cases was abortion successful within a 6-hour infusion (Karim and Filshie, 1970). Roth-Brandel et al. (1970) also infused PGE_1 (1–10 μg per minute for 6 hours on 2 days) and found similar effects as with $PGF_{2\alpha}$, but in this case 2 out of 5 women aborted. $PGF_{2\alpha}$ was also administered by subcutaneous injection to 5 women (5 mg every 3 hours 5 or 6 times a day for 2 days), and this dosage regimen induced one abortion in 4 patients (9–28 weeks pregnant) with PGE_1 and PGE_2. The infusion rate was 2–5 μg per minute, and a total dose of 2–5 mg was required for successful abortion. Wiqvist and Bygdeman (1970) have also demonstrated that infusion of $PGF_{2\alpha}$ (20–300 μg per minute) for up to 2 days during the first weeks of pregnancy caused abortion in all of 7 cases. Vomiting or diarrhea in 4 patients were the only side effects. At this stage of pregnancy, oxytocin has little effect on the uterus, whereas $PGF_{2\alpha}$ caused strong contractions.

The implications of the effects of the prostaglandins on the uterus and corpus luteum are obvious in terms of contraception and in the safe termination of early pregnancy, especially where amniocentesis has established the existence of cytogenic or other defects of the fetus.

B. *Fallopian Tubes*

The mechanism of action of prostaglandins on the fallopian tubes remains to be determined since, as Pickles (1967) has emphasized, "Different authors have used different methods on different species, making direct comparison a little difficult."

Prostaglandins have an antifertility effect by delaying transportation of the fertilized ovum through the rat oviduct (Nutting and Cammarata, 1969). A mixture of prostaglandins (mainly PGE_2 and $PGF_{2\alpha}$ 0.5 mg twice a day) injected on the first 6–7 days of pregnancy reduced the number of implantation sites and those that were present were beginning to resorb; delayed nidation was also observed in 3 of 5 rats.

These observations have been confirmed using pure $PGF_{2\alpha}$ and have been extended to studies in the rabbit (Gutknecht et al., 1969). $PGF_{2\alpha}$ was found to be completely effective in preventing or terminating pregnancy in the rat when given at 2 mg per day s.c. over any consecutive 3-day period from day 4 through day 13 after coitus. $PGF_{2\alpha}$ was ineffective when given orally at 10 times the subcutaneous dose. Exogenous progestagen treatment reversed the effect of $PGF_{2\alpha}$, suggesting that the $PGF_{2\alpha}$ effect in the rat was caused by inhibiting endogenous progesterone formation. Since $PGF_{2\alpha}$ also terminated luteal activity in pseudopregnant rats, this excluded the fetal or placental tissue playing a role in the antifertility effect.

It is unlikely that $PGF_{2\alpha}$ is acting through inhibition of estrogen secretion. $PGF_{2\alpha}$ had little effect on developing follicles in the guinea pig (Blatchley and Donovan, 1969), and Gutknecht et al. (1969) demonstrated that exogenous progesterone will maintain pregnancy better in $PGF_{2\alpha}$-treated animals than in ovariectomized rats. More recent studies in which estrogens have been measured directly after $PGF_{2\alpha}$ administration to rats (Behrman et al., 1971) and hamsters (Tillson and Thorneycroft, unpublished observations) also indicate that $PGF_{2\alpha}$ has no effect on peripheral estrogen levels.

C. Kidney

It is well recognized that expansion of the extracellular fluid by saline loading causes urinary sodium excretion which is accompanied by a normal glomerular filtration rate and secretion of aldosterone. The sodium excretion results from inhibition of the reabsorption of sodium in the proximal tubule, but the identity of the substance responsible for this effect is still unknown (Rector et al., 1968). Interest was aroused in the prostaglandins as a possible candidate for this hormonelike material ("third factor") following isolation of potent vasodepressor lipid fractions from the kidney medulla ("medullin"), which was subsequently identified with prostaglandins (Lee et al., 1966; Daniels et al., 1967). PGE_1 (0.01–2.0 μg/minute) infused into the left renal artery of the anesthetized dog increased sodium excretion, free water clearance, and renal plasma flow and decreased p-aminohippurate uptake (Johnston et al., 1967). There were no changes in the contralateral kidney or in glomerular filtration rate and mean aortic pressure. These observations were confirmed by Vander (1968). Other vasodilators (dopamine, bradykinin, and acetylcholine) produced similar results, but the prostaglandins are the only substances endogenous to the kidney that have these effects.

It was considered that the natriuretic effects of PGE_1 may result from a direct effect of PGE_1 on the tissues, for it is known that PGE_1 will stimulate sodium movements in isolated frog skin (Ramwell and Shaw, 1970) and inhibit vasopressin-induced transport of water across the toad bladder (Orloff et al., 1965) and isolated rabbit collecting tubules (Orloff and Grantham, 1967). Johnston et al. (1967) attempted to demonstrate a direct inhibitory effect of PGE_1 on the tubules by infusing vasopressin in normal and water-loaded dogs. They were unsuccessful, however, because of simultaneous changes in renal hemodynamics and solute excretion. Fichman (1969) reported that in man PGA$_1$ (0.3–3.0 µg/kg per minute for 10–60 minutes) failed to alter the effect of antidiuretic hormone (ADH) on water excretion, but it did inhibit proximal tubular reabsorption of sodium. In the dog PGA$_1$ (1.7–2.4 µg/minute) has been reported to decrease Na$^+$ excretion, but in this study there was decreased glomerular filtration rate and decreased blood pressure (Carr, 1968). Perfusion of PGE$_2$ (0.64 µg/minute per dog) resulted in an initial decrease in renal blood flow which was followed by an increase (Lee, 1968). These observations were correlated with decreased medullary flow and subsequent increased cortical flow, suggesting that the natriuretic and diuretic effects of prostaglandin on the kidney may be the result of a redistribution of blood flow from outer medulla to cortex.

Lee and his collaborators (Lee et al., 1969) extended these studies to include PGA$_2$ (0.05 µg/kg/minute) which caused an increase in blood flow and significant natriuresis whether infused intravenously or intraaortically. PGA$_2$, PGA$_1$, PGE$_1$, and PGE$_2$ (1×10^{-4} M), all of which have natriuretic properties, also decreased the uptake of p-aminohippurate when rabbit kidney cortex slices were incubated *in vitro* (Lee and Ferguson, 1969). Bricker et al. (1968) had previously demonstrated that a factor from saline-expanded plasma inhibited the uptake of p-aminohippurate by rabbit kidney cortical slices and exhibited a chromophore at 280 nm as do the PGB compounds. Recently an isomerase capable of forming PGB compounds has been described in blood (Jones, 1970).

On the basis of these findings, it was suggested that prostaglandins might be identified with the natriuretic hormone (Lee et al., 1969; Lee and Ferguson, 1969). It was envisaged that on expansion of the extracellular fluid the prostaglandins may be released from the renal medulla into the renal vein and return via the renal artery to the renal cortex and enhance sodium excretion, possibly by redistribution of intrarenal blood flow. The only prostaglandins capable of such an action may be the PGA series (Lee et al., 1969) since, unlike PGE compounds, they are not significantly metabolized by passage through the lungs (McGiff et al., 1969b; Piper et al., 1970). In the one report to date, PGE$_{2\alpha}$ (0.05 µg/kg/minute) did not cause diuresis in pregnant women (Roberts et al., 1970).

Before PGA$_2$ or PGA$_1$ can be recognized as the physiological natriuretic hormone, its presence in saline-loaded plasma must be demonstrated; satisfactory methods for bioassay of small amounts of PGA compounds have only recently been developed (Horton and Jones, 1969)

However, certain studies suggest that prostaglandin is not the natriuretic hormone since the mode of action of the natriuresis is different with the two substances. Thus, natriuretic effect of the prostaglandins is often associated with an increased glomerular filtration rate unlike the natural natriuretic factor. Furthermore, Fichman (1969) was also able to observe an increase in natriuresis with PGA_1 in patients already excreting large amounts of sodium (i.e., patients with high circulating endogenous natriuretic hormone).

Release of PGE compounds from the kidney has been detected following stimulation of natriuresis and diuresis with norepinephrine in the cat (Fujimoto and Lockett, 1969). When norepinephrine was infused, renal lymph flow was doubled, as was the prostaglandin content of the lymph. The increase in diuresis and natriuresis was not blocked by α- or β-adrenergic antagonists. Furthermore, the natriuretic effects of norepinephrine seen after administration of α- and β-adrenergic blocking drugs resembled those of a PGE_1 infusion (0.1 µg/kg per minute). Angiotensin II infused intravenously also enhanced renal lymph flow but only increased the prostaglandin content of renal lymph to a small degree when compared with norepinephrine. McGiff et al. (1969a) showed that, in the dog, infusion of angiotensin II into the renal artery increased the release of prostaglandin-like substances.

As stated previously, certain lipids extracted from the kidney medulla have antihypotensive and vasoactive properties, and some of these lipids have been identified with prostaglandins. PGE_2, $PGF_{2\alpha}$, and PGA_2 have been positively identified in rabbit renal medulla (Daniels et al., 1967; Lee et al., 1966), and since the prostaglandins are potent vasodilator substances, the possibility of utilizing these compounds for treatment of hypertension has been investigated.

PGE_2 (15–29 µg/kg per day), PGA_1 (50–100 µg/kg per day), and $PGF_{1\alpha}$ (15–30 µg/kg per day) given orally completely suppressed acute canine renoprival hypertension for up to 2 days, but thereafter there was some increase in blood pressure; PGA_1 was also effective at a lower dose level (5 µg/kg per day). Less conclusive data indicated that prostaglandins also lowered the arterial pressure in experimental renal hypertension (Muirhead et al., 1967). Recently Lee et al. (1970) reported that lower doses of PGA_1 (0.1–2.1 µg/kg per minute) did not affect blood pressure but did increase renal plasma flow, glomerular filtration rate, urinary flow, and urinary sodium and potassium excretion. In 6 hypertensive patients the decrease in blood pressure brought about by higher doses of PGA_1 was associated with normal renal blood flow and normal sodium excretion (see also Carr, 1970).

Lee (1968) has previously suggested that a deficiency of prostaglandins in the renal medulla might result in an augmented outer medullary flow associated with reduced cortical blood flow. The cortical vasoconstriction could result in a release of renal pressor substances into the systemic circulation with the production of sustained hypertension.

In support of this hypothesis, McGiff et al. (1969a) observed an increased release of prostaglandin and angiotensin-like substances from the renal vein of the dog after constriction of the renal artery. The contralateral kidney also showed an increased release of prostaglandin-like substances in response to the ischemia. Since an infusion of angiotensin II into the renal artery of a normal dog reproduced the effects of the ischemia, it was suggested that the increase in prostaglandin-like substances was mediated by the release of angiotensin from the ischemic kidney. The increase in the prostaglandin E content of renal lymph on norepinephrine infusion (Fujimoto and Lockett, 1969) is further evidence that prostaglandins may have a physiological role in the control of blood pressure.

V. Exocrine Hormone Interaction

Information on the action of prostaglandins on the formation, secretion, and action of the exocrine hormones is sparse. What work has been done has been directed to studying the effect of prostaglandins on the glands themselves, particularly with respect to the gastric mucosa. Nothing is yet reported concerning the interaction of prostaglandins with enterogastrone or cholecystokinin.

A. Pancreas

The volume and bicarbonate content of dog pancreatic juice following secretin or secretin-pancreozymin stimulation was inhibited by PGE_1 (1–50 µg/kg or 1–5 µg/kg per minute, i.v.); 5 µg/kg per minute completely suppressed secretion. On the other hand, enzyme secretion was stimulated at doses greater than 1 µg/kg (Rudick et al., 1970).

B. Stomach

The release of PGE_1, PGE_2, $PGF_{1\alpha}$, and $PGF_{2\alpha}$ from the serosal surface of the isolated rat stomach, together with increased biosynthesis and release of PGE_2 and $PGF_{2\alpha}$ on vagal or transmural stimulation was reported by Coceani et al. (1967). Release of prostaglandins is unlikely to result from prior muscular contractions since hexamethonium or tetrodotoxin effectively inhibited muscle contraction without modification of prostaglandin release (Bennett et al., 1967). On perfusion of the mucosal surface of the rat stomach *in vivo*, the same four prostaglandins were identified in the perfusates, and in these studies stimulation of gastric acid secretion with i.v. pentapeptide or vagal stimulation resulted in an increased release of PGE_1 (Shaw and Ramwell, 1968b). Studies with the isolated perfused rat stomach (Bennett et al., 1967) indicated that the prostaglandin content of gastric tissue was equivalent to 3.2 ± 0.63 µg of PGE_1 per gram wet weight and that the concentration in the mucosa was 4–6 times that of the muscle. A similar distribution of activity between mucosa and muscle was noted in human gastric tissue, where the principal prostaglandin was identified with PGE_2 (0.01–2.4 µg/gm wet weight) (Bennett et al., 1968a).

The finding that prostaglandins not only are present in gastric tissue, but also modify activity of gastric and intestinal smooth muscle (Chawla and Eisenberg, 1969; Bennett et al., 1968a,b) has led to the suggestion that prostaglandins may function as local hormones to regulate gastric movements.

In frog, rat, dog, and man, prostaglandins have been shown to effectively inhibit H^+ secretion by the gastric mucosa. In the anesthetized rat, PGE_1 (0.1–1.0 µg/minute) perfused across the gastric mucosa inhibited basal H^+ secretion and that induced by i.v. administration of histamine or pentapeptide. The effect of PGE_1 was readily reversible and could be repeated after a second administration (Shaw and Ramwell, 1968b). In the Shay rat, PGE_1 (200–300 µg s.c. in 2 hours or 0.5–1.0 mg/kg s.c. per minute) inhibited by some 50% the acid accumulation during the 4 hours after ligation of the pylorus. In these studies PGE_1 also reduced the volume of gastric juice secreted and the output of mucus and pepsin (Robert et al., 1968a). In the conscious dog with either an innervated (Pavlov) or a denervated (Heidenhain) pouch, or gastric fistula, PGE_1 has been found to reduce titratable acidity, pepsin, and volume of secretion. PGE_1 was effective administered intravenously (0.5–2 µg/kg per minute) or subcutaneously and inhibited acid secretion induced by administration of food, histamine, pentagastrin, 2-deoxyglucose, or reserpine (Robert et al., 1967, 1968b; Robert, 1968). Preliminary studies in man did not reveal any inhibitory effect of orally administered PGE_1 (10–40 µg/kg) against pentapeptide-induced H^+ secretion (Horton et al., 1968). Conversely PGA_1 (0.5–0.6 µg/kg i.v. per hour) reduced H^+ secretion by 18% and volume of gastric juice by 30% within 15 minutes (Wilson et al., 1970).

PGE_1 (1–2 µg/kg s.c. per minute) also effectively inhibits ulcer formation, and the incidence of perforation in the Shay rat and at the same concentration also reduced steroid-induced ulcer formation (Robert et al., 1968a).

Since there is a direct correlation between gastric secretion and mucosal blood flow, and PGE₁ is known to modify blood flow through vascular beds, Jacobson (1970) has examined the effect of PGE₁ on the mucosal circulation in the dog. Using the aminopyrine clearance technique, he calculated the ratio of mucosal blood flow to the rate of gastric secretion. After stimulation of H⁺ secretion with histamine or gastrin, PGE₁ was found to decrease secretion prior to a decrease in the measured ratio of blood flow to secretion. From these results Jacobson concluded that PGE₁ was likely to have a direct effect on the oxyntic cell.

Supporting the possibility of a direct action of PGE₁ on the gastric mucosa was the finding that PGE₁ (10^{-7} M) will inhibit the H⁺ response of the isolated frog gastric mucosa to histamine or pentapeptide (Way and Durbin, 1969), while higher concentrations of PGE₁ (2.8×10^{-6} to 2.8×10^{-5} M) alone will stimulate H⁺ secretion (Shaw and Ramwell, 1969). These findings negate implication of the vascular system in the response to PGE₁. Furthermore, PGE₁ has recently been reported to modify cyclic AMP accumulation in the guinea pig gastric mucosa (Perrier and Laster, 1970). Although the role of cyclic AMP in hormone-induced acid secretion has not been defined, we have the possibility that PGE₁ may modulate hormone activity in gastric tissue as in other tissues via changes in intracellular cyclic AMP.

VI. Actions on Lipid and Carbohydrate Metabolism

The significance of prostaglandins in regulating lipid metabolism was appreciated at an early stage due to the work of Steinberg et al. (1963). As a result, this aspect of prostaglandin action is better understood than most so far, although there have been problems arising from differences in species and techniques (see Bergström et al., 1968).

Prostaglandins inhibit lipolysis in rat, dog, rabbit, and human whether induced by catecholamines, theophylline, TSH, GH, and dexamethasone, ACTH, ADH, glucagon, or triiodothyronine. PGE₁ inhibits the basal release of glycerol in rat and some human adipose tissues at concentrations (1–100 ng/ml) which makes it the most potent antilipolytic agent known. In all situations, including brown as well as white fat, PGE₁ inhibits hormone-induced release of free fatty acids. There are only quantitative differences between the various prostaglandins, the order of potency being PGE₂ > PGE₁ = dihomo PGE₁ > PGF₁α > PGA₁ > PGF₁β.

The site of action of PGE₁ in inhibiting lipolysis is not clear. Steinberg and Vaughan (1967) showed that PGE₁ suppresses activation of the hormone-sensitive triglyceride lipase and that PGE₁ was ineffective against cyclic AMP induced lipolysis. Butcher and his colleagues

(Butcher et al., 1967; Butcher and Sutherland, 1967; Butcher and Baird, 1968) found that PGE_1 inhibited hormonal-induced cyclic AMP formation both in fat pads and isolated cells. These authors, and Steinberg and Vaughan (1967), concluded that prostaglandins act on adenyl cyclase. In contrast, Paoletti et al. (1967) suggested that PGE_1 acts by activating the phosphodiesterase since by using a phosphodiesterase inhibitor (theophylline), they were able to demonstrate competition between the lipolytic effect of this compound and the antilipolytic action of PGE_1. Previously Krishna et al. (1966) had shown that nicotinic acid increases phosphodiesterase activity and Butcher and Sutherland (1967) also considered such a mechanism as a possibility for insulin action.

The physiological significance of these results lies in the discovery that fat pads contain prostaglandins and that biosynthesis readily occurs. Moreover, prostaglandin release is related to lipolysis in that efflux is increased by nerve stimulation, lipolytic agents and inhibited by insulin (Shaw and Ramwell, 1968a). Previously, Berti et al. (1967) had shown that only 1 ng of PGE_1 was effective in blocking lipolysis induced by sympathetic stimulation. Thus arose the concept that the endogenous prostaglandins in adipose tissue regulate fat pad homeostasis by being formed as a consequence of stimulation and then act back to curtail the duration and intensity of hormone action (Ramwell and Shaw, 1967).

There has been much discussion on the "insulin-like" effects of PGE_1. Vaughan (1967) showed that PGE_1 had a slight but significant effect on glucose uptake; PGA_1 was ineffective. PGE_1 also resembled insulin in stimulating ^{14}C incorporation from glucose into glyceride fatty acids and into glycogen. Crawford and Haessler (1968) obtained evidence that PGE_1 promotes fatty acid reesterification and also lipid synthesis from acetate and glucose. More recently Blecher et al. (1969) have shown that PGE_1 does not inhibit epinephrine-stimulated uptake and oxidation of glucose, although epinephrine-induced lipolysis is inhibited. The general conclusion is that the insulin-like effects of PGE_1 are small and are unlikely to have a significant effect in vivo.

Administration of PGE_1 in vivo has been shown to inhibit epinephrine, norepinephrine, ACTH, and cold-induced elevations of plasma free fatty acids and glycerol. Large doses of PGE_1 in rabbits, guinea pigs, and rats lowers basal free fatty acids. Small doses (i.v.) in man increase plasma fatty acids and glycerol due to sympathetic stimulation brought about by another property of PGE_1, namely vasodepression. Other vasodepressor agents which have no antilipolytic effect increase free fatty acids, e.g., PGA_1 and nitroglycerine. These increases were antagonized by using ganglionic blocking agents (see Bergström et al., 1968). The effects of PGE_1 on basal lipolysis are complicated by species differences, for in dog and man, PGE_1 increases FFA, an effect due to sympathetic activation due to vasodepressin (Bergström et al., 1966a,b; Carlson et al., 1968). Other mechanisms have been considered, including facilitation of sympathetic ganglionic transmission. Most of the effects of PGE_1 in raising plasma glucose are ascribable to catecholamine release from the adrenal medulla (Paoletti et al., 1968). On the other hand, PGE_1 may stimulate cyclic AMP formation and glycogenolysis in the liver (Böhle and May, 1968). The isolated rat liver releases both prostaglandins and glucose on glucagon stimulation (Ramwell, 1969; Ramwell and Shaw, 1970); epinephrine failed to release prostaglandins which may be due to its weaker action in stimulating cyclic AMP formation.

Paoletti (1968) reported that PGE_1 was more active than 48/80 in releasing both heparin-^{35}S and histamine-^{3}H from mast cells; this effect of PGE_1 was calcium dependent. Whether the increased lipoprotein lipase activity seen in rat heart after PGE_1 administration is due to an action on mast cells remains to be determined.

VII. Conclusions

The emergence of the close relationship between the pharmacological effects of prostaglandins and cyclic AMP may appear to complicate the already difficult problem of elucidating hormone action. However, knowledge of the presence in the target tissue of substances such as the prostaglandins whose formation is modulated on hormonal stimulation provides the basis for an entirely unsuspected concept pertaining to regulation of hormonal activity. The difficulties encountered in relating levels of circulating hormones to tissue responses and in interpretation of stimulus-response temporal patterns are well recognized. Some of these problems may be simplified if within the target tissue one can envisage compounds functioning as feedback regulating mechanisms capable of controlling the hormonal response at the cellular level.

As described earlier, prostaglandins attenuate humoral responses in stomach, renal tubules, cerebellar Purkinje cells, and adipocytes. The list of tissues where prostaglandins mimic humoral action is much longer. A prominent feature of both prostaglandin and adenyl cyclase action is the responsiveness of these systems to changes in calcium ion concentration. This point has been discussed with respect to readily displaceable calcium ions acting as the transducent between receptor activation and cyclic AMP formation (Ramwell and Shaw, 1970). However, a single basis for two such divergent mechanisms is difficult to conceive, and it is possibly easier to think in terms of two cellular sites of prostaglandin action: one leading to activation of adenyl cyclase with a concomitant increase in cyclic AMP, and the other perhaps associated with activation of cyclic AMP metabolism which would lead to decreased hormonal response (Shaw *et al.*, 1971; Shio *et al.*, 1971). The situation may be closely analogous to that described by Robison and his colleagues who, from the known pharmacological effects of α and β adrenergic agonists, suggested that α agonists should decrease tissue cyclic AMP formation while β agonists should increase cyclic AMP. They were able to provide a substantial body of evidence to support this concept by use of specific α and β antagonists. It is presently not possible to predict whether prostaglandins will increase or decrease cellular cyclic AMP levels, and no specific prostaglandin antagonists are yet available. Caution must be exercised in extending the analogy between the prostaglandins and the catecholamines, for the prostaglandins are readily formed in mast cells, and any theory of hormone regulation must account for the situation where prostaglandins are formed in response to hormones and then modify hormone action at a site subsequent to the hormone receptor or discriminator level; evidence indicates some possible interaction with the catalytic site of adenyl cyclase. Precise localization of prostaglandin action and realization of their potential implications awaits morphological studies of the link between a hormone receptor and the catalytic unit of adenyl cyclase and clarification of the sequence of molecular events which control adenyl cyclase and phosphodiesterase activity. Another area where information is required is the link between hormone receptor activation and increased acid hydrolase, which results in release of prostaglandin precursor. As considered previously, this is generally considered to be the rate-limiting step in prostaglandin formation. The suggestion has been made by a number of workers that the hydrolase is identifiable with phospholipase A.

In conclusion, it is clear now that any discussion of hormone action without consideration of the prostaglandins will be incomplete.

References

Ahn, C. S., and Rosenberg, I. N. (1970). *Endocrinology* **86**, 870.
Aldridge, R. R., Barrett, S., Brown, J. B., Funder, J. W., Goding, J. R., Kaltenbach, C. C., and Mole, B. J. (1970). *J. Reprod. Fert.* **21**, 369.
Avanzino, G. L., Bradley, P. B., and Wolstencroft, J. H. (1966). *Brit. J. Pharmacol. Chemother.* **27**, 157.
Beck, L., Pollard, A. A., Harbo, J. N., and Silver, T. M. (1968). *In* "Prostaglandin," Symp. Worcester Found. Exp. Biol. (P. W. Ramwell and J. E. Shaw, eds.), pp. 295–307. Wiley (Interscience), New York.
Bedwani, J. R., and Horton, E. W. (1968). *Life Sci.* **7**, 389.

Behrman, H. R., Yoshinaga, K., and Greep, R. O. (1971). *Ann. N.Y. Acad. Sci.* **180**, 426.
Bennett, A., Friedmann, C. A., and Vane, J. R. (1967). *Nature (London)* **216**, 873.
Bennett, A., Murray, J. G., and Wyllie, J. H. (1968a). *Brit. J. Pharmacol. Chemother.* **32**, 339.
Bennett, A., Eley, K. G., and Scholes, G. B. (1968b). *Brit. J. Pharmacol.* **34**, 630.
Bergström, S., Carlson, L. A., and Oro, L. (1966a). *Acta Physiol. Scand.* **67**, 141.
Bergström, S., Carlson, L. A., and Oro, L. (1966b). *Acta Physiol. Scand.* **67**, 185.
Bergström, S., Carlson, L. A., and Weeks, J. R. (1968). *Pharmacol. Rev.* **20**, 1.
Berti, F., Lentati, R. L., Usardi, M. M., and Paoletti, R. (1967). *Protoplasma* **63**, 143.
Blatchley, F. R., and Donovan, B. T. (1969). *Nature (London)* **221**, 1065.
Blecher, M., Merlino, N. S., Ro'Ane, J. R., and Flynn, P. D. (1969). *J. Biol. Chem.* **244**, 3423.
Böhle, E., and May, B. (1968). In "Prostaglandin," Symp. Worcester Found. Exp. Biol. (P. W. Ramwell and J. E. Shaw, eds.), pp. 115–129. Wiley (Interscience), New York.
Bradley, P. B., Samuels, G. M. R., and Shaw, J. E. (1969). *Brit. J. Pharmacol.* **37**, 151.
Breckenridge, B. (1970). *Annu. Rev. Pharmacol.* **10**, 19.
Bricker, N. S., Klahr, S., Purkerson, M., Schultze, R. G., Avioli, L. V., and Birge, S. J. (1968). *Nature (London)* **219**, 1058.
Burke, G. (1970). *Amer. J. Physiol.* **218**, 1445.
Butcher, R. W., and Baird, C. E. (1968). *J. Biol. Chem.* **243**, 1713.
Butcher, R. W., and Sutherland, E. W. (1967). *Ann. N.Y. Acad. Sci.* **139**, 849.
Butcher, R. W., Pike, J. E., and Sutherland, E. W. (1968). In "Prostaglandins," Nobel Symp. 2 (S. Bergström and B. Samuelsson, eds.), pp. 133–138. Almqvist & Wiksell, Uppsala.
Bygdeman, M., Kwon, S. U., Kukherjee, T., and Wiqvist, N. (1968). *Amer. J. Obstet. Gynecol.* **102**, 317.
Carlson, L. A., Ekelund, L., and Oro, L. (1968). *Acta Med. Scand.* **183**, 423.
Carpenter, M. P., and Wiseman, B. (1970). *Fed. Proc. Fed. Amer. Soc. Exp. Biol.* **29**, 248. (Abstr.)
Carr, A. A. (1968). In "Prostaglandin," Symp. Worcester Found. Exp. Biol. (P. W. Ramwell and J. E. Shaw, eds.), pp. 163–174. Wiley (Interscience), New York.
Carr, A. A. (1970). *Amer. J. Med. Sci.* **259**, 21.
Cehovic, G., Lewis, U. J., and VanderLaan, W. P. (1970). *Abstr. 52nd Meet. Endocrine Soc., St. Louis*, p. 150.
Chawla, R. C., and Eisenberg, M. M. (1969). *Proc. Soc. Exp. Biol. Med.* **132**, 1081.
Coceani, F., and Wolfe, L. S. (1965). *Can. J. Physiol. Pharmacol.* **43**, 445.
Coceani, F., Pace-Asciak, C., Volta, F., and Wolfe, L. S. (1967). *Amer. J. Physiol.* **213**, 1056.
Crawford, J. D., and Haessler, H. A. (1968). In "Prostaglandin," Symp. Worcester Found. Exp. Biol. (P. W. Ramwell and J. E. Shaw, eds.), pp. 103–114. Wiley (Interscience), New York.

Daniels, E. G., Hinman, J. W., Leach, B. E., and Muirhead, E. E. (1967). *Nature* (*London*) **215**, 1298.
de Wied, D., Witter, A., Versteeg, D. H. G., and Mulder, A. H. (1969). *Endocrinology* **86**, 561.
Dorrington, J. H., and Baggett, B. (1969). *Endocrinology* **84**, 989.
DuCharme, D. W., Weeks, J. R., and Montgomery, R. G. (1968). *J. Pharmacol. Exp. Ther.* **160**, 1.
Duda, P., Horton, E. W., and McPherson, A. (1968). *J. Physiol.* (*London*) **196**, 151.
Edwards, W. G., Jr., Strong, C. G., and Hunt, J. C. (1969). *J. Lab. Clin. Med.* **74**, 389.
Eik-Nes, K. B. (1969). *Gen. Comp. Endocrinol. Suppl.* **2**, 87.
Embrey, M. P. (1970). *Brit. Med. J.* **ii**, 256.
Fain, J. N. (1968). *In* "Prostaglandin," Symp. Worcester Found. Exp. Biol. (P. W. Ramwell and J. E. Shaw, eds.), pp. 67–77. Wiley (Interscience), New York.
Fain, J. N. (1970). *Abstr. 52nd Meet. Endocrine Soc.*, St. Louis, p. 47.
Fichman, M. P. (1969). *Clin. Res.* **17**, 429.
Field, J. B., Zor, U., and Kaneko, T. (1969). *Abstr. 51st Meet. Endocrine Soc.* New York, p. 98.
Flack, J. D., Jessup, R., and Ramwell, P. W. (1969). *Science* **163**, 691.
Fujimoto, S., and Lockett, M. F. (1969). *Proc. Int. Congr. Pharmacol., 4th, Basel* p. 122. (Abstr.)
Funder, J. W., Blair-West, J. R., Coghlan, J. P., Denton, D. A., Scoggins, B. A., and Wright, R. D. (1969). *Aust. J. Exp. Biol. Med. Sci.* **47**, P11.
Garay, G. L., and Martin, J. M. (1970). *Abstr. 52nd Meet. Endocrine Soc.*, St. Louis, p. 46.
Grant, J. K. (1968). *J. Endocrinol.* **41**, 111.
Grimley, P. M., Deftos, L. J., Weeks, J. R., and Rabson, A. S. (1969). *J. Nat. Cancer Inst.* **42**, 663.
Gutknecht, G. D., Cornette, J. C., and Pharriss, B. B. (1969). *Biol. Reprod.* **1**, 367.
Hansson, E., and Samuelsson, B. (1965). *Biochim. Biophys. Acta* **106**, 379.
Hoffer, B. J., Siggins, G. R., and Bloom, F. E. (1969). *Science* **166**, 1418.
Holmes, S. W. (1970). *Brit. J. Pharmacol.* **38**, 653.
Holmes, S. W., and Horton, E. W. (1968). *J. Physiol.* (*London*) **195**, 731.
Horton, E. W. (1964). *Brit. J. Pharmacol. Chemother.* **22**, 189.
Horton, E. W., and Jones, R. L. (1969). *J. Physiol.* (*London*) **200**, 56P.
Horton, E. W., and Main, I. H. M. (1967). *Brit. J. Pharmacol. Chemother.* **30**, 568.
Horton, E. W., Main, I. H. M., Thompson, C. J., and Wright, P. M. (1968). *Gut* **9**, 655.
Jacobson, E. D. (1970). *Proc. Soc. Exp. Biol. Med.* **133**, 516.
Johnston, H. H., Herzog, J. P., and Lauler, D. P. (1967). *Amer. J. Physiol.* **213**, 939.
Jones, R. L. (1970). *Biochem. J.* **119**, 64P.
Kakiuchi, S., and Rall, T. W. (1968). *Mol. Pharmacol.* **4**, 367.
Kaltenbach, C. C., Barrett, S., Funder, J. W., Mole, B. J., Aldridge, R. R., and Goding, J. R. (1969). *Proc. Meet. Soc. Study Reprod., 2nd, Davis*, 1969, 1. (Abstr.)
Karim, S. M. M. (1966). *J. Obstet. Gynaecol. Brit. Commonw.* **73**, 903.
Karim, S. M. M. (1968). *Brit. Med. J.* **iv**, 618.
Karim, S. M. M., and Devlin, J. (1967). *J. Obstet. Gynaecol. Brit. Commonw.* **74**, 230.

Karim, S. M. M., and Filshie, G. M. (1970). *Clin. Res.* **18**, 314.
Karim, S. M. M., Hillier, K., and Devlin, J. (1968a). *J. Pharm. Pharmacol.* **20**, 749.
Karim, S. M. M., Trussell, R. R., Patel, R. C., and Hillier, K. (1968b). *Brit. Med. J.* iv, 621.
Kataoka, K., Ramwell, P. W., and Jessup, S. J. (1967). *Science* **157**, 1187.
Kirton, K. T., Pharriss, B. B., and Forbes, A. D. (1970a). *Proc. Soc. Exp. Biol. Med.* **133**, 314.
Kirton, K. T., Pharriss, B. B., and Forbes, A. D. (1970b). *Biol. Reprod.* **3**, 163.
Krishna, G., Weiss, B., Davies, J. I., and Hynie, S. (1966). *Fed. Proc. Fed. Amer. Soc. Exp. Biol.* **25**, 719.
Lee, J. B. (1968). *In* "Prostaglandin," Symp. Worcester Found. Exp. Biol. (P. W. Ramwell and J. E. Shaw, eds.), pp. 131–146. Wiley (Interscience), New York.
Lee, J. B., and Ferguson, J. F. (1969). *Nature* (*London*) **222**, 1185.
Lee, J. B., Gougoutas, J. Z., Takman, B. H., Daniels, E. G., Grostic, M. F., Pike, J. E., Hinman, J. W., and Muirhead, E. E. (1966). *J. Clin. Invest.* **45**, 1036.
Lee, J. B., McGiff, J. C., and Frawley, T. F. (1969). *Abstr. 51st Meet. Endocrine Soc., New York*, p. 60.
Lee, J. B., McGiff, J. C., Kannegiesser, H., Aykent, Y. Y., Mudd, J. G., and Frawley, T. F. (1970). *Ann. Int. Med.* **74**, 703.
Leier, D. J., and Jungmann, R. A. (1970). *Abstr. 52nd Meet. Endocrine Soc., St. Louis*, p. 85.
Lewis, G. P., and Matthews, J. (1969). *J. Physiol.* (*London*) **202**, 95P.
McCracken, J. A., Glew, M. E., and Scaramuzzi, R. J. (1970). *J. Clin. Endocrinol. Metab.* **30**, 544.
McGiff, J. C., Crowshaw, K., Terragno, N. A., Lonigro, A. J., Strand, J. C., Williamson, Sr., Ng, K. K. F., and Lee, J. B. (1969a). *Circulation Suppl.* **III**, 144.
McGiff, J. C., Terragno, N. A., Strand, J. C., Lee, J. B., Lonigro, A. J., and Ng, K. K. F. (1969b). *Nature* (*London*) **223**, 742.
Macho, L., and Palkovic, M. (1965). *Physiol. Bohemoslov.* **14**, 563.
MacLeod, R. M., and Lehmeyer, J. E. (1970). *Clin. Res.* **18**, 366.
Maier, R., and Staehelin, M. (1968). *Acta Endocrinol.* (*Copenhagen*) **58**, 619.
Margoulies, M., Coninx, P., and Plomteux, G. (1969). *In* "Protein and Polypeptide Hormones," Proc. Int. Symp., Liege (M. Margoulies, ed.), pp. 467–471. Excerpta Med. Found., Amsterdam.
Marsh, J. M. (1970). *Fed. Proc. Fed. Amer. Soc. Exp. Biol.* **29**, 387. (Abstr.)
Marsh, J. M., and Savard, K. (1966). *Steroids* **8**, 133.
Mazer, R. S., and Wright, P. A. (1968). *Endocrinology* **83**, 1065.
Milton, A. S., and Wendlandt, S. (1970). *J. Physiol.* (*London*) **207**, 76P.
Muirhead, E. E., Leach, B. E., Brown, G. B., Daniels, E. G., and Hinman, J. W. (1967). *J. Lab. Clin. Med.* **70**, 986.
Nutting, E. F., and Cammarata, P. S. (1969). *Nature* (*London*) **222**, 287.
Onaya, T., and Solomon, D. H. (1969). *Abstr. 51st Meet. Endocrine Soc., New York*, p. 99.
Onaya, T., and Solomon, D. H. (1970). *Endocrinology* **86**, 423.
Orloff, J., and Grantham, J. (1967). *In* "Prostaglandins," Nobel Symp. 2 (S. Bergström and B. Samuelsson, eds.), pp. 143–146. Almqvist & Wiksell, Uppsala.
Orloff, J., Handler, J. S., and Bergström, S. (1965). *Nature* (*London*) **205**, 397.

Paoletti, R. (1968). USAF Sch. of Aerospace Med., Aerospace Med. Div. (AFSC), Brooks Air Force Base, Texas.
Paoletti, R., Lentati, R. L., and Korolkiewicz, Z. (1966). In "Prostaglandins," Nobel Symp. 2 (S. Bergström and B. Samuelsson, eds.), pp. 147–159. Almqvist & Wiksell, Uppsala.
Paoletti, R., Puglisi, L., and Usardi, M. M. (1968). *Advan. Exp. Med. Biol.* **2**, 425.
Peng, T. C., Six, K. M., and Munson, P. L. (1970). *Endocrinology* **86**, 202.
Perrier, C. V., and Laster, L. (1970). *J. Clin. Invest.* **49**, 73a.
Pharriss, B. B., and Wyngarden, L. J. (1969). *Proc. Soc. Exp. Biol. Med.* **130**, 92.
Pharriss, B. B., Wyngarden, L. J., and Gutknecht, G. D. (1968). In "Gonadotropins, 1968," Proc. Workshop Conf. (E. Rosemberg, ed.), pp. 121–129. Geron-X, Inc., Los Altos, California.
Pharriss, B. B., Cornette, J. C., and Gutknecht, G. D. (1970). *J. Reprod. Fert. Suppl.* **10**, 97.
Phillis, J. W., and Tebecis, A. K. (1968). *Nature (London)* **217**, 1076.
Pickles, V. R. (1957). *Nature (London)* **180**, 1198.
Pickles, V. R. (1967). *Biol. Rev. Cambridge Phil. Soc.* **42**, 614.
Pickles, V. R. (1969). *Nature (London)* **224**, 221.
Pickles, V. R., Hall, W. J., Best, F. A., and Smith, G. N. (1965). *J. Obstet. Gynaecol. Brit. Commonw.* **72**, 185.
Piper, P. J., Vane, J. R., and Wyllie, J. H. (1970). *Nature (London)* **225**, 600.
Ramwell, P. W. (1969). *Proc. Int. Congr. Pharmacol.*, 4th, Basel, p. 12. (Abstr.)
Ramwell, P. W., and Shaw, J. E. (1966). *Amer. J. Physiol.* **211**, 125.
Ramwell, P. W., and Shaw, J. E. (1967). In "Prostaglandins," Nobel Symp. 2 (S. Bergström and B. Samuelsson, eds.), pp. 283–292. Almqvist & Wiksell, Uppsala.
Ramwell, P. W., and Shaw, J. E. (1970). *Recent Progr. Horm. Res.* **26**, 139.
Ramwell, P. W., Shaw, J. E., Douglas, W. W., and Poisner, A. M. (1966a). *Nature (London)* **210**, 273.
Ramwell, P. W., Shaw, J. E., and Jessup, R. (1966b). *Amer. J. Physiol.* **211**, 998.
Rector, F. C., Martinez, M. M., Kurtzman, N. A., Sellman, J. C., Oerther, F., Seldin, D. W., and Nunn, A. C. (1968). *J. Clin. Invest.* **47**, 761.
Robert, A. (1968). In "Prostaglandin," Symp. Worcester Found. Exp. Biol. (P. W. Ramwell and J. E. Shaw, eds.), pp. 47–54. Wiley (Interscience), New York.
Robert, A., Nezamis, J. E., and Phillips, J. P. (1967). *Amer. J. Dig. Dis.* **12**, 1073.
Robert, A., Nezamis, J. E., and Phillips, J. P. (1968a). *Gastroenterology* **55**, 481.
Robert, A., Phillips, J. P., and Nezamis, J. E. (1968b). *Gastroenterology* **54**, 1263.
Roberts, G., Anderson, A., McGarry, J., and Turnbull, A. C. (1970). *Brit. Med. J.* **ii**, 152.
Rodesch, F., Neve, P., Willems, C., and Dumont, J. E. (1969). *Eur. J. Biochem.* **8**, 26.
Roth-Brandel, U., Bygdeman, M., Wiqvist, N., and Bergström, S. (1970). *Lancet* **i**, 190.
Rudick, J., Gonda, M., and Janowitz, H. D. (1970). *Fed. Proc. Fed. Amer. Soc. Exp. Biol.* **29**, 445. (Abstr.)
Samuelsson, B. (1965). *J. Amer. Chem. Soc.* **87**, 3011.
Sandler, M., Williams, E. D., and Karim, S. M. M. (1969). In "Prostaglandins, Peptides and Amines" (P. Mantegazza and E. W. Horton, eds.), pp. 3–7. Academic Press, New York.

Shaw, J. E., and Ramwell, P. W. (1967). In "Prostaglandins," Nobel Symp. 2 (S. Bergström and B. Samuelsson, eds.), pp. 293–299. Almqvist & Wiksell, Uppsala.
Shaw, J. E., and Ramwell, P. W. (1968a). *J. Biol. Chem.* **243**, 1498.
Shaw, J. E., and Ramwell, P. W. (1968b). In "Prostaglandin," Symp. Worcester Found. Exp. Biol. (P. W. Ramwell and J. E. Shaw, eds.), pp. 55–56. Wiley (Interscience), New York.
Shaw, J. E., and Ramwell, P. W. (1969). *Proc. Int. Congr. Pharmacol., 4th, Basel,* p. 109. (Abstr.)
Shaw, J. E., Gibson, W. J., Jessup, S. J., and Ramwell, P. W. (1971). *Ann. N.Y. Acad. Sci.* **180**, 241.
Shio, H., Shaw, J. E., and Ramwell, P. W. (1971). *Ann. N.Y. Acad. Sci.* In press.
Speroff, L., and Ramwell, P. W. (1970a). *Amer. J. Obstet. Gynecol.* **107**, 1111.
Speroff, L., and Ramwell, P. W. (1970b). *J. Clin. Endocrinol. Metab.* **30**, 345.
Steinberg, D., and Vaughan, M. (1967). In "Prostaglandins," Nobel Symp. 2 (S. Bergström and B. Samuelsson, eds.), pp. 109–121. Almqvist & Wiksell, Uppsala.
Steinberg, D., Vaughan, M., Nestel, P., and Bergström, S. (1963). *Biochem. Pharmacol.* **12**, 764.
Sutherland, E. W., Rall, T. W., and Menon, T. (1962). *J. Biol. Chem.* **237**, 1220.
Vander, A. J. (1968). *Amer. J. Physiol.* **214**, 218.
Vaughan, M. (1967). In "Prostaglandins," Nobel Symp. 2 (S. Bergström and B. Samuelsson, eds.), pp. 139–142. Almqvist & Wiksell, Uppsala.
Vogt, W., Bartels, J., Kunze, H., and Meyer, U. (1969). *Proc. Int. Congr. Pharmacol. 4th, Basel,* p. 378. (Abstr.)
von Euler, U. S., and Eliasson, R., eds. (1967). "Prostaglandins." Academic Press, New York.
Way, L., and Durbin, R. P. (1969). *Nature (London)* **221**, 874.
Weeks, J. R. (1969). *Proc. Int. Congr. Pharmacol., 4th, Basel,* p. 12. (Abstr.)
Weiss, B., and Costa, E. (1968). *Biochem. Pharmacol.* **17**, 2107.
Williams, E. D., Karim, S. M. M., and Sandler, M. (1968). *Lancet* **i**, 22.
Wilson, D. W., Phillips, C., and Levine, R. (1970). *Clin. Res.* **18**, 468.
Wiqvist, N., and Bygdeman, M. (1970). *Lancet* **i**, 889.
Wiqvist, N., Bygdeman, M., Kwon, S. U., Mukherjee, T., and Roth-Brandel, U. (1968). *Amer. J. Obstet. Gynecol.* **102**, 327.
Wolfe, L. S., Coceani, F., and Pace-Asciak, C. (1967). *Pharmacologist* **9**, 171.
Zor, U., Kaneko, T., Schneider, H. P. G., McCann, S. M., Lowe, I. P., Bloom, G., Borland, B., and Field, J. B. (1969a). *Proc. Nat. Acad. Sci. U.S.* **63**, 918.
Zor, U., Bloom, G., Lowe, I. P., and Field, J. B. (1969b). *Endocrinology* **84**, 1082.
Zor, U., Kaneko, T., Schneider, H. P. G., McCann, S. M., and Field, J. B. (1970). *J. Biol. Chem.* **245**, 2883.

EFFECTS OF OVARIAN HORMONES AT THE SUBCELLULAR LEVEL

Elwood V. Jensen and Eugene R. DeSombre

THE BEN MAY LABORATORY FOR CANCER RESEARCH
THE UNIVERSITY OF CHICAGO
CHICAGO, ILLINOIS

I. Introduction	229
II. Estrogens	231
A. Early Effects of Estrogens on Cellular Processes	231
B. Estrogen–Receptor Interactions	235
III. Progestins	250
A. Early Effects of Progestins on Cellular Processes	250
B. Progestin–Receptor Interactions	251
IV. Hormone–Receptor Interaction Pattern and Its Biochemical Significance	259
References	263

I. Introduction

Although the steroid sex hormones exert some influence on a great many tissues of the vertebrate organism, a principal action, usually taken as a measure of biological activity, is the induction and maintenance of growth and function in tissues of the reproductive tract. For some reason these tissues lack the capacity for development unless they are continually exposed to the hormone. Whether such "hormone-dependency" is a phenomenon of deletion or acquisition has not been established. During the process of differentiation, the hormone-dependent tissues may lose some important component or property which must be restored to them before optimal growth can occur. On the other hand, they may acquire some mechanism of biosynthetic restraint which must be removed or neutralized by the hormone's action. Because of current concepts in microbial molecular biology, it is attractive to consider that cells of hormone-dependent tissues may contain inhibitors of specific genetic function and that the hormone acts in some way to switch on these repressed genes. Experimental evidence, however, has not established that gene derepression is the initial event leading to the multiplicity of biochemical alterations associated with overall hormonal response. For the present, considerations of the mechanism of sex hormone action must recognize that the primary event may be of either a positive (restorative) or a negative (derepressive) nature.

The action of humoral agents at the subcellular level may be studied from two standpoints: (1) what the hormone does to the tissue and (2) what the tissue does with the hormone. During the past decade, considerable information relevant to endocrine mechanisms has been acquired from both types of experimental approach. The influence of administered sex hormones on the rate of incorporation of labeled precursors into cellular constituents, both *in vivo* and *in vitro*, has demonstrated many rapid biochemical responses in dependent tissues of hormone-deprived animals. The sensitivity of these responses to what presumably are selective inhibitors of biosynthesis, such as cycloheximide, puromycin, and actinomycin D, has provided some insight as to their chronological interrelation. Determination of the uptake and chemical fate of physiological amounts of radioactive hormones in various tissues of experimental animals has led to the recognition that target tissues contain unique amounts of characteristic extranuclear proteins, now generally called hormone "receptors," which associate with the steroid and accompany it to its ultimate site of fixation in the nucleus. It is presumed that the hormone–receptor interaction and the acceleration of biosynthetic processes are closely interrelated.

In the following presentation, an attempt is made to summarize the principal early biochemical responses in target tissues to estrogenic and progestational hormones, to describe the nature of the hormone–receptor interaction and, finally, to consider the possible role of the receptor proteins in eliciting a biochemical response.

II. Estrogens

A. Early Effects of Estrogens on Cellular Processes

As reviewed in more detail elsewhere (Mueller, 1960; 1965; Hechter and Halkerston, 1964; Segal and Scher, 1967; Hamilton, 1968; Williams-Ashman and Reddi, 1971), the estrogenic hormones exert a marked influence on the levels and metabolism of a great many cellular components in target tissues. Although it is generally considered that most of these effects are secondary phenomena resulting from the initial stimulation of some key biochemical process, it is entirely possible that estrogens exert more than one primary effect on the target cell. In particular, the estrogen-induced release of uterine histamine (Spaziani and Szego, 1958; Szego, 1965), which appears to be involved in the rapid onset of hyperemia and water imbibition, is difficult to correlate with the findings regarding estrogen–receptor interaction and genome activation and may well represent a separate hormonal action which augments the overall biological effect.

In an effort to elucidate the initial step or steps in the estrogenic stimulation of uterine growth, investigators have attempted to establish the chronological sequence of biochemical events *in vivo*, both by determining the earliest detectable response and by studying the effect of presumably selective inhibitors of RNA and protein synthesis on the various estrogen-induced alterations in the immature or ovariectomized rat uterus. Although an increase in the uterine content of phospholipid (Mueller, 1960) and glycogen (Bitman *et al.*, 1965) can be detected 1–2 hours after estrogen administration, the total RNA and protein levels do not rise until after 6 and 12 hours, respectively, with an increase in DNA coming much later (Mueller, 1960; Billing *et al.*, 1969c). By determining the incorporation of labeled precursors, it can be demonstrated that the rate of overall protein synthesis is accelerated between 2 and 4 hours after hormone administration (Mueller *et al.*, 1961; Noteboom and Gorski, 1963) whereas an increase in the rate of RNA synthesis, particularly in the nucleus, can be detected at 1 hour (Gorski and Nicolette, 1963; Hamilton, 1964; Gorski and Nelson, 1965). Uteri excised 2 hours after estrogen injection show an enhanced ability to incorporate labeled precursors into phospholipid and RNA *in vitro*, but this stimulatory effect is lost as the uterine segments are maintained under *in vitro* conditions (Aizawa and Mueller, 1961; Gorski and Nicolette, 1963).

Examination of only the rapidly labeled nuclear RNA reveals a striking enhancement of tritiated uridine incorporation, which is detectable at 2 minutes after estrogen injection, reaches a maximum of five to six times the control level at 20 minutes, and then declines as increased incorporation of the labeled precursor into microsomal RNA becomes evident (Hamilton et al., 1965, 1968; Means and Hamilton, 1966). This rapidly stimulated RNA appears to be a ribosomal or preribosomal type of nucleolar origin, which then passes from the nucleus to the cytoplasm. Certain other investigators, however, have failed to confirm this early effect of estrogen on the synthesis of RNA in the nucleus (Joel and Hagerman, 1969; Billing et al., 1969b; Greenman, 1970). Because the estrogen treatment also causes an increased influx of tritiated uridine, presumably by an effect on cell permeability related to the water imbibition phenomenon, there is some uncertainty, also recognized by the original investigators (Hamilton et al., 1968), as to whether the extremely rapid estrogen-induced labeling of nuclear RNA *in vivo* may be an artifact due to a change in the specific activity of the intracellular uridine pool rather than an actual stimulation of RNA synthesis.

Apart from the question about the significance of the 20-minute labeling phenomenon, there is general agreement that an enhanced capacity for RNA synthesis, evident 1–2 hours after hormone administration, is certainly an important response of the uterus to estrogen and is probably conducive to the increased rate of total protein synthesis that follows. This is substantiated by the increased RNA polymerase activity observed in uterine nuclei isolated from estrogen-treated animals 1–4 hours after hormone administration (Noteboom and Gorski, 1963; Gorski, 1964; Hamilton et al., 1965, 1968; Nicolette and Mueller, 1966; Gorski and Morgan, 1967; Nicolette et al., 1968; Barry and Gorski, 1971). After estrogen stimulation, the RNA produced either *in vivo* or in isolated uterine nuclei appears to be of a ribosomal type and is different in composition from that produced in the absence of estrogen as indicated by nearest-neighbor frequency analysis and hybridization experiments (Barton and Liao, 1967; Teng and Hamilton, 1968; Hamilton et al., 1968; Trachewsky and Segal, 1968; Billing et al., 1969a). The appearance of new species of RNA after estrogen stimulation has been demonstrated also in the rabbit uterus and hen oviduct, as well as in the liver of the rabbit, the hen, and the lizard (Church and McCarthy, 1970; Hahn et al., 1969a,b). Possibly relevant to the synthesis of new species of RNA are observations of the stimulation by estrogen of tRNA methylase activity in the uterus, but not the liver, of the ovariectomized pig (Sharma and Borek, 1970) and in the chick oviduct (Hacker, 1969).

Once the new population of uterine RNAs has been produced under the influence of estrogen, they appear to possess the ability to initiate uterine growth without need for the hormone. When instilled into the uterine lumen of ovariectomized rats, RNA isolated from rat uteri excised 4 or 12 hours after estrogen administration was found to induce hypertrophy of the uterine endometrium similar to that evoked by estrogen itself (Segal *et al.*, 1965; Unhjem *et al.*, 1968). Similarly, protein synthesis in the uteri of immature rats is stimulated following intrauterine application of RNA from the uteri of estrogen-treated but not of nontreated rats (Fencl and Villee, 1971). The foregoing effects on the uterus are not seen with RNA obtained from liver or vagina, and they are abolished by treatment of the uterine RNA with ribonuclease.

The mechanism by which estrogen effects an increase in the rate of RNA synthesis in the uterine nucleus has been the subject of extensive interest and investigation. It is not clear whether this stimulation results from an effect of the hormone on chromatin template activity, RNA polymerase activity, RNA transport from nucleus to cytoplasm, or a combination of factors; evidence supporting all these possibilities has been reported. Uterine chromatin, isolated from estrogen-treated rats, shows increased DNA template activity when assayed in an RNA polymerase system using a bacterial enzyme (Barker and Warren, 1966; Teng and Hamilton, 1968), and that from rabbit endometrium an even greater enhancement, demonstrable 10 minutes after hormone injection, when assayed with the enzyme obtained from endometrial nuclei (Church and McCarthy, 1970). It has been suggested (Teng and Hamilton, 1969) that the activation of chromatin may involve synthesis of new acidic proteins which overcome an inhibitory effect on transcription by the uterine histones. On the other hand, careful analysis of the incorporation of nucleotides into RNA by nuclei isolated from estrogen-stimulated rats indicates that the increased rate of precursor incorporation does not involve the synthesis of more RNA chains, as would be the case if new template sites were being made available, but rather it appears to result from the production of longer chains, suggesting an effect on the activity of the enzyme (Barry and Gorski, 1971). Changes in selective transport of nuclear RNA to the cytoplasm have been observed in the rabbit uterus after estrogen stimulation (Church and McCarthy, 1970).

That the overall uterotropic effect, accompanied by an increase in various biosynthetic activities, is not a simple phenomenon resulting directly from stimulation of general RNA synthesis was recognized very early by the finding that the estrogen-induced enhancement of RNA synthesis, determined either *in vivo* or in isolated uterine nuclei, is abolished not only by injection of actinomycin D (Ui and Mueller, 1963), but also by inhibitors of protein synthesis, such as puromycin or cyclohexmide* (Mueller et al., 1961; Noteboom and Gorski, 1963; Gorski and Axman, 1964; Gorski and Morgan, 1967). All these inhibitors also block the early stimulation of phospholipid synthesis (Mueller et al., 1961; Gorski et al., 1965) and glucose metabolism (Nicolette and Gorski, 1964; Gorski and Morgan, 1967; Smith and Gorski, 1968). These observations suggest that all these biochemical responses observed 1–2 hours after estrogen administration are secondary phenomena resulting from the activation of some earlier process which is sensitive to inhibitors of both RNA and protein synthesis.

The need for some type of continued protein synthesis in the estrogenic stimulation of nuclear RNA polymerase activity is indicated by two interesting observations concerning the influence of various treatments of the whole uterine tissue during the period between excision from the hormone-treated animals and preparation of the nuclei for polymerase assay (Nicolette and Mueller, 1966; Nicolette et al., 1968). Incubation of the uterine tissue at either 37°C or 4°C maintains the estrogen-induced activation, but incubation at 23°C leads to a decrease in stimulated nuclear RNA polymerase activity which can be gradually restored by increasing the temperature to 37°C. The resulting conclusion that polymerase activation requires continued availability of a protein which is stable at 4°C, consumed at 23°C and continuously resynthesized at 37°C is supported by the further observation that incubation of the tissue at 37°C with cycloheximide likewise results in a decrease in RNA polymerase activity in the nuclei from the estrogen-treated but not from the control uteri, and that this activity, along with protein-synthesizing ability, can be restored by incubation in fresh medium to wash out the cycloheximide.

On the basis of all the foregoing observations, it is evident that during the first hour after estrogen administration there are changes in the metabolism of uterine RNA, lipid, and glucose, which precede the overall stimulation of protein synthesis. Because of their sensitivity both to actinomycin D and to puromycin and cycloheximide, these early changes appear to require the synthesis of RNA and protein in amounts too small to contribute to the overall labeling pattern. But such specific uterine protein, synthesized rapidly in response to estrogen, has been detected by starch gel electrophoresis of cytosol from immature rat uteri which have been either excised from animals injected with radioactive leucine or incubated with the labeled amino acid *in vitro* (Notides and Gorski, 1966). By the use of different isotopes to label the proteins

* The effect of cycloheximide on the 20-minute incorporation of uridine into rapidly labeled nuclear RNA is difficult to evaluate because under the conditions of these experiments cycloheximide causes a marked increase of labeling in uteri of animals receiving no estrogen (Hamilton et al., 1968).

of the control and the treated animals, respectively, the sensitivity of the detection procedure has been substantially increased; these later experiments indicate that the ability to synthesize the specific protein is inhibited by actinomycin D and that the effect is detectable 30–40 minutes after estrogen administration, reaching a maximum in 1–2 hours, after which it declines (Mayol and Thayer, 1970; Barnea and Gorski, 1970; DeAngelo and Gorski, 1970). The specific protein synthesis appears to result from the production of a new messenger RNA, which is not sensitive to puromycin or cycloheximide and shows indirect evidence of being present 15 minutes after estrogen administration (DeAngelo and Gorski, 1970). Acrylamide-gel electrophoresis indicates that the new protein consists of at least two components with isoelectric points, as determined by electrofocusing, of between 3.5 and 4 (Mayol and Thayer, 1970). The capacity for synthesizing the new protein can be induced by incubating the uteri with hyperphysiological (Mayol and Thayer, 1970) or nearly physiological (Katzenellenbogen and Gorski, 1971) levels of estradiol *in vitro,* so that this phenomenon, along with the action of transformed estrogen–receptor complex on isolated uterine nuclei described in Section IV, represent the only confirmed examples of an early biochemical effect elicited by estrogen *in vitro.*

Very recently it was reported (Barker, 1971) that the administration of estrogen to ovariectomized rats which have received an intraluminal application of a labeled amino acid mixture results in the rapid incorporation of isotope into an acidic protein (pI 4–5) found in the arginine-rich histone fraction (F3) of the uterus. Increased synthesis of the specific protein, accompanied by a reduction in the total amount of these histones, is detectable 15 minutes after estrogen administration and does not appear to be sensitive to actinomycin D.

The relation of the two types of estrogen-induced protein to each other, to the protein synthesis which appears to be required for RNA polymerase activation in uterine nuclei (Nicolette *et al.*, 1968), and to the estrogen–receptor interaction described in Section IV remains to be established. It seems probable, however, that this rapid induction phenomenon, which at least in one case is demonstrable in an *in vitro* system, will provide important insight into the molecular mechanism of estrogen action.

B. Estrogen–Receptor Interactions

1. Binding of Estrogens by Target Tissues *in Vivo* and *in Vitro*

The presence in estrogen-responsive tissues of characteristic hormone-binding components, now called estrogen "receptors" or "estrophiles," was first indicated by the striking affinity of these tissues for

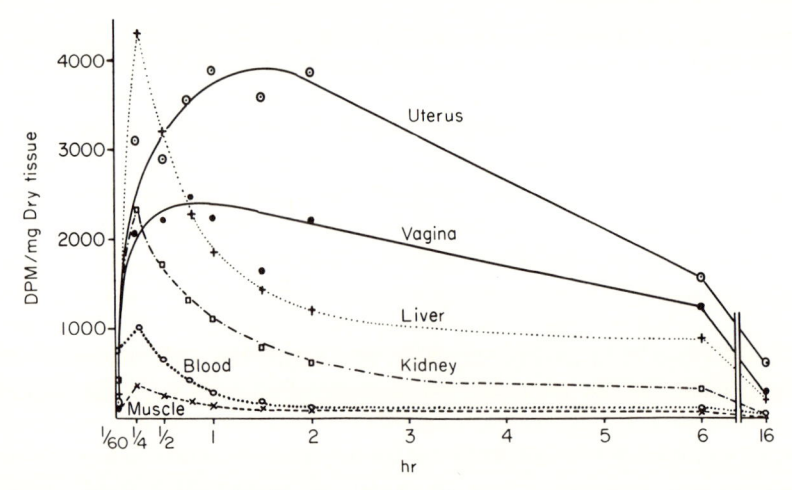

Fig. 1. Tissue tritium levels after single subcutaneous injection of 98 ng (11.5 µCi) of estradiol-6,7-³H in 0.5 ml of saline to immature rats. Each point is based on 6 animals. From Jensen and Jacobson (1960).

the hormone *in vivo*. After the administration of physiological amounts of tritiated estradiol to immature rats (Jensen, 1960; Jensen and Jacobson, 1960; Gupta, 1960) or tritiated hexestrol to young goats and sheep (Glascock and Hoekstra, 1959), the uterus, vagina, and anterior pituitary were found to take up and retain the radioactive hormone against a marked concentration gradient with the blood (Fig. 1). Although extensive metabolic transformation of administered estradiol occurs in such tissues as the liver, and the blood contains a great mixture of both free and conjugated metabolites, only unchanged estradiol is taken up and bound by the uterus of the immature[*] rat (Jensen and Jacobson, 1962) or mouse (Stone, 1964). The resulting conclusion that estradiol initiates uterine growth without itself undergoing metabolic transformation has proved consistent with much subsequent evidence.

Studies by a number of investigators have provided further information about the biological fate of estrogenic hormones in the reproductive tract of the mouse (Stone, 1963; Stone *et al.*, 1963; Stone and Martin, 1964; Stone and Baggett, 1965a; Terenius, 1965; Folman and Pope, 1969), the rat (Roy *et al.*, 1964; Talwar *et al.*, 1964; Noteboom and Gorski,

[*] Although the immature rat uterus appears to be unable to oxidize estradiol to estrone, the uterus of the adult rat (Pack and Brooks, 1970; Wenzel *et al.*, 1970) and the rabbit (Jütting *et al.*, 1967; Jungblut *et al.*, 1967b), as well as human endometrium (Sweat *et al.*, 1967; Gurpide and Welch, 1969), can convert estradiol to estrone, either *in vivo* or *in vitro*.

1965; King and Gordon, 1966; Jensen et al., 1966; Brecher and Wotiz, 1967; Kato and Villee, 1967b; Callantine et al., 1968; DeHertogh et al., 1971a,b), and the human (Davis et al., 1963; Brush et al., 1967). Although estradiol is specifically bound in all regions of the uterus, the concentration is higher in the endometrium than in the myometrium (Alberga and Baulieu, 1965, 1968; Flesher, 1965; Jensen, 1965b; King and Gordon, 1966). The binding sites appear to possess stereospecificity, inasmuch as the uptake of tritiated estradiol by the rat uterus is inhibited by an excess of nonradioactive estradiol, but not by its 17-epimer, estradiol-17α (Noteboom and Gorski, 1965). Studies of estradiol incorporation as a function of dose indicate that the interaction of estrogens with target tissues in the immature rat consists of two distinct phenomena: an uptake process, which is not saturable with considerably hyperphysiological amounts of administered hormone, and a retention process, which becomes saturated as the dose exceeds the physiological level (Jensen et al., 1967a).

Binding of estradiol by the uterus appears to be influenced by the hormonal state of the animal. Although the binding capacity and receptor content of the adult rat uterus are less than those of the immature animal (Eisenfeld and Axelrod, 1966; Hughes et al., 1969; Feherty et al., 1970) and gradually decrease with age (Lee and Jacobson, 1971), removal of the ovaries is followed by a significant decrease in receptor concentration (McGuire and Lisk, 1968; Hughes et al., 1969). Variation in uterine receptor content with ovarian cycle (Feherty et al., 1970; DeHertogh et al., 1971b; Lee and Jacobson, 1971) provides further indication of hormonal control of receptor capacity.

Although the uptake by hypothalamus is quite low in comparison to pituitary, uterus, or vagina, careful investigation by both biochemical methods (Eisenfeld and Axelrod, 1965, 1967; Kato and Villee, 1967a; McGuire and Lisk, 1969; Kahwanago et al., 1970; Attramadal and Aakvaag, 1970) and by autoradiography (Michael, 1965; Stumpf, 1968b; Pfaff, 1968; Attramadal, 1970) has demonstrated the presence of receptor sites for estradiol in hypothalamic tissue. Specific estrogen binding is observed in mammary glands of the rat (Sander, 1968; Sander and Attramadal, 1968a), the mouse (Puca and Bresciani, 1968b, 1969a), and the human (Desphande et al., 1967) and in certain hormone-dependent mammary tumors in the rat (King et al., 1965b, 1966; Jensen, 1965b; Mobbs, 1966, 1968, 1969; Jungblut et al., 1967a; Jensen et al., 1967c; Sander and Attramadal, 1968b; Kyser, 1970) and in the human (Demetriou et al., 1964; Braunsberg et al., 1967; Deshpande et al., 1967; Johansson et al., 1970). The presence of estrogen receptors in human breast cancer tissue appears to be a requirement for response of the patient to such ablative endocrine therapy as adrenalectomy or hypophysectomy (Folca et al., 1961; Jensen et al., 1971b).

The uptake of estradiol by target tissues is markedly decreased by simultaneous administration of one of several chemically similar compounds, known from previous work to block the uterine growth response to estrogens. This phenomenon of binding inhibition was first observed with MER-25 or ethamoxytriphetol (Jensen, 1962) and subsequently with the more potent antagonists, clomiphene (Roy et al., 1964; Wyss et al., 1968b; Kahwanago et al., 1970), Upjohn 11,100A or nafoxidine (Jensen, 1965a,b) and Parke-Davis CI-628, originally called CN-55,945-27 (Callantine, 1967). Inasmuch as these reagents have no effect on the low levels of estrogen which appear in the nontarget tissues (Jensen et al., 1966), they appear to be selective inhibitors of the interaction of estrogen with receptor sites and have proved to be of considerable value in distinguishing specific from nonspecific binding. The quantitative correlation between the reduction in estrogen uptake and the inhibition of uterine growth following the administration of varying doses of nafoxidine (Jensen, 1965b) provides evidence that estrogen–receptor interaction plays an important role in the uterotropic process.

Although the binding of estradiol to uterine receptor sites is sensitive to antiestrogens of the MER-25 type, it is not inhibited by puromycin or actinomycin D (Jensen, 1965a,b), substances also known to block the overall growth response to estrogens as well as the early acceleration of many biochemical processes in the uterus (Mueller et al., 1961; Ui and Mueller, 1963). This observation suggests that the interaction of the steroid with the receptor is an early step in the uterotropic process, preceding the acceleration of those biosynthetic reactions which are sensitive to actinomycin D or puromycin.

In contrast to their striking incorporation of estradiol, rat uterus, vagina, and anterior pituitary exhibit little affinity for estrone. When estrone is administered to the immature rat, a part of it is reduced to estradiol which accumulates in the uterus in approximately one-tenth the amount that would result from a similar dose of estradiol itself (Jensen and Jacobson, 1962). Hexestrol, 17α-methylestradiol, 17α-ethynylestradiol, and, to a lesser extent, estriol all show marked uptake and retention by target tissues, and each is incorporated without chemical transformation (Jensen, 1965b; Jensen et al., 1966); mestranol, on the other hand, does not bind to receptors but undergoes gradual demethylation, probably in the liver, to furnish 17α-ethynylestradiol, which accumulates in the uterine tissue. Thus the physiological interaction with target tissues appears to require the presence of free hydroxyl or phenolic groups at both extremities of the estrogen molecule.

When excised uterine tissue is exposed to dilute solutions of tritiated estradiol at physiological temperatures *in vitro,* an association of hormone with receptor takes place which shows all the principal characteristics of the *in vivo* phenomenon (Jungblut *et al.,* 1965; Stone and Baggett, 1965b; Terenius, 1966; Jensen *et al.,* 1966, 1967b; Maurer and Chalkley, 1967; Wyss *et al.,* 1968b). This interaction *in vitro* does not require the presence either of oxygen or of added nutrients. If an inhibitor of specific estradiol binding, such as nafoxidine, CI-628, or clomiphene, is present in the incubation medium, the uptake of estradiol by uterine tissue is reduced to the low level observed with diaphragm or other nontarget tissues, which represents nonspecific binding not sensitive to the inhibitor (Fig. 2). Using an *in vitro* system, a dependence of estrogen binding on sulfhydryl groups can be demonstrated (Terenius, 1967; Jensen *et al.,* 1967b,d; Shyamala and Gorski, 1969; Steggles and King, 1970). Treatment of uterine tissue with sulfhydryl-blocking reagents before exposure to estradiol prevents specific hormone uptake, whereas such treatment of uteri previously exposed to estradiol, either *in vivo* or *in vitro,* causes rapid release of the bound hormone.

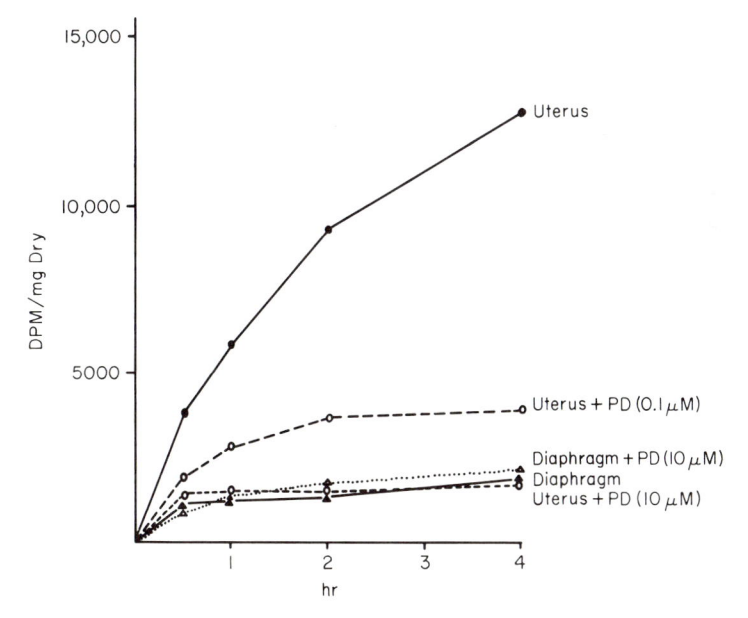

Fig. 2. Tritium levels in slit uterine horns and hemidiaphragms of immature rats after stirring in 0.12 nM estradiol-6,7-^{3}H (57 Ci/mmole) at 37°C in Krebs-Ringer-Henseleit glucose buffer, pH 7.3, in the presence and in the absence of an estrogen antagonist, Parke-Davis CI-628 (PD). Each point is the median value of 5 specimens.

The foregoing studies of the biochemical fate of estrogenic hormones *in vivo* and *in vitro* establish the principal characteristics of the specific interaction of estrogens with the estrophilic components of intact target tissues and provide a basis for evaluating the significance of estrogen-binding phenomena in broken-cell systems. The sensitivity to sulfhydryl reagents and to selective inhibitors, such as nafoxidine and Parke-Davis CI-628, affords valuable criteria for distinguishing the physiological estrogen–receptor interaction from artifacts of nonspecific binding to macromolecules or organelle surfaces.

2. Estrogen–Receptor Complexes and Their Intracellular Localization

Cell fractionation experiments, confirmed by autoradiographic investigations, indicate two sites of estrogen binding in target tissues. When uterine homogenates from estradiol-treated rats are subjected to differential centrifugation, either in sucrose or in hypotonic medium, the incorporated hormone appears principally in two fractions, the high speed supernatant, or cytosol, and the heavy or nuclear-myofibrillar sediment (Talwar *et al.*, 1964; Noteboom and Gorski, 1965; Jensen, 1965a; King and Gordon, 1966; Baulieu *et al.*, 1967; Jensen *et al.*, 1967a). Although some investigators originally reported that the cytosol radioactivity is predominant, our own studies and those of Gorski indicate that, up to 6 hours after estradiol administration, most of the labeled steroid appears in the nuclear fraction, with a smaller amount (20–30%) in the cytosol. Similar results are obtained with anterior pituitary (King *et al.*, 1965a); in rat mammary tumor a somewhat greater proportion of hormone (85–90%) is bound in the nucleus (Kyser, 1970). If the binding inhibitor, nafoxidine, is administered in amounts sufficient partially to inhibit the uptake of estradiol, the ratio of nuclear to cytosol radioactivity in the uterus remains essentially unchanged, suggesting a relation between the two sites of binding (Jensen *et al.*, 1967a).

Autoradiographic localization of tritiated estradiol in rat uterus, using a dry mount technique which minimizes steroid translocation during tissue processing (Stumpf and Roth, 1966), demonstrates a distribution pattern similar to that obtained by cell fractionation (Stumpf, 1968a, 1969; Jensen *et al.*, 1967a,b, 1969a). In all regions of the uterus, most of the radioactive hormone is seen in the nucleus; the extranuclear radioactivity varies from 15–20% of the total in the epithelial glands and myometrium to 35–40% in the lamina propria, strengthening the conclusion that the radioactivity of the cytosol represents extranuclear estradiol.

The correlation of the results of autoradiography with those of cell fractionation provides reassurance that the high estradiol content of the nucleus is not an artifact of redistribution taking place during cell disruption. The autoradiography also indicates that little if any estradiol is bound in the nucleolus (Stumpf, 1969).

The radioactive estradiol taken up by the immature rat uterus is associated with a different form of the receptor substance in the cytosol than in the nucleus. The fact that the hormone in the cytosol is bound to a macromolecule was first indicated by its failure to be included on gel filtration through Sephadex (Talwar et al., 1964). A valuable procedure for characterizing the receptor substances became available with the observation (Toft and Gorski, 1966) that on ultracentrifugation in a sucrose gradient the cytosol complex sediments as a discrete band (Fig. 3A) with a coefficient* originally believed to be 9.5 S but later found to be about 8 S (Erdos, 1968; Rochefort and Baulieu, 1968). In the presence of sodium or potassium chloride at concentrations of 0.2 M or higher, the 8 S complex is reversibly transformed into a more slowly sedimenting entity (Erdos, 1968; Korenman and Rao, 1968; Rochefort and Baulieu, 1968), which, in salt-containing sucrose gradients, migrates just behind bovine plasma albumin (Fig. 3B), or about 4 S (Jensen et al., 1969b). Although this 4 S moiety has been generally considered to be a subunit of the 8 S complex, one cannot exclude the possibility that it is the intact 8 S complex which, in the presence of salt, undergoes extensive conformational change.

The major part of the uterine estradiol, which is found in the nuclear fraction, appears to be associated with chromatin (King et al., 1966; Maurer and Chalkley, 1967; Teng and Hamilton, 1968). The bound hormone can be solubilized, unaccompanied by detectable DNA, by extraction with 0.3 M KCl at pH 7.5 (Jungblut et al., 1967b; Jensen et al., 1967b), or, more effectively, with 0.4 M KCl at pH 8.5 (Puca

* The sedimentation coefficient figures of 8, 5, and 4 S are convenient approximations based on the sedimentation peaks of crude mixtures in sucrose gradients in relation to those of standard proteins, such as yeast alcohol dehydrogenase (7.4 S), γ-globulin (7.0 S), and bovine plasma albumin (4.6 S). The sedimentation rate of the cytosol complex in low salt varies with the degree of dilution. With cytosol from a 20% homogenate, the complex sediments significantly faster than γ-globulin (Fig. 3A) and slightly faster than ADH; after 10-fold dilution, the complex sediments about the same as γ-globulin. The actual sedimentation coefficient of the nuclear complex in salt-containing gradients is probably close to 5.8 S. In salt-containing sucrose gradients, the cytosol complex from calf uterus sediments a little faster than that from rat uterus. Precise values for the sedimentation coefficients of these complexes must await determination in the analytical ultracentrifuge after the receptor proteins have been isolated in purified form.

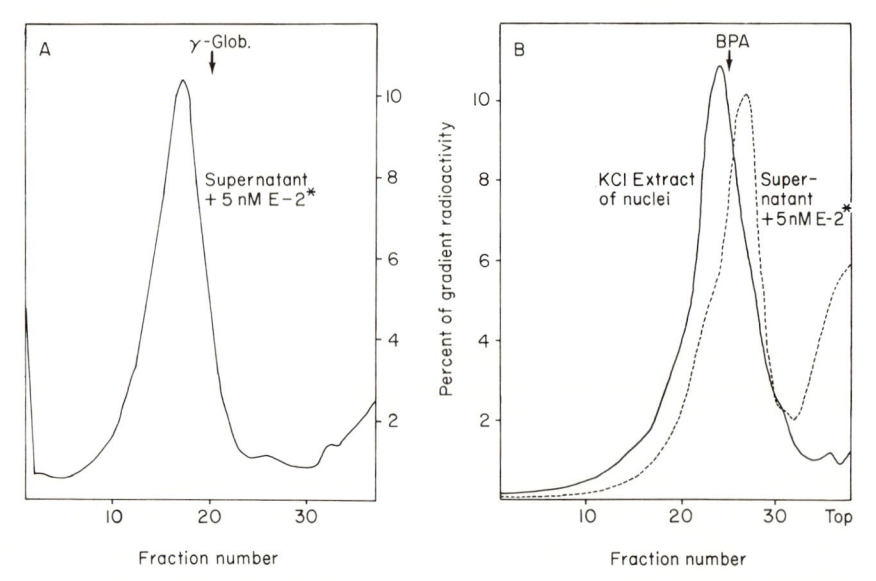

Fig. 3. Sedimentation pattern of radioactive estradiol–receptor complexes obtained from immature rat uteri. Panel A: Uterine cytosol from untreated animals made 5 nM in estradiol-³H and centrifuged in a 10–30% sucrose gradient at 308,000 g for 12 hours at 1°C. Panel B: Cytosol plus 5 nM added estradiol-³H and nuclear extract from uteri excised from immature rats 1 hour after subcutaneous injection of 100 ng (20.8 μCi) of estradiol-³H centrifuged in a 5–20% sucrose gradient containing 400 mM KCl at 284,500 g for 12 hours at 2°C. Total counts per minute on gradient: (A) 30,240; (B) cytosol, 35,380; nuclear extract, 6035. B is from Jensen et al. (1969b). BPA and γ-Glob. indicate positions of bovine plasma albumin and γ-globulin markers.

and Bresciani, 1968a), to yield an estradiol–receptor complex which is easily distinguished from the 4 S unit of the cytosol complex in that it sediments at about 5 S, somewhat faster than bovine plasma albumin (Fig. 3B). In our early experiments (Jensen et al., 1967b), as well as in certain studies of others (Puca and Bresciani, 1968a; Steggles and King, 1970), the nuclear extract was found to sediment at about 5 S whether or not salt is present in the sucrose gradient. More recently we, as well as others (Korenman and Rao, 1968), have found consistently that the complex in the nuclear extract aggregates to a 8–9 S form unless salt is present. The reason for this variable behavior of the nuclear complex under low-salt conditions is not clear.

The uterus of the adult rat differs from that of the immature rat in that a portion of its cytosol receptor sediments in the 4 S form in the absence of salt (Steggles and King, 1969, 1970). A similar phenomenon is observed with cytosol from adult human and monkey uteri (Wyss *et al.*, 1968a) and sheep endometrium (Zimmering *et al.*, 1970), as well as from some, but not all, receptor-containing human breast cancers (Jensen *et al.*, 1971b). After ovariectomy or hypophysectomy, the cytosol receptor pattern is similar to that of the immature rat (Steggles and King, 1970), suggesting a hormonal influence on the properties of the cytosol receptor protein as well as on the total binding capacity discussed earlier.

When immature rat or calf uteri are incubated with dilute solutions of tritiated estradiol at 37°C *in vitro*, the intracellular distribution of uterine radioactivity, as well as the formation of 8 S and 5 S complexes, is quite similar to that observed after hormone administration *in vivo* (Jungblut *et al.*, 1967b; Jensen *et al.*, 1967b, 1969a). But if the tissue is exposed to hormone at 2°C, the major portion (70–75%) of the radioactive steroid appears as 8 S complex in the cytosol fraction and is seen in the extranuclear region on autoradiography (Jensen *et al.*, 1968, 1969a,b; Gorski *et al.*, 1968; Shyamala and Gorski, 1969; Rochefort and Baulieu, 1969). When such uteri, rich in extranuclear 8 S complex, are warmed briefly to 37°C, redistribution of the steroid takes place within the tissue to yield predominantly nuclear bound steroid, extractable as 5 S complex, as determined both by fractionation and by autoradiographic techniques. These observations indicate that radioactive estradiol, which associates with the extranuclear receptor in the cold, can be transferred to its nuclear binding site by a process which is temperature dependent.

The 8 S estradiol–receptor complex, or its 4 S modification, is formed directly, even in the cold, simply by adding tritiated estradiol to the cytosol fraction of uteri not previously exposed to hormone (Toft *et al.*, 1967; Jungblut *et al.*, 1967b; Jensen *et al.*, 1967b). As in the whole tissue, this interaction in the isolated cytosol is prevented by the presence of nafoxidine or CI-628 (Jensen *et al.*, 1969c, 1971b). The total cytosol receptor content of a tissue can be readily estimated by adding an excess of tritiated estradiol to the cytosol and determining the amount of bound hormone. This can be done by measuring the radioactivity present in the 8 S sedimentation peak (Toft *et al.*, 1967; Jensen *et al.*, 1968), adsorbed by hydroxyapatite (Erdos *et al.*, 1970) or by powdered glass in the presence of magnesium ions (Clark and Gorski, 1969; Notides, 1970), precipitated by protamine (Steggles and King, 1970) or remaining in solution after removal of unbound steroid by Sephadex gel filtration (Talwar *et al.*, 1968; Puca and Bresciani, 1969b; Lee and Jacobson, 1971) or adsorption on charcoal (Korenman, 1968, 1969; Méšter *et al.*, 1970). The sedimentation method, although somewhat more laborious, is by far the most accurate and should be used to calibrate other assay procedures.

Using the sucrose gradient technique, it can be demonstrated that immature rat uterus contains a minimum of 100 fmoles of 8 S binding capacity per milligram of wet tissue, corresponding to an average of about 100,000 cytosol receptor sites per uterine cell (Jensen et al., 1968). Lower values reported in the literature probably reflect losses of the labile receptor protein during homogenization and assay procedures. All rat tissues examined appear to contain some of the 8 S binding protein, but target tissues show a much higher content than nontarget tissues (Jensen et al., 1969c). Thus, the difference between target and nontarget tissues, with respect to receptor protein, appears to be quantitative rather than qualitative.

3. Cytosol Dependence of Nuclear Binding

In contrast to the 8 S receptor protein which is a component of the uterine cytosol of hormone-deprived animals, there is no evidence for the presence of the 5 S binding protein in the uterine nucleus before estradiol administration. No 5 S complex is formed either by addition of estradiol to an extract of uterine nuclei or by direct treatment of the nuclei themselves, although it is readily produced when estradiol is incubated either with whole uterine homogenate (Fig. 4) or with purified nuclei or washed nuclear sediment in the presence of the cytosol fraction (Jensen et al., 1967b, 1968, 1969c; Musliner et al., 1970). As is nuclear binding in whole uterine tissue, this production of the 5 S complex in isolated nuclei is temperature dependent. Exposure of uterine nuclei to cytosol and estradiol at 2°C results in a small uptake of radioactivity which, on salt extraction, sediments as 4 S complex, whereas incubation at temperatures of 25–37°C gives a much higher incorporation of radioactivity which is extracted predominantly or exclusively as 5 S complex, depending on the length of the incubation period. If, before mixing with nuclei, the cytosol is heated to 45°C, which destroys the ability of the receptor protein to bind estradiol, no 5 S complex is obtained in the nuclei, demonstrating clearly an important role of the intact cytosol complex in the origin of the 5 S nuclear complex.

More recently it has been found that a 5 S complex, similar in most respects* to that observed in the nuclear extract, is produced by warming a cytosol–estradiol mixture in the absence of nuclei (Brecher et al., 1970;

---

* The estradiol–receptor complex obtained by warming a mixture of estradiol and uterine cytosol sediments slightly faster in salt-containing sucrose gradients than does the complex extracted from the nucleus (Jensen et al., 1971a). Whether this small but consistent discrepancy in sedimentation rate represents a difference in composition of the two "5 S" complexes, or whether it results from a difference in protein milieu between cytosol and nuclear extract, is not certain.

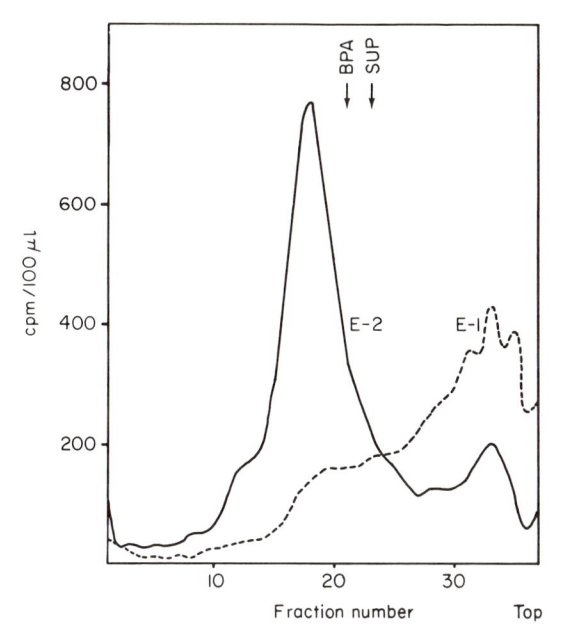

Fig. 4. Sedimentation pattern of KCl extracts of nuclear sediment after incubation of a 10% rat uterine homogenate in 10 mM Tris, pH 8.2, for 30 minutes at 25°C in the presence of 5 nM estradiol-^{3}H(E-2) or estrone-^{3}H(E-1). Centrifugation in a 5–20% sucrose gradient containing 400 mM KCl at 250,000 g for 16 hours at 4°C. BPA and SUP indicate respective positions of bovine plasma albumin marker and 4 S form of the cytosol (supernatant) complex.

Jensen et al., 1971a). This observation suggests that the 4 S binding unit of the cytosol complex is first converted to a 5 S form which then associates with an "acceptor" site in the uterine nucleus.* The temperature dependence of 5 S complex formation in cytosol alone is similar to that observed on incubation with nuclei, and in both cases the rate of 5 S complex production is accelerated with increasing pH, over the range 6.5–8.5, and retarded by the presence of EDTA. Both processes require the presence of estradiol and will not take place with estrone. Although estrone forms a typical 8 S complex and 4 S binding unit when added to uterine cytosol in the cold, after warming with estrone the 4 S unit remains essentially unchanged (Jensen et al., 1971a). If nuclei are present during this incubation, they incorporate a significant

---

* The ability of preformed 5 S cytosol complex both to bind to isolated uterine nuclei and to stimulate their RNA polymerase activity on exposure at 0° (page 261) strongly suggests that the temperature-dependent step is the 4 S to 5 S conversion of the cytosol binding unit.

amount of radioactive estrone, but none of this can be extracted as 5 S complex (Fig. 4). The failure of estrone to promote the 4 S to 5 S conversion of the cytosol binding unit explains the previous finding that, after incubation of immature rat uteri with estrone *in vitro*, 8 S complex is present in the cytosol fraction, but no 5 S complex can be extracted from the nuclei (Jensen *et al.*, unpublished observations). Diethylstilbestrol, hexestrol, estriol, and 17α-ethynylestradiol all promote the 4 S to 5 S transformation, whereas quinestrol (17α-ethynylestradiol 3-cyclopentyl ether) does not (Pakula *et al.*, 1972), confirming the previous demonstration (page 238) of the need for hydroxyl or phenolic groups at both extremities of the hormone molecule.

The participation of the extranuclear receptor protein in the formation of the nuclear estrogen–receptor complex is further indicated by the disappearance of cytosol receptor as estradiol reacts with uterine tissue *in vivo* to become localized in the nucleus. Not only is the total 8 S receptor content of the cytosol less after a large dose of estradiol than after a smaller one (Jensen *et al.*, 1968), but after the injection of a physiological dose of hormone, there is a progressive fall in cytosol receptor level for 4 hours, after which the receptor content is gradually restored, apparently by resynthesis (Jensen *et al.*, 1969b).

Uterine nuclei appear to contain a specific acceptor site which binds the 5 S estradiol–receptor complex. On incubation with estradiol in uterine cytosol, uterine nuclei show a greater uptake of radioactive hormone than do liver, diaphragm, or kidney nuclei, and with uterine nuclei more of the hormone can be extracted as 5 S complex. In the case of diaphragm nuclei, some unexplained transformation takes place to yield an extracted complex sedimenting more slowly than the 4 S binding unit; this is sometimes accompanied by a second entity which sediments at about 4.5 S (Jensen *et al.*, 1969c; Musliner *et al.*, 1970).

4. Properties and Purification of Estrogen Receptor Proteins

The estrogen receptor substances of uterine tissue appear to be mainly protein in composition, inasmuch as both the 8 S cytosol complex (Toft and Gorski, 1966) and the 5 S nuclear complex (Jensen *et al.*, 1971a) are destroyed by the action of proteases but not by nucleases. The 8 S complex binds to ribonuclease to form a more rapidly sedimenting species (Jensen *et al.*, 1969c); this phenomenon probably reflects a general ability of the cytosol complex to associate with basic proteins and peptides as indicated by its precipitation with protamine or polylysine (King *et al.*, 1969; Steggles and King, 1970). The presence of a lipid moiety in the cytosol receptor is suggested by the transformation of the 8 S complex to a 4 S form under the action of lipase (Erdos,

1968), while the possibility that it contains phosphorus is indicated by an apparently successful attempt to label the 8 S receptor protein with ^{32}P by the intraluminal instillation of radioactive orthophosphate *in vivo* (Hughes *et al.*, unpublished observations).

Despite a report to the contrary (Puca and Bresciani, 1970), bound estradiol is clearly liberated from the 8 S cytosol complex by organic mercurials (Jensen *et al.*, 1967d), provided that the uteri have been previously washed to remove contaminants, probably of serum origin, which have a tendency to aggregate with the cytosol complex under the action of these reagents. In contrast, the nuclear complex is not as readily cleaved by sulfhydryl reagents. Although in some instances we have observed partial or total release of bound estradiol, in other experiments, both in our laboratory and elsewhere (Puca and Bresciani, 1970), treatment of the nuclear extract with organic mercurials or N-ethylmaleimide was found to produce a more rapidly sedimenting complex (10–12 S), accompanied by highly aggregated material. This difference between the cytosol and nuclear complexes in reactivity toward sulfhydryl reagents suggests that sulfhydryl groups may become inaccessible during the 4 S to 5 S transformation of the estrogen-binding receptor unit.

The association of estradiol with uterine receptor proteins is an extremely strong interaction. Studies of estradiol binding as a function of hormone concentration—using Sephadex gel filtration (Puca and Bresciani, 1969b; Erdos *et al.*, 1969; Lee and Jacobson, 1971), adsorption on charcoal (Korenman, 1970; Méster *et al.*, 1970) powdered glass (Clark and Gorski, 1969; Notides, 1970), or hydroxyapatite (Erdos *et al.*, 1970; Best-Belpomme *et al.*, 1970), protamine precipitation (Steggles and King, 1970), sucrose gradient centrifugation (Toft *et al.*, 1967), or equilibrium dialysis (Erdos *et al.*, 1968; Baulieu and Raynaud, 1970) to distinguish bound from unbound steroid—have indicated the association constant for the 8 S cytosol complex from uteri of various species to be in the range of 10^9 to 10^{10} M^{-1}. By the gel filtration technique, the K_A of the nuclear complex from calf uteri was likewise found to be 10^9 M^{-1} (Puca and Bresciani, 1969b), although the cytosol receptor of human uterus, after warming with estradiol at 37°C, which presumably transforms the binding unit to a 5 S form, shows a value of 10^{12} (Hähnel, 1971). In our own laboratory, such nonequilibrium procedures as gel filtration or charcoal adsorption give values of 10^{10} or below for the rat or calf cytosol complex, but a kinetic dialysis technique (Jensen *et al.*, unpublished observations) indicates a K_A of about 2×10^{11} M^{-1}. Similarly, calculations based on association–dissociation kinetics indicate the association constant of the calf cytosol complex to be about 10^{12} M^{-1} (Best-Belpomme *et al.*, 1970). These higher values are in agreement with estimates calculated from the uptake and retention of estradiol by rat uteri *in vivo* (Bush, 1965; DeHertogh *et al.*, 1971a) and *in vitro* (Alberga and Baulieu, 1968).

The remarkably tight binding of estradiol to receptor appears to result from an extremely low rate of dissociation (Ellis and Ringold, 1971; Truong and Baulieu, 1971). This may explain the fact that, once the complex is formed, the tritiated estradiol does not readily exchange *in vitro*, even in the presence of a large excess of unlabeled hormone, and that the complex can be studied and purified without need for the continued presence of unbound hormone. The nuclear complex, in which the binding appears as strong or stronger than in the cytosol complex, is readily dissociated at 45°C; the liberated estradiol can be removed by filtration through Sephadex to yield the uncomplexed 5 S receptor protein, which then can react again with estradiol (Puca and Bresciani, 1968a, 1969b).

Whether the 8 S form of the cytosol receptor, observed in low salt, represents a more compact or otherwise less buoyant modification of an asymmetric 4 S protein, an aggregate of 4 S estrogen-binding units or a 4 S unit associated with a nonbinding moiety is not certain. Both in our laboratory and elsewhere (Vonderhaar *et al.*, 1970b), it has been found that the radioactive complex obtained from the 4 S sedimentation peak of a salt-containing sucrose gradient runs more slowly (about 7 S) than the original complex when it is recentrifuged in a salt-free gradient. This phenomenon has been interpreted as evidence for a partial separation of binding and nonbinding components by sedimentation difference (Vonderhaar *et al.*, 1970b). However, the same degree of dilution of the original cytosol without centrifugation causes a similar decrease in the sedimentation rate of the cytosol complex, invalidating any conclusions regarding centrifugal separation of receptor components, except that a nonreaggregable 4 S subunit cannot be prepared by differential sedimentation of the salt-dissociated 8 S complex.

In crude uterine cytosol, the 8 S complex is a rather unstable substance, tending both to decompose and to form large aggregates with other cytosol components. In combination with estradiol, the receptor becomes somewhat more stable toward decomposition, but its tendency to aggregate is enhanced, especially in the presence of magnesium or manganese ions (Brecher *et al.*, 1969). The binding of the 8 S complex to powdered glass in the presence of Mg^{2+} forms the basis of an ingenious assay for the cytosol receptor (Clark and Gorski, 1969).

Because of its instability and tendency toward aggregation, isolation of the purified cytosol receptor protein has proved difficult. Attempted purification by affinity chromatography, using estradiol linked to benzyl cellulose, polystyrene, or Agarose (Jungblut et al., 1967b; Jensen et al., 1967b; Vonderhaar and Mueller, 1969; Cuatrecasas, 1970), has not been successful. Although such columns remove the estrogen-binding capacity of uterine cytosol, the receptor cannot be recovered again in an active form.

Purification of the binding unit of the cytosol receptor by conventional techniques was facilitated by the observation (DeSombre et al., 1969; Jensen et al., 1969c) that addition of calcium ions and salt to uterine cytosol, prepared in the presence of EDTA, yields a "stabilized" 4 S binding unit which does not revert to the 8 S form when the salt is removed and which is highly resistant to aggregation. With mature rat uteri, loss in the ability to re-form the 8 S complex in low salt also takes place on aging of the salt-dissociated cytosol complex in the cold or after incubation of the cytosol at 37°C (Vonderhaar et al., 1970a,b).

Although the calcium-stabilized 4 S complex no longer will undergo transformation to the 5 S form, either in the presence or the absence of uterine nuclei, it represents the fundamental binding unit of the cytosol complex, so that information concerning its composition and structure should provide insight into the nature of at least part of the receptor molecule. By ammonium sulfate precipitation, Sephadex G-200 filtration and DEAE-cellulose chromatography, the calcium stabilized 4 S complex of calf uterine cytosol, obtained by high speed centrifugation, has been purified about 5000-fold and that from low-speed cytosol about 1000-fold, corresponding to purities of about 5% and 1%, respectively, if there is one estradiol bound per 4 S unit. The partially purified 4 S complex shows an apparent molecular weight (Sephadex G-200 elution) of about 75,000 and an isoelectric point of 6.4, in contrast to respective values of 200,000 and 5.8 observed with the 8 S cytosol complex (DeSombre et al., 1969). Subsequent studies, involving determination of Stokes radii, indicate molecular weights of 236,000 for the 8 S complex and 61,000 for the stabilized 4 S complex, as well as isoelectric points of 6.6–7.0 and 6.2, respectively (Puca et al., 1971). The product from low speed cytosol has been further purified by acrylamide gel electrophoresis to yield a material showing a single radioactive protein band by amido black staining, probably the first time the receptor protein has been detected by any criterion except the radioactivity of the steroid bound to it (DeSombre et al., 1971a).

Under most conditions, the 5 S complex, extracted by KCl from the nucleus, undergoes aggregation to a 8–9 S form when the salt is removed. Unlike the binding unit of the cytosol complex, the nuclear complex is not stabilized toward this aggregation by treatment with calcium ions. However, after ammonium sulfate precipitation followed by gel filtration in the presence of KCl, the nuclear complex loses its tendency to aggregate in low salt and can be further purified by ion-exchange chromatography and/or acrylamide gel electrophoresis at pH 8.8, where it moves considerably faster than the calcium-stabilized 4 S complex of the cytosol. In this way the nuclear complex, prepared by incubating estradiol and calf uterine cytosol with preextracted calf uterine nuclei, has been obtained in substantially purified form. This partially purified nuclear complex shows clear differences from the stabilized 4 S complex both in sedimentation and electrophoretic properties (DeSombre *et al.*, 1971b).

III. Progestins

A. *Early Effects of Progestins on Cellular Processes*

Although a wealth of information is available regarding the gross biological and morphological responses to progestins in tissues of the reproductive tract, systematic investigations of the early hormonal effects on biochemical processes have been relatively few. Much of the detailed information concerning the early effects of progestins in target tissue cells have been obtained from experiments with the estrogen-prestimulated chick oviduct, since in this organ progestins induce the synthesis of a specific protein, avidin (O'Malley *et al.*, 1967, 1969). This hormone-specific induction has been observed after the administration of progesterone or other progestational hormones (O'Malley *et al.*, 1967) to diethylstilbestrol-treated chicks *in vivo* (Korenman and O'Malley, 1968), to minced oviduct tissue *in vitro* (O'Malley, 1967), as well as to oviduct cells maintained in tissue culture (O'Malley and Kohler, 1967a,b). The stimulation of avidin synthesis, detectable 10 hours after hormone treatment *in vivo* or 6 hours *in vitro*, takes place under conditions where there is no increase in other major oviduct proteins, such as ovalbumin and lysozyme (O'Malley, 1967).

During the induction of avidin, progesterone does not increase the incorporation of tritiated thymidine into DNA, and, based on experiments involving partial blockage of DNA synthesis by hydroxyurea, which does not inhibit or delay avidin synthesis, its action does not appear to require new synthesis of DNA (O'Malley and McGuire, 1968). New DNA-dependent RNA synthesis is required for the hormonal effect, as shown by the fact that actinomycin D, administered at the same time as the progesterone, causes a 90% reduction in the stimulation of avidin synthesis without inhibiting general protein synthesis (O'Malley et al., 1969). It is interesting that when actinomycin D is administered 6 hours after progesterone, an increased rather than a decreased rate of avidin synthesis is observed (O'Malley and McGuire, 1968). This phenomenon of "superinduction" is similar to that described for glucocorticoid action in hepatoma cells *in vitro* (Tomkins et al., 1969).

Although no change in the total RNA content follows the *in vitro* exposure of oviduct tissue to the hormone, there is a significant initial decrease in the specific activity of rapidly labeled nuclear RNA which is followed by a marked rise in its specific activity prior to the appearance of avidin (O'Malley et al., 1969). A similar fall and subsequent rise are seen in the RNA polymerase activity of isolated oviduct nuclei, measured either in the presence or the absence of ammonium sulfate, after administration of progesterone to chicks *in vivo*, whether or not they have been prestimulated with estrogen (McGuire and O'Malley, 1968).

The action of progesterone appears to increase chromatin template activity and to induce the synthesis of new species of RNA, as determined by DNA-RNA hybridization and nearest neighbor frequency analysis of the resulting RNA (O'Malley and McGuire, 1969; O'Malley et al., 1968, 1969). These effects on RNA synthesis occur before any influence on avidin production is evident.

On the basis of the foregoing experimental observations, it appears that, by an as yet unknown mechanism, the progestational hormones bring about the expression of new regions of DNA template giving rise to new species of RNA which are involved in the synthesis of avidin. The relation of these effects to the progesterone–receptor interactions, described in the next section, still remains to be established.

B. Progestin–Receptor Interactions

1. Binding of Progestins by Target Tissues *in Vivo* and *in Vitro*

The first attempts to demonstrate specific progesterone binding gave no evidence for the presence of characteristic progestin receptors in uterus or other target tissues. The observation that the ability of the ovariectomized mouse vagina to retain locally administered progesterone is markedly increased after treatment with estrogen (Podratz and Katzman, 1968) suggested that the level of progesterone-binding substances in target tissues may be enhanced by estrogen stimulation. Subsequent experiments have firmly established the estrogen dependence of progesterone binding, and during the past two years, rapid progress has been made in the study of progesterone–receptor interactions, both *in vivo* and *in vitro*.

In comparison to estrogens, considerably fewer studies with progesterone have been carried out in the whole animal, inasmuch as investigators have tended to proceed directly to *in vitro* incubations of tissue segments and to binding studies with cell fractions. A few careful *in vivo* investigations have been carried out, which provide a basis of reference for evaluating binding phenomena in cell-free systems.

The ovariectomized guinea pig uterus shows a small uptake and retention of progesterone *in vivo*; this incorporation is increased 7-fold (Fig. 5) by pretreatment of the animal with estrogen (Falk and Bardin, 1970). In the same tissue, estrogen priming significantly increases the concentration of uterine receptor molecules (Milgrom *et al.*, 1970). Although concentration of progesterone above the blood level is not observed in the chick oviduct, specific progesterone binding to macromolecules can be demonstrated both *in vivo* and *in vitro*, with a binding capacity after diethylstilbestrol pretreatment which is twenty times greater than that observed in oviducts from chicks not treated with estrogen (O'Malley *et al.*, 1969, 1970). In the ovariectomized rabbit, the incorporation of progesterone by uterus *in vivo* is greater than that

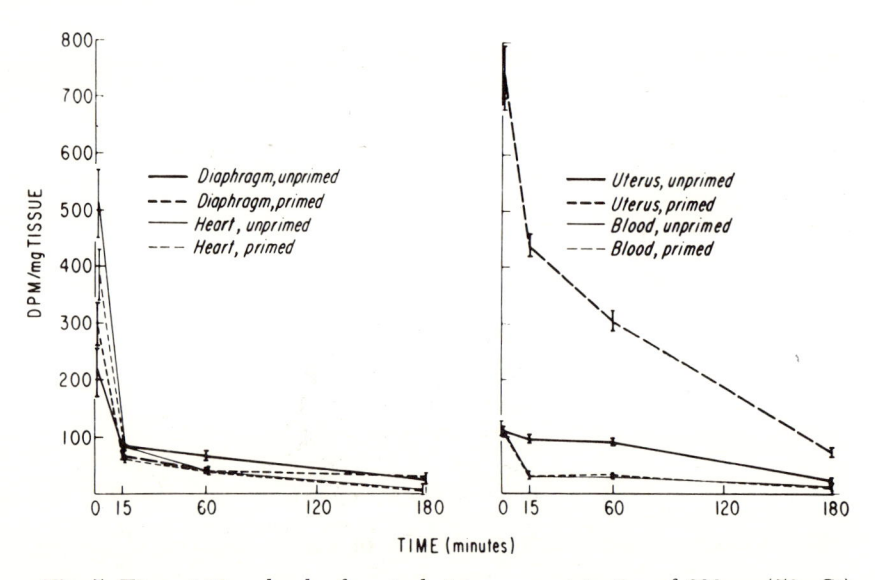

Fig. 5. Tissue tritium levels after single intravenous injection of 286 ng (50 μCi) of progesterone-1,2-^{3}H to castrate guinea pigs. Estrogen-primed animals received 1 μg of estrone twice daily for 2 days. Each point is the mean of 10 animals. From Falk and Bardin (1970).

by thigh muscle; the uptake in uterus but not in muscle is increased 2- to 4-fold by preliminary administration of estradiol (Wiest and Rao, 1971). The binding of progesterone by the uterus and vagina is increased by estrogen pretreatment in the ovariectomized hamster and varies with the ovarian cycle in the intact hamster (Reuter et al., 1970). Progesterone uptake *in vitro* has been observed in uterine segments from immature rats, in which case estrogen prestimulation apparently is not required for substantial progesterone binding to occur (McGuire and DeDella, 1971). The effect of estrogen priming on the properties of the receptor molecules is described in the next section.

The specificity of progesterone binding, as defined by the limited capacity of binding sites, is demonstrated both *in vivo* (Falk and Bardin, 1970) and *in vitro* (McGuire and DeDella, 1971) by the diminution of radioactive progesterone uptake by the presence of unlabeled progesterone but not of estradiol, testosterone, or cortisol. Similarly, tritiated cortisol does not show selective uptake by the uterine issue of the estrogen-primed guinea pig (Falk and Bardin, 1970).

Although the progesterone administered undergoes extensive metabolic transformation in the whole animal (Falk and Bardin, 1970) and is readily reduced to 5α-pregnane-3, 20-dione by isolated uterine nuclei of estrogen-treated castrate rats (Armstrong and King, 1970), the steroid taken up and specifically bound by target tissues appears to be chiefly progesterone itself. One and 3 hours after tritiated progesterone injection, unchanged progesterone comprises 88 and 72%, respectively, of the radioactivity present in the estrogen-primed guinea pig uterus (Falk and Bardin, 1970); the remainder of the uterine radioactivity may reflect the level of other radioactive substances in the blood plasma (Fig. 5). Up to 2 hours after progesterone administration to the estrogen-primed ovariectomized rabbit, most of the nuclear and nearly all of the extranuclear steroid bound in the uterus can be identified as progesterone (Wiest and Rao, 1971). However, 4 hours after injection of progesterone into the ovariectomized rat, most of the uterine radioactivity is found to be a polar unconjugated progesterone metabolite, present at seven times the plasma level (Reel et al., 1969; McGuire and DeDella, 1971). The uterine concentration of this substance is not sensitive to estrogen pretreatment, and its relation to specific progesterone–receptor interaction is not clear.

On incubation with rat uterine tissue *in vitro*, progesterone appears to be incorporated without chemical change (McGuire and DeDella, 1971). The same is true for brief *in vitro* treatment of chick oviduct (O'Malley et al., 1970), although on incubations of 1 hour or longer extensive conversion of progesterone to polar metabolites takes place

(O'Malley et al., 1969). It would appear that target tissues can actively metabolize progesterone, but that the initial interaction of progesterone with receptor substances takes place without metabolic transformation of the steroid. This conclusion is substantiated by studies in cell-free systems to be described later.

2. Progestin–Receptor Complexes and Their Intracellular Localization

Cell fractionation experiments indicate that, in target tissues of the estrogen-prestimulated animal, progesterone is specifically bound both in the cytosol and in the nucleus. However, the predominantly nuclear localization seen with the estrogens is not evident with progesterone. In the chick oviduct, somewhat more radioactive steroid appears in the cytosol than in the nuclear fraction, especially 1–8 minutes after progesterone injection (O'Malley et al., 1970, 1971a). In the ovariectomized rabbit uterus, approximately equal amounts of cytosol and nuclear radioactivity are obtained, with little steroid observed in the mitochondrial or microsomal fractions (Wiest and Rao, 1971). Only a few preliminary attempts at autoradiographic localization of progestins in target tissues have been reported; these have indicated cytoplasmic rather than nuclear

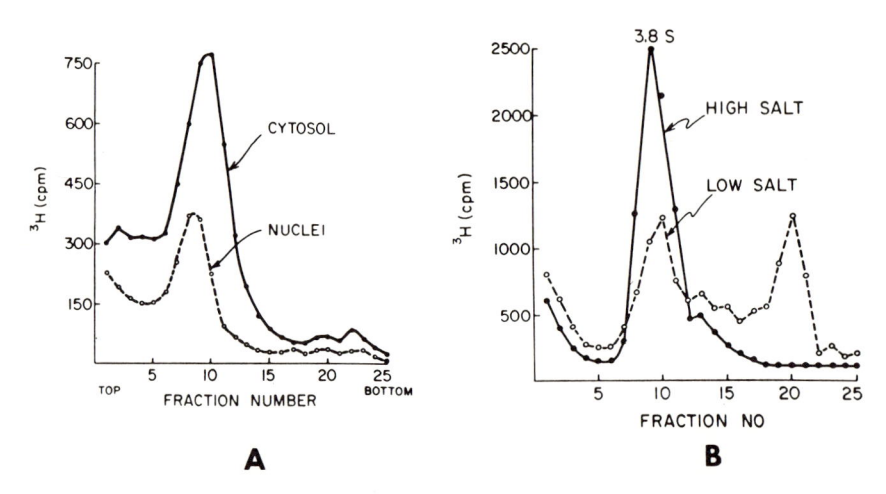

Fig. 6. Sedimentation patterns of radioactive progesterone–receptor complexes obtained from chick oviduct. Panel A: Cytosol and nuclear extract from tissue excised 8 minutes after intravenous injection of 845 ng (90 μCi) of progesterone-³H centrifuged in a 5–20% sucrose gradient containing 300 mM KCl at 204,000 g for 16 hours at 1°C. Panel B: Oviduct cytosol from untreated chicks made 10 nM in progesterone-³H and centrifuged under similar conditions in a 5–20% sucrose gradient in the presence and the absence of 300 mM KCl. From O'Malley et al. (1970).

localization in the rat uterus for both progesterone (Rogers et al., 1966) and norethynodrel (Stumpf, 1968a).

As in the case of estrogens, progesterone binding in the nucleus, but not the cytosol, is markedly temperature dependent. After exposure of chick oviduct segments to tritiated progesterone at 0°C *in vitro*, the incorporated radioactivity appears almost exclusively in the cytosol; when these tissues containing extranuclear progesterone are then incubated at 37°C, the nuclear radioactivity steadily increases until at 30 minutes 75% of the radioactivity has shifted to the nucleus (O'Malley et al., 1970, 1971a).

The progesterone present in both the cytosol and nuclear fractions of target tissue cells is bound to macromolecules which can be characterized by the technique of sucrose gradient ultracentrifugation. As in the case of estrogen, the progesterone–receptor complex present in the nucleus is solubilized by extraction with 0.3 or 0.4 M KCl. That the complex actually is intranuclear is indicated by its failure to be released when the outer nuclear membrane is removed by Triton X-100 (O'Malley et al., 1971a). After administration of the hormone *in vivo* (Fig. 6A) or exposure of tissue segments to progesterone at 37°C *in vitro*, the complexes of both the cytosol and the nuclear extract from chick oviducts sediment at about 4 S in sucrose gradients containing KCl (O'Malley et al., 1970, 1971a). The cytosol complex can be prepared in higher yield by direct addition of tritiated progesterone to the supernatant fraction (Fig. 6B); this product sediments at 3.8 S in salt-containing gradients, but as a mixture of 5 S and 8 S components in salt-free gradients (O'Malley et al., 1970, 1971b; Sherman et al., 1970). The cytosol complex of chick oviduct also can be recognized by its elution from Agarose columns; by this technique, no receptor can be detected in the cytosol of chick lung or spleen (Sherman et al., 1970).

Not only is the total amount of cytosol receptor increased by estrogen pretreatment (O'Malley et al., 1970; Milgrom et al., 1970; Rao and Wiest, 1971), but the sedimentation behavior of the cytosol complex in low-salt sucrose gradients is markedly influenced by this prestimulation. With the ovariectomized rabbit uterus which has not been primed with estrogen, the progesterone–receptor complex of the cytosol sediments at about 4 S in low salt, either after administration of progesterone *in vivo* (Wiest and Rao, 1971) or direct addition of the hormone to the cytosol (McGuire and DeDella, 1971). After estrogen pretreatment, followed by injection of tritiated progesterone *in vivo*, the uterine cytosol shows sedimentation peaks at both 8 S and 4 S in salt-free gradients but a single 4 S peak in gradients containing KCl (Wiest and Rao, 1971). The nuclear extract from these uteri shows a 4 S sedimentation peak, even in low salt. With the ovariectomized guinea pig not primed with estrogen, the complex formed by adding tritiated progesterone to the uterine cytosol sediments at 4–5 S, whereas, after estrogen priming, the cytosol complex, obtained either after progesterone injection *in vivo* or addition of the hormone to the cytosol, sediments at 6.7 S in the absence of salt, shifting to 4.3 S in salt-containing sucrose gradients (Milgrom *et al.*, 1970).

Thus, it would appear that, in rabbit and guinea pig uterus and probably in chick oviduct, estrogen prestimulation causes the 4 S binding unit of the cytosol progesterone receptor to convert partly or entirely to a form which sediments more rapidly in low salt gradients. This is the converse of its effect on the estrogen receptor of rat uterus, where the cytosol complex of the immature or ovariectomized rat sediments at 8 S in low salt but that of the animal with functioning ovaries exists partially in a 4 S form (Steggles and King, 1970). The influence of estrogen on the progesterone complex is not a direct effect on the receptor protein, inasmuch the addition of estradiol to rabbit cytosol does not alter the sedimentation pattern of the 4 S and 8 S peaks (Wiest and Rao, 1971).

The presence of specific progesterone–receptor complexes in extracts of rat uterine tissue has not been established with certainty. After incubation of tritiated progesterone with segments of traumatized pseudopregnant rat uterus at 37°C (Reel *et al.*, 1970) or addition of the hormone to uterine cytosol from estrogen-primed castrated rats (Milgrom and Baulieu, 1970), the cytosol contains progesterone as a 4 S complex. But in contrast to the interactions of progesterone with chick oviduct or rabbit and guinea pig uterus, which are neither shared nor inhibited by cortisol, rat uterine cytosol forms a 4 S complex with cortisol as well as with progesterone, raising the question whether the complex in rat uterus might involve corticoid binding proteins from the blood. Although the progesterone and cortisol complexes are reported to possess different thermal stabilities (Reel *et al.*, 1970), the marked similarities in their properties observed by others (Milgrom and Baulieu, 1970), including precipitation by antibodies to rat serum, renders the significance of these complexes open to question until more experimental work has been done.

Binding to the receptor substances of chick oviduct and guinea pig or rabbit uterus is specific for progesterone and other progestational compounds, such as norethindrone, norethynodrel, medroxyprogesterone acetate, and chlormadinone, and in general is not seen with cortisol, aldosterone, estrogens, or androgens (O'Malley *et al.*, 1970; Milgrom *et al.*, 1970; McGuire and DeDella, 1971; Wiest and Rao, 1971). From its ability to compete with progesterone binding, 5α-pregnane-3, 20-dione shows significant affinity for progesterone receptors in oviduct (O'Malley et al., 1970) and guinea pig uterus (Milgrom et al., 1970) but is less tightly bound in rabbit uterus (Wiest and Rao, 1971). Only with the cytosol receptor of chick oviduct does testosterone appear to compete for progesterone binding sites (Sherman et al., 1970).

3. Cytosol Dependence of Nuclear Binding

In similarity with the estrogen–receptor interaction, the cytosol progesterone–receptor complex is formed directly on mixing the hormone with the cytosol fraction of target tissues, and there is no evidence for the presence of any receptor substance in the nucleus before the tissue has been exposed to progesterone. Incubation of chick oviduct nuclei with tritiated progesterone in buffer gives no extractable progesterone complex unless oviduct cytosol is also present, in which case the 4 S nuclear complex is readily formed (O'Malley et al., 1971a). In contrast to the marked temperature dependence of nuclear progesterone binding observed with whole oviduct tissue *in vitro*, the interaction of oviduct nuclei with progesterone and cytosol gives a better yield of 4 S nuclear complex at 0°C than at 23°C or 37°C (O'Malley et al., 1970, 1971a). This result may reflect thermal instability of the receptor proteins in the cell-free system.

The participation of the progesterone–receptor complex of oviduct cytosol in the formation of the nuclear complex is further indicated both by the cytosol specificity of the nuclear binding and by the depletion of cytosol receptor content which takes place when whole oviduct tissue interacts with progesterone *in vitro* (O'Malley et al., 1971a). If lung or liver cytosol is substituted for oviduct cytosol, no 4 S complex is formed in oviduct nuclei.

When lung or liver nuclei are incubated with tritiated progesterone and oviduct cytosol, radioactive hormone is taken up, but none of this is extracted as 4 S complex (O'Malley et al., 1971a). Thus, oviduct nuclei appear to possess characteristic acceptor sites for the cytosol complex which are not present in lung and liver nuclei. This nuclear acceptor site appears to be associated with the chromatin; experiments in which the separated constituents of the chromatin from different tissues are reassembled in various combinations indicate that the specificity of the nuclear acceptor site for the cytosol progesterone–receptor complex lies in the acidic nuclear proteins rather than in the histones or the DNA (Spelsberg et al., 1971; O'Malley et al., 1971b).

4. Properties and Purification of Progesterone Receptor Proteins

Like the estrogen receptors, the progesterone-binding substances of target tissues appear to be thermolabile, sulfhydryl-containing proteins. The cytosol complexes of chick oviduct (Sherman et al., 1970) and rabbit uterus (Wiest and Rao, 1971) are cleaved by treatment with pronase, but not by RNase or DNase; the oviduct complex, as well as that of guinea pig uterus (Milgrom et al., 1970), is destroyed by warming to 60°C or by exposure to p-hydroxymercuribenzoate in the cold.

From the ratio of bound-to-free steroid after sedimentation in sucrose gradients, the dissociation constant of the cytosol complex of chick oviduct has been estimated as 8×10^{-10} M (Sherman et al., 1970) and that of the guinea pig uterus as 5×10^{-10} M (Milgrom et al., 1970). Using charcoal to separate free from bound steroid, a K_D of about 2×10^{-10} M is obtained for rabbit oviduct (Rao and Wiest, 1971). The concentration of cytosol binding sites reported for chick oviduct and guinea pig uterus can be expressed as approximately 75 and 20 fmoles per milligram of fresh tissue, respectively. These values are in the same range as those reported for estradiol receptor sites in rat uterus. The cytosol progesterone complex can also be assayed by the binding to glass powder in the presence of magnesium ions (O'Malley et al., 1971b) in a manner similar to the estrogen receptor (Clark and Gorski, 1969).

The nuclear complex of chick oviduct also is destroyed by warming to 60°C or by treatment with pronase or N-ethylmaleimide (O'Malley et al., 1971a). Unlike the estrogen complexes, the nuclear and cytosol progesterone–receptor complexes of chick oviduct cannot be differentiated in the presence of KCl, either by sedimentation or by elution behavior on Agarose columns. By the latter criterion, the apparent molecular weights of both complexes are approximately 100,000 (O'Malley et al., 1971a).

On gel filtration, ion-exchange chromatography, acrylamide-gel electrophoresis and isoelectric focusing, the progesterone–receptor complex of chick oviduct cytosol is resolved into two components; these differ with respect to molecular size and charge, with isoelectric points of 4.0 and 4.5, respectively (O'Malley et al., 1971b). By the sequence of ammonium sulfate precipitation, gel filtration with Agarose, ion-exchange chromatography on DEAE-cellulose and sucrose gradient centrifugation, the cytosol complex, stabilized by the presence of thioglycerol, has been purified approximately 2500-fold.

IV. Hormone–Receptor Interaction Pattern and Its Biochemical Significance

On the basis of a variety of self-consistent experimental evidence described in the foregoing sections, it appears that estrogens and progestins interact with their respective target tissues by similar two-step mechanisms in which the hormone first binds to an extranuclear receptor protein, which is a characteristic component of hormone-dependent tissues. By a temperature-dependent process, the steroid–receptor complex is translocated to the nucleus, where it associates with a specific acceptor site, again characteristic of the target tissue, and in some way causes the acceleration of certain nuclear biosynthetic processes. In the case of estrogens, nuclear transfer is either accompanied (Fig. 7, pathway I) or preceded (Fig. 7, pathway II) by conversion of the receptor binding unit from a 4 S to a 5 S form; with progesterone, no characteristic alteration of the receptor during nuclear transfer has yet been demonstrated.

A relation between the cytosol and nuclear estrogen–receptor complexes in rat uterine tissue was first suggested by observations that nafoxidine inhibits cytosol and nuclear binding to the same degree (Jensen et al., 1967a), by considerations that the cytosol protein, which is present in excess amount and can associate directly with estradiol, might serve as the nonsaturable "uptake receptor" for subsequent nuclear retention (Jensen et al., 1967b), and by the finding that more radioactivity is bound to uterine nuclei on incubation with tritiated estradiol in the presence of uterine cytosol than in its absence (Brecher et al., 1967).

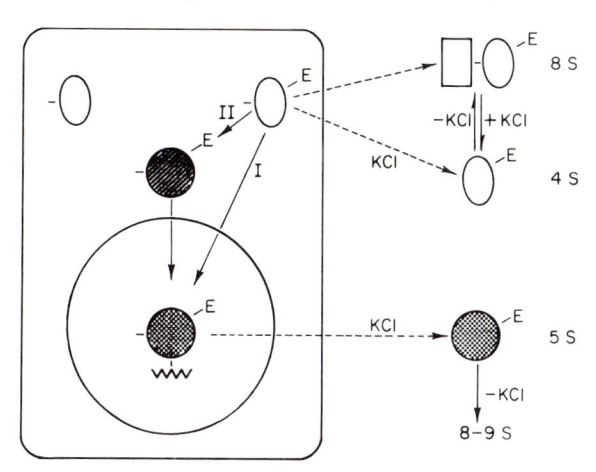

Fig. 7. Two-step interaction pattern of estrogen (E) with receptors in uterine cells.

The present two-step interaction mechanism (Fig. 7), modified in certain details (Jensen *et al.*, 1971a) from its original proposal (Gorski *et al.*, 1968; Jensen *et al.*, 1968) on the basis of subsequent information concerning the 4 S binding unit and its transformation to a 5 S form, rests principally on three pieces of experimental evidence: the cytosol requirement for 5 S complex production in isolated uterine nuclei, the temperature-induced shift of extranuclear 8 S estradiol to nuclear 5 S estradiol in uterine tissue *in vitro*, and the striking temporary depletion of cytosol receptor protein which takes place *in vivo* as estradiol becomes bound in rat uterine nuclei. An analogous mechanism for the interaction of progesterone with chick oviduct is likewise indicated by the requirement for oviduct cytosol in nuclear complex formation, the temperature dependence of nuclear binding, and the depletion of cytosol receptor content when oviduct tissue reacts with progesterone *in vitro* (O'Malley *et al.*, 1970, 1971a). In the case of progesterone, there is evidence that the specificity of the nuclear acceptor site involves the acidic protein components of the oviduct chromatin (Spelsberg *et al.*, 1971).

How the steroid induces the receptor protein to move to the nucleus, and how the hormone leaves the nucleus and the cell once its function is completed, are important questions about which little is known. It has been suggested (Jungblut *et al.*, 1970) that the cytosol receptor is not free in the cytoplasm but is a part of the cell membrane or endoplasmic reticulum, from which it is extracted during homogenization, and that elements of this structure accompany the hormone–receptor complex in its transfer to the nucleus. Recent photomicroscopic evidence indicates that lysosomes of uterine cells are induced to migrate to the nucleus after stimulation with estrogen *in vivo*, suggesting that these structures may function as carriers of the extranuclear estradiol–receptor complex (Smith and Szego, 1971). The nuclear turnover of estradiol appears to be considerably more rapid than would be implied by the overall radioactivity retention pattern, as indicated by the fact that, in the immature rat, the depletion of uterine cytosol receptor content after the injection of a physiological dose of estradiol is four to five times greater than can be accounted for by the estradiol present in the nucleus (Jensen *et al.*, 1971a). It is possible that, on leaving the nucleus, estradiol encounters more extranuclear receptor and repeats the interaction cycle, so that each estradiol molecule may effect the transfer of several receptor molecules to the nucleus before it finally escapes from the cell.

In considering how the foregoing sequence of steroid–receptor interactions might be related to the hormone-induced acceleration of biosynthetic reactions in the target cell nucleus, one must recognize two alternative possibilities: the protein may be needed to carry the hormone to the nucleus or the steroid may serve to promote nuclear transfer of the protein (Jensen et al., 1969b,c, 1971a). Although the receptor system may be simply a transport device to deliver the hormone to the proper nuclear location, where it leaves the receptor and exerts its action by some undefined mechanism, it is attractive to consider that the receptor protein itself may play a role in some key nuclear process and that the function of the steroid is to enable the protein to reach its action site. The presence of increased amounts of extranuclear receptor in the hormone-responsive tissues may reflect the inability of this protein to penetrate the nucleus in such tissues until association with the steroid promotes its conversion to an active form (pathway II, Fig. 7).

That the transformed receptor protein may be the active species in estrogen action is suggested by the effect of the 5 S, but not the 4 S, complex in enhancing RNA synthesis in isolated uterine nuclei. Recently it was observed (Raynaud-Jammet and Baulieu, 1969) that nuclei, isolated in sucrose from heifer endometrium, show a significant increase in their ability to incorporate radioactive nucleotide into RNA *in vitro* after they have been incubated with uterine cytosol containing estradiol but not with cytosol or estradiol alone. It was then shown (Mohla et al., 1971a,b) that this enhancement of RNA synthetic capacity takes place only under conditions which permit transformation of the receptor from the 4 S to the 5 S form. Calf endometrium nuclei are activated by incubation for 30 minutes at 25°C with cytosol containing estradiol, but not with cytosol and estrone, which, as discussed earlier, can not effect 4 S to 5 S conversion. No effect of cytosol plus estradiol is seen after incubation with nuclei at 0°C unless the hormone–cytosol mixture has previously been warmed to effect transformation, in which case activation of the nuclei is effected in the cold. The 5 S estradiol receptor complex extracted by KCl from previously treated uterine nuclei is fully active in stimulating fresh nuclei. The tissue specificity of the phenomenon is indicated by the fact that, after incubation with estradiol in rat uterine cytosol, nuclei from immature rat uterus show markedly increased synthetic capacity, whereas the already high levels of RNA synthesis in rat liver and kidney nuclei are not changed by incubation with estradiol, either in their own cytosols or in uterine cytosol.

The foregoing enhancement of RNA synthetic capacity in uterine nuclei involves significant increase in "soluble" as well as "aggregate" RNA polymerase activity, indicating that at least part of the phenomenon is independent of any effect on chromatin template function (Mohla et al., 1971b). This conclusion is also indicated by experiments in which the hormone–receptor mixture is added directly to the RNA polymerase assay system (Beziat et al., 1970; Hough et al., 1970; Arnaud et al., 1971a). Under these conditions, the salt-dissociated cytosol complex (presumably transformed from the 4 S to the 5 S form, inasmuch as complexing with estradiol is effected at 37°C), as well as the 5 S complex extracted from the nucleus, causes a significant increase in the activity of the aggregate enzyme prepared from heifer endometrium nuclei, although the soluble enzyme apparently is not stimulated. In subsequent studies it was shown that it is the RNA polymerase of the uterine nucleolus which is affected by the addition of cytosol complex (Arnaud et al., 1971b).

The degree of enhancement of RNA synthetic capacity of uterine nuclei when they are treated with the estradiol–receptor complex *in vitro* is comparable to that observed when the hormone is administered *in vivo* (Gorski, 1964; Nicolette et al., 1968; Hamilton et al., 1968) and is considerably greater than that which would correspond to new messenger for a single protein species. Thus, the relation of this effect to the formation of the induced proteins discussed in Section II,A is not clear. Still the tissue and steroid specificity associated with this nuclear stimulation suggests that the phenomenon may be of physiological significance and that it may provide a valuable system for evaluating the biological activity of purified receptor proteins, when these become available, leading to a more detailed understanding of the mechanism of estrogen action.

The two-step sequence, involving nuclear transfer of an extranuclear receptor protein, represents a general pattern of interaction, not only for estrogenic and progestational hormones, but for other classes of steroid hormones as well. As summarized in more detail elsewhere (Jensen et al., 1971a), recent studies of Liao, Mainwaring, Baulieu, Sekeris, Tomkins, Munck, and Edelman have demonstrated that target tissues for androgens, glucocorticoids, and mineralocorticoids likewise possess extranuclear receptor proteins, specific for the particular steroid hormone, which show remarkable similarities in their general properties. In all cases, the hormone forms an initial complex with the receptor protein, which, by a temperature-dependent process, is then transferred to the nucleus, where hormonal action appears to be initiated.

It is tempting to speculate that the two-step steroid–receptor interaction mechanism may represent one of two general patterns for hormonal control in mammalian cells. In the case of certain catecholamine and peptide hormones, it appears likely that a primary action of the hormone is to activate an adenyl cyclase system at the cell membrane to generate a cyclic nucleotide, which then serves as a second messenger carrying out a specific action somewhere in the cell (Sutherland and Robison, 1966). In the case of the steroid hormones, it is possible that it is the hormone-activated receptor protein, present in unique amounts in the particular target tissue, which delivers the regulatory message. When receptor proteins are isolated in pure form and the details of the hormone-dependent thermal transformation are elucidated, we should have a much clearer understanding of the fundamental mechanism of steroid hormone action.

References

Aizawa, Y., and Mueller, G. C. (1961). *J. Biol. Chem.* 236, 381.
Alberga, A., and Baulieu, E. E. (1965). *C. R. Acad. Sci., Ser. D* 261, 5226.
Alberga, A., and Baulieu, E. E. (1968). *Mol. Pharmacol.* 4, 311.
Armstrong, D. T., and King, E. R. (1970). *Fed. Proc. Fed. Amer. Soc. Exp. Biol.* 29, 250.
Arnaud, M., Beziat, Y., Guilleux, J. C., Hough, A., Hough, D., and Mousseron-Canet, M. (1971a). *Biochim. Biophys. Acta* 232, 117.
Arnaud, M., Beziat, Y., Guilleux, J. C., and Mousseron-Canet, M. (1971b). *C. R. Acad. Sci., Ser. D* 272, 635.
Attramadal, A. (1970). *Z. Zellforsch. Mikrosk. Anat.* 104, 572.
Attramadal, A., and Aakvaag, A. (1970). *Z. Zellforsch. Mikrosk. Anat.* 104, 582.
Barker, K. L. (1971). *Biochemistry* 10, 284.
Barker, K. L., and Warren, J. C. (1966). *Proc. Nat. Acad. Sci. U.S.* 56, 1298.
Barnea, A., and Gorski, J. (1970). *Biochemistry* 9, 1899.
Barry, J., and Gorski, J. (1971). *Biochemistry* 10, 2384.
Barton, R. W., and Liao, S. (1967). *Endocrinology* 81, 409.
Baulieu, E. E., and Raynaud, J. P. (1970). *Eur. J. Biochem.* 13, 293.
Baulieu, E. E., Alberga, A., and Jung, I. (1967). *C. R. Acad. Sci., Ser. D* 265, 454.
Best-Belpomme, M., Fries, J., and Erdos, T. (1970). *Eur. J. Biochem.* 17, 425.
Beziat, Y., Guilleux, J. C., and Mousseron-Canet, M. (1970). *C. R. Acad. Sci., Ser. D* 270, 1620.
Billing, R. J., Barbiroli, B., and Smellie, R. M. S. (1969a). *Biochem. J.* 112, 563.
Billing, R. J., Barbiroli, B., and Smellie, R. M. S. (1969b). *Biochim. Biophys. Acta* 190, 52.
Billing, R. J., Barbiroli, B., and Smellie, R. M. S. (1969c). *Biochim. Biophys. Acta* 190, 60.
Bitman, J., Cecil, H. C., Mench, M. L., and Wren, T. R. (1965). *Endocrinology* 76, 63.
Braunsberg, H., Irvine, W. T., and James, V. H. T. (1967). *Brit. J. Cancer* 21, 714.
Brecher, P. I., and Wotiz, H. H. (1967). *Steroids* 9, 431.
Brecher, P. I., Vigersky, R., Wotiz, H. S., and Wotiz, H. H. (1967). *Steroids* 10, 635.
Brecher, P. I., Pasquina, A., and Wotiz, H. H. (1969). *Endocrinology* 85, 612.

Brecher, P. I., Numata, M., DeSombre, E. R., and Jensen, E. V. (1970). *Fed. Proc. Fed. Amer. Soc. Exp. Biol.* **29**, 249.
Brush, M. G., Taylor, R. W., and King, R. J. B. (1967). *J. Endocrinol.* **39**, 599.
Bush, I. E. (1965). *Proc. Int. Congr. Endocrinol., 2nd, London, 1964,* p. 1324.
Callantine, M. R. (1967). *Clin. Obstet. Gynecol.* **10**, 74.
Callantine, M. R., Clemens, C. E., and Shih, Y. (1968). *Proc. Soc. Exp. Biol. Med.* **128**, 382.
Church, R. B., and McCarthy, B. J. (1970). *Biochim. Biophys. Acta* **199**, 103.
Clark, J., and Gorski, J. (1969). *Biochim. Biophys. Acta* **192**, 508.
Cuatrecasas, P. (1970). *J. Biol. Chem.* **245**, 3059.
Davis, M. E., Wiener, M., Jacobson, H. I., and Jensen, E. V. (1963). *Amer. J. Obstet. Gynecol.* **87**, 979.
DeAngelo, A. B., and Gorski, J. (1970). *Proc. Nat. Acad. Sci. U.S.* **66**, 693.
DeHertogh, R., Ekka, E., Vanderheyden, I., and Hoet, J. J. (1971a). *Endocrinology* **88**, 165.
DeHertogh, R., Ekka, E., Vanderheyden, I., and Hoet, J. J. (1971b). *Endocrinology* **88**, 175.
Demetriou, J. A., Crowley, L. G., Kushinsky, S., Donovan, A. J., Kotin, P., and Macdonald, I. (1964). *Cancer Res.* **24**, 926.
DeSombre, E. R., Puca, G. A., and Jensen, E. V. (1969). *Proc. Nat. Acad. Sci. U.S.* **64**, 148.
DeSombre, E. R., Chabaud, J. P., Puca, G. A., and Jensen, E. V. (1971a). *J. Steroid Biochem.* **2**, 95.
DeSombre, E. R., Ikeda, M., Tanaka, S., Smith, S., and Jensen, E. V. (1971b). *Abstr. 53rd Meet. Endrocrine Soc., San Francisco,* p. 149.
Desphande, N., Jensen, V., Bulbrook, R. D., Berne, T., and Ellis, F. (1967). *Steroids* **10**, 219.
Eisenfeld, A. J., and Axelrod, J. (1965). *J. Pharmacol. Exp. Ther.* **150**, 469.
Eisenfeld, A. J., and Axelrod, J. (1966). *Endocrinology* **79**, 38.
Eisenfeld, A. J., and Axelrod, J. (1967). *Biochem. Pharmacol.* **16**, 1781.
Ellis, D. J., and Ringold, H. J. (1971). In "Biochemical Endocrinology: III. The Sex Steroids: Molecular Mechanisms" (K. W. McKerns, ed.). Appleton, New York. In press.
Erdos, T. (1968). *Biochem. Biophys. Res. Commun.* **32**, 338.
Erdos, T., Gospodarowicz, D., Bessada, R., and Fries, J. (1968). *C. R. Acad. Sci., Ser. D* **266**, 2164.
Erdos, T., Bessada, R., and Fries, J. (1969). *FEBS Lett.* **5**, 161.
Erdos, T., Best-Belpomme, M., and Bessada, R. (1970). *Anal. Biochem.* **37**, 244.
Falk, R. J., and Bardin, C. W. (1970). *Endocrinology* **86**, 1059.
Feherty, P., Robertson, D. M., Waynforth, H. B., and Kellie, A. E. (1970). *Biochem. J.* **120**, 837.
Fencl, M. M., and Villee, C. A. (1971). *Endocrinology* **88**, 279.
Flesher, J. W. (1965). *Steroids* **5**, 737.
Folca, P. J., Glascock, R. F., and Irvine, W. T. (1961). *Lancet* ii, 796.
Folman, Y., and Pope, G. S. (1969). *J. Endocrinol.* **44**, 203.
Glascock, R. F., and Hoekstra, W. G. (1959). *Biochem. J.* **72**, 673.
Gorski, J. (1964). *J. Biol. Chem.* **239**, 899.
Gorski, J., and Axman, M. C. (1964). *Arch. Biochem. Biophys.* **105**, 517.
Gorski, J., and Morgan, M. S. (1967). *Biochim. Biophys. Acta* **149**, 282.
Gorski, J., and Nelson, N. J. (1965). *Arch. Biochem. Biophys.* **110**, 284.

Gorski, J., and Nicolette, J. A. (1963). *Arch. Biochem. Biophys.* **103**, 418.
Gorski, J., Noteboom, W. D., and Nicolette, J. A. (1965). *J. Cell. Comp. Physiol.* **66**, Suppl., 91.
Gorski, J., Toft, D., Shyamala, G., Smith, D., and Notides, A. (1968). *Recent Progr. Horm. Res.* **24**, 45.
Greenman, D. L. (1970). *Endocrinology* **87**, 716.
Gupta, G. N. (1960). Ph.D. Thesis, Dep. of Biochem., Univ. of Chicago, Chicago, Illinois.
Gurpide, E., and Welch, M. (1969). *J. Biol. Chem.* **244**, 5159.
Hacker, B. (1969). *Biochim. Biophys. Acta* **186**, 214.
Hahn, W. E., Schjeide, O. A., and Gorbman, A. (1969a). *Proc. Nat. Acad. Sci. U.S.* **62**, 112.
Hahn, W. E., Church, R. B., and Gorbman, A. (1969b). *Endocrinology* **84**, 738.
Hähnel, R. (1971). *Steroids* **17**, 105.
Hamilton, T. H. (1964). *Proc. Nat. Acad. Sci. U.S.* **51**, 83.
Hamilton, T. H. (1968). *Science* **161**, 649.
Hamilton, T. H., Widnell, C. C., and Tata, J. R. (1965). *Biochim. Biophys. Acta* **108**, 168.
Hamilton, T. H., Widnell, C. C., and Tata, J. R. (1968). *J. Biol. Chem.* **243**, 408.
Hechter, O., and Halkerston, I. D. K. (1964). In "The Hormones (G. Pincus, K. V. Thimann, and E. B. Astwood, eds.), Vol. V, pp. 697–825. Academic Press, New York.
Hough, D., Arnaud, M., and Mousseron-Canet, M. (1970). *C. R. Acad. Sci., Ser. D* **271**, 603.
Hughes, A., Smith, S., DeSombre, E. R., and Jensen, E. V. (1969). *Fed. Proc. Fed. Amer. Soc. Exp. Biol.* **28**, 703.
Jensen, E. V. (1960). *Proc. Int. Congr. Biochem., 4th, Vienna, 1958,* Vol. 15, p. 144.
Jensen, E. V. (1962). *Recent Progr. Horm. Res.* **18**, 461.
Jensen, E. V. (1965a). *Proc Int. Congr. Endocrinol., 2nd, London, 1964,* p. 420.
Jensen, E. V. (1965b). *Proc. Can. Cancer Res. Conf.* **6**, 143.
Jensen, E. V., and Jacobson, H. I. (1960). In "Biological Activities of Steroids in Relation to Cancer" (G. Pincus and E. P. Vollmer, eds.), pp. 161–178. Academic Press, New York.
Jensen, E. V., and Jacobson, H. I. (1962). *Recent Progr. Horm. Res.* **18**, 387.
Jensen, E. V., and Jacobson, H. I., Flesher, J. W., Saha, N. N., Gupta, G. N., Smith, S., Colucci, V., Shiplacoff, D., Neumann, H. G., DeSombre, E. R., and Jungblut, P. W. (1966). In "Steroid Dynamics" (G. Pincus, T. Nakao, and J. F. Tait, eds.), pp. 133–157. Academic Press, New York.
Jensen, E. V., DeSombre, E. R., and Jungblut, P. W. (1967a). *Proc. Int. Congr. Horm. Steroids, 2nd, Milan, 1966,* pp. 492–500.
Jensen, E. V., DeSombre, E. R., Hurst, D. J., Kawashima, T., and Jungblut, P. W. (1967b). *Arch. Anat. Microsc. Morphol. Exp.* **56**, Suppl., 547.
Jensen, E. V., DeSombre, E. R., and Jungblut, P. W. (1967c). In "Endogenous Factors Influencing Host-Tumor Balance" (R. W. Wissler, T. L. Dao, and S. Wood, Jr., eds.), pp. 15–30. Univ. of Chicago Press, Chicago, Illinois.
Jensen, E. V., Hurst, D. J., DeSombre, E. R., and Jungblut, P. W. (1967d). *Science* **158**, 385.
Jensen, E. V., Suzuki, T., Kawashima, T., Stumpf, W. E., Jungblut, P. W., and DeSombre, E. R. (1968). *Proc. Nat. Acad. Sci. U.S.* **59**, 632.
Jensen, E. V., DeSombre, E. R., Jungblut, P. W., Stumpf, W. E., and Roth, L. J.

(1969a). In "Autoradiography of Diffusible Substances" (L. J. Roth and W. E. Stumpf, eds.), pp. 81–97. Academic Press, New York.
Jensen, E. V., Suzuki, T., Numata, M., Smith, S., and DeSombre, E. R. (1969b). *Steroids* **13**, 417.
Jensen, E. V., Numata, M., Smith, S., Suzuki, T., Brecher, P. I., and DeSombre, E. R. (1969c). *Develop. Biol. Suppl.* **3**, 151.
Jensen, E. V., Numata, M., Brecher, P. I., and DeSombre, E. R. (1971a). *Biochem. Soc. Symp.* **32**, 133.
Jensen, E. V., Block, G. E., Smith, S., Kyser, K., and DeSombre, E. R. (1971b). *Nat. Cancer Inst. Monogr.* **34**. In press.
Joel, P. B., and Hagerman, D. D. (1969). *Biochim. Biophys. Acta* **195**, 328.
Johansson, H., Terenius, L., and Thorén, L. (1970). *Cancer Res.* **30**, 692.
Jütting, G., Thun, K. J., and Kuss, E. (1967). *Eur. J. Biochem.* **2**, 146.
Jungblut, P. W., Morrow, R. I., Reeder, G. L., and Jensen, E. V. (1965). *Abstr. 47th Meet. Endocrine Soc., New York*, p. 56.
Jungblut, P. W., DeSombre, E. R., and Jensen, E. V. (1967a). *Abh. Deut. Akad. Wiss. Berlin, Kl. Med.* p. 109.
Jungblut, P. W., Hätzel, I., DeSombre, E. R., and Jensen, E. V. (1967b). *Colloq. Ges. Physiol. Chem.* **18**, 58.
Jungblut, P. W., McCann, S., Görlich, L., Rosenfeld, G. C., and Wagner, R. (1970). In "Research on Steroids" (C. Conti, ed.), Vol. 4, pp. 213-232. Pergamon-Vieweg, Braunschweig.
Kahwanago, I., Heinrichs, W. L., and Herrmann, W. L. (1970). *Endocrinology* **86**, 1319.
Kato, J., and Villee, C. A. (1967a). *Endocrinology* **80**, 567.
Kato, J., and Villee, C. A. (1967b). *Endocrinology* **80**, 1133.
Katzenellenbogen, B. S., and Gorski, J. (1971). *Fed. Proc. Fed. Amer. Soc. Exp. Biol.* **30**, 1214.
King, R. J. B., and Gordon, J. (1966). *J. Endocrinol.* **34**, 431.
King, R. J. B., Gordon, J., and Inman, D. R. (1965a). *J. Endocrinol.* **32**, 9.
King, R. J. B., Cowan, D. M., and Inman, D. R. (1965b). *J. Endocrinol.* **32**, 83.
King, R. J. B., Gordon, J., Cowan, D. M., and Inman, D. R. (1966). *J. Endocrinol.* **36**, 139.
King, R. J. B., Gordon, J., and Steggles, A. W. (1969). *Biochem. J.* **114**,649.
Korenman, S. G. (1968). *J. Clin. Endocrinol. Metab.* **28**, 127.
Korenman, S. G. (1969). *Steroids* **13**, 163.
Korenman, S. G. (1970). *Endocrinology* **87**, 1119.
Korenman, S. G., and O'Malley, B. W. (1968). *Endocrinology* **83**, 11.
Korenman, S. G., and Rao, B. R. (1968). *Proc. Nat. Acad. Sci. U.S.* **61**, 1028.
Kyser, K. A. (1970). Ph.D. Thesis, Dep. of Physiol., Univ. of Chicago, Chicago, Illinois.
Lee, C., and Jacobson, H. I. (1971). *Endocrinology* **88**, 596.
McGuire, J. L., and DeDella, C. (1971). *Endocrinology* **88**, 1099.
McGuire, J. L., and Lisk, R. D. (1968). *Proc. Nat. Acad. Sci. U.S.* **61**, 497.
McGuire, J. L., and Lisk, R. D. (1969). *Neuroendocrinology* **4**, 289.
McGuire, W. L., and O'Malley, B. W. (1968). *Biochim. Biophys. Acta* **157**, 187.
Maurer, H. R., and Chalkley, G. R. (1967). *J. Mol. Biol.* **27**, 431.
Mayol, R. F., and Thayer, S. A. (1970). *Biochemistry* **9**, 2484.
Means, A. R., and Hamilton, T. H. (1966). *Proc. Nat. Acad. Sci. U.S.* **56**, 1594.
Méšter, J., Robertson, D. M., Feherty, P., and Kellie, A. E. (1970). *Biochem. J.* **120**, 831.

Michael, R. P. (1965). *Brit. Med. Bull.* **21**, 87.
Milgrom, E., and Baulieu, E. E. (1970). *Endocrinology* **87**, 276.
Milgrom, E., Atger, M., and Baulieu, E. E. (1970). *Steroids* **16**, 741.
Mobbs, B. (1966). *J. Endocrinol.* **36**, 409.
Mobbs, B. (1968). *J. Endocrinol.* **41**, 339.
Mobbs, B. (1969). *J. Endocrinol.* **44**, 463.
Mohla, S., DeSombre, E. R., and Jensen, E. V. (1971a). *Fed. Proc. Fed. Amer. Soc. Exp. Biol.* **30**, 1214.
Mohla, S., DeSombre, E. R., and Jensen, E. V. (1971b). *Biochem. Biophys. Res. Commun.* In press.
Mueller, G. C. (1960). In "Biological Activities of Steroids in Relation to Cancer" (G. Pincus and E. P. Vollmer, eds.), pp. 129–145. Academic Press, New York.
Mueller, G. C. (1965). In "Mechanisms of Hormone Action" (P. Karlson, ed.), pp. 228–239. Academic Press, New York.
Mueller, G. C., Gorski, J., and Aizawa, Y. (1961). *Proc. Nat. Acad. Sci. U.S.* **47**, 164.
Musliner, T. A., Chader, G. J., and Villee, C. A. (1970). *Biochemistry* **9**, 4448.
Nicolette, J. A., and Gorski, J. (1964). *Arch. Biochem. Biophys.* **107**, 279.
Nicolette, J. A., and Mueller, G. C. (1966). *Biochem. Biophys. Res. Commun.* **24**, 851.
Nicolette, J. A., Lemahieu, M. A., and Mueller, G. C. (1968). *Biochim. Biophys. Acta* **166**, 403.
Noteboom, W. D., and Gorski, J. (1963). *Proc. Nat. Acad. Sci. U.S.* **50**, 250.
Noteboom, W. D., and Gorski, J. (1965). *Arch. Biochem. Biophys.* **111**, 559.
Notides, A. C. (1970). *Endocrinology* **87**, 987.
Notides, A., and Gorski, J. (1966). *Proc. Nat. Acad. Sci. U.S.* **56**, 230.
O'Malley, B. W. (1967). *Biochemistry* **6**, 2546.
O'Malley, B. W., and Kohler, P. O. (1967a). *Biochem. Biophys. Res. Commun.* **28**, 1.
O'Malley, B. W., and Kohler, P. O. (1967b). *Proc. Nat. Acad. Sci. U.S.* **58**, 2359.
O'Malley, B. W., and McGuire, W. L. (1968). *J. Clin. Invest.* **47**, 654.
O'Malley, B. W., and McGuire, W. L. (1969). *Endocrinology* **84**, 63.
O'Malley, B. W., McGuire, W. L., and Middleton, P. A. (1967). *Endocrinology* **81**, 677.
O'Malley, B. W., McGuire, W. L., and Middleton, P. A. (1968). *Nature (London)* **218**, 1249.
O'Malley, B. W., McGuire, W. L., Kohler, P. O., and Korenman, S. G. (1969). *Recent Progr. Horm. Res.* **25**, 105.
O'Malley, B. W., Sherman, M. R., and Toft, D. O. (1970). *Proc. Nat. Acad. Sci. U.S.* **67**, 501.
O'Malley, B. W., Toft, D. O., and Sherman, M. R. (1971a). *J. Biol. Chem.* **246**, 1117.
O'Malley, B. W., Sherman, M. R., Toft, D. O., Spelsberg, T. C., Schrader, W. T., and Steggles, A. W. (1971b). In "Advances in the Biosciences 7," Schering Workshop Steroid Horm. "Receptors" (G. Raspé, ed.), pp. 213–231. Pergamon, Oxford.
Pack, B. A., and Brooks, S. C. (1970). *Endocrinology* **87**, 924.
Pakula, S., Brecher, P. I., DeSombre, E. R., and Jensen, E. V. (1972). To be published.
Pfaff, D. W. (1968). *Endocrinology* **82**, 1149.
Podratz, K. C., and Katzman, P. A. (1968). *Fed. Proc. Fed. Amer. Soc. Exp. Biol.* **27**, 497.

Puca, G. A., and Bresciani, F. (1968a). *Nature* (*London*) **218**, 967.
Puca, G. A., and Bresciani, F. (1968b). *Eur. J. Cancer* **3**, 475.
Puca, G. A., and Bresciani, F. (1969a). *Endocrinology* **85**, 1.
Puca, G. A., and Bresciani, F. (1969b). *Nature* (*London*) **223**, 745.
Puca, G. A., and Bresciani, F. (1970). *Nature* (*London*) **225**, 1251.
Puca, G. A., Nola, E., Sica, V., and Bresciani, F. (1971). *In* "Advances in the Biosciences 7," Schering Workshop Steroid Horm. "Receptors" (G. Raspé, ed.), pp. 97–113. Pergamon, Oxford.
Rao, B. R., and Wiest, W. G. (1971). *Fed. Proc. Fed. Amer. Soc. Exp. Biol.* **30**, 1213.
Raynaud-Jammet, C., and Baulieu, E. E. (1969). *C. R. Acad. Sci., Ser. D* **268**, 3211.
Reel, J. R., Lee, S., and Callantine, M. R. (1969). *Abstr. 51st Meet. Endocrine Soc., New York*, p. 113.
Reel, J. R., VanDewark, S. D., Shih, Y., and Callantine, M. R. (1970). *Abstr. 52nd Meet. Endocrine Soc., St. Louis*, p. 83.
Reuter, L. A., Ciaccio, L. A., and Lisk, R. D. (1970). *Fed. Proc. Fed. Amer. Soc. Exp. Biol.* **29**, 250.
Rochefort, H., and Baulieu, E. E. (1968). *C. R. Acad. Sci., Ser. D* **267**, 662.
Rochefort, H., and Baulieu, E. E. (1969). *Endocrinology* **84**, 108.
Rogers, A. W., Thomas, G. H., and Yates, K. M. (1966). *Exp. Cell Res.* **40**, 668.
Roy, S., Mahesh, V. B., and Greenblatt, R. B. (1964). *Acta Endocrinol.* (*Copenhagen*) **47**, 669.
Sander, S. (1968). *Acta Endocrinol.* (*Copenhagen*) **58**, 49.
Sander, S., and Attramadal, A. (1968a). *Acta Endocrinol.* (*Copenhagen*) **58**, 235.
Sander, S., and Attramadal, A. (1968b). *Acta Pathol. Microbiol. Scand.* **74**, 169.
Segal, S. J., and Scher, W. (1967). *In* "Cellular Biology of the Uterus" (R. M. Wynn, ed.), pp. 114–150. Appleton, New York.
Segal, S. J., Davidson, O. W., and Wada, K. (1965). *Proc. Nat. Acad. Sci. U.S.* **54**, 782.
Sharma, O. K., and Borek, E. (1970). *Biochemistry* **9**, 2507.
Sherman, M. R., Corvol, P. L., and O'Malley, B. W. (1970). *J. Biol. Chem.* **245**, 6085.
Shyamala, G., and Gorski, J. (1969). *J. Biol. Chem.* **244**, 1097.
Smith, D. E., and Gorski, J. (1968). *J. Biol. Chem.* **243**, 4169.
Smith, R. E., and Szego, C. M. (1971). *Abstr. 53rd Meet. Endocrine Soc., San Francisco*, p. 151.
Spaziani, E., and Szego, C. M. (1958). *Endocrinology* **63**, 669.
Spelsberg, T. C., Steggles, A. W., and O'Malley, B. W. (1971). *J. Biol. Chem.* **246**, 4188.
Steggles, A. W., and King, R. J. B. (1969). *Acta Endocrinol.* (*Copenhagen*), Suppl. **138**, 36.
Steggles, A. W., and King, R. J. B. (1970). *Biochem. J.* **118**, 695.
Stone, G. M. (1963). *J. Endocrinol.* **27**, 281.
Stone, G. M. (1964). *Acta Endocrinol.* (*Copenhagen*) **47**, 433.
Stone, G. M., and Baggett, B. (1965a). *Steroids* **6**, 277.
Stone, G. M., and Baggett, B. (1965b). *Steroids* **5**, 809.
Stone, G. M., and Martin, L. (1964). *Steroids* **3**, 699.
Stone, G. M., Baggett, B., and Donnelly, R. B. (1963). *J. Endocrinol.* **27**, 271.

Stumpf, W. E. (1968a). *Endocrinology* **83**, 777.
Stumpf, W. E. (1968b). *Science* **162**, 1001.
Stumpf, W. E. (1969). *Endocrinology* **85**, 31.
Stumpf, W. E., and Roth, L. J. (1966). *J. Histochem. Cytochem.* **14**, 274.
Sutherland, E. W., and Robison, G. A. (1966). *Pharmacol. Rev.* **18**, 145.
Sweat, M. L., Bryson, M. J., and Young, R. B. (1967). *Endocrinology* **81**, 167.
Szego, C. M. (1965). *Fed. Proc. Fed. Amer. Soc. Exp. Biol.* **24**, 1343.
Talwar, G. P., Segal, S. J., Evans, A., and Davidson, O. W. (1964). *Proc. Nat. Acad. Sci. U.S.* **52**, 1059.
Talwar, G. P., Sapori, M. L., Biswas, D. K., and Segal, S. J. (1968). *Biochem. J.* **107**, 765.
Teng, C. S., and Hamilton, T. H. (1968). *Proc. Nat. Acad. Sci. U.S.* **60**, 1410.
Teng, C. S., and Hamilton, T. H. (1969). *Proc. Nat. Acad. Sci. U.S.* **63**, 465.
Terenius, L. (1965). *Acta Endocrinol. (Copenhagen)* **50**, 584.
Terenius, L. (1966). *Acta Endocrinol. (Copenhagen)* **53**, 611.
Terenius, L. (1967). *Mol. Pharmacol.* **3**, 423.
Toft, D., and Gorski, J. (1966). *Proc. Nat. Acad. Sci. U.S.* **55**, 1574.
Toft, D., Shyamala, G., and Gorski, J. (1967). *Proc. Nat. Acad. Sci. U.S.* **57**, 1740.
Tomkins, G. M., Gelehrter, T. D., Granner, D., Martin, D., Jr., Samuels, H. H., and Thompson, E. B. (1969). *Science* **166**, 1474.
Trachewsky, D., and Segal, S. J. (1968). *Eur. J. Biochem.* **4**, 279.
Truong, H., and Baulieu, E. E. (1971). *Biochim. Biophys. Acta* **237**, 167.
Ui, H., and Mueller, G. C. (1963). *Proc. Nat. Acad. Sci. U.S.* **50**, 256.
Unhjem, O., Attramadal, A., and Sölna, J. (1968). *Acta Endocrinol. (Copenhagen)* **58**, 227.
Vonderhaar, B. K., and Mueller, G. C. (1969). *Biochim. Biophys. Acta* **176**, 626.
Vonderhaar, B. K., Kim, U. H., and Mueller, G. C. (1970a). *Biochim. Biophys. Acta* **208**, 517.
Vonderhaar, B. K., Kim, U. H., and Mueller, G. C. (1970b). *Biochim. Biophys. Acta* **215**, 125.
Wenzel, M., Mützel, W., and Hieronimus, B. (1970). *Biochem. J.* **120**, 899.
Wiest, W. G., and Rao, B. R. (1971). In "Advances in the Biosciences 7," Schering Workshop Steroid Horm. "Receptors" (G. Raspé, ed.), pp. 251–264. Pergamon, Oxford.
Williams-Ashman, H. G., and Reddi, A. H. (1971). *Annu. Rev. Physiol.* **33**, 31.
Wyss, R. H., Heinrichs, W. L., and Herrmann, W. L. (1968a). *J. Clin. Endocrinol. Metab.* **28**, 1227.
Wyss, R. H., Karsznia, R., Heinrichs, W. L., and Herrmann, W. L. (1968b). *J. Clin. Endocrinol. Metab.* **28**, 1824.
Zimmering, P. E., Kahn, I., and Lieberman, S. (1970). *Biochemistry* **9**, 2498.

AUTHOR INDEX

Numbers in italics refer to the pages on which the complete references are listed.

A

Aakvaag, A., 237, *263*
Abdou, N. I., 133, *145*
Abel, J. J., 86, *115*
Abrahams, V. A., 94, *115*
Abrams, R. M., 51, *79*
Acher, R., 84, 86, *115*, *120*
Ackerman, G. A., 124, *145*
Adams, D. D., 176, 177, 180, 182, 183, 187, 188, 193, *195*, *197*
Adamson, A. R., 93, *116*
Adamsons, H., 98, *117*
Ahn, C. S., 207, *223*
Aisenberg, A. C., 133, *145*
Aizawa, Y., 231, 234, 238, *263*, *267*
Albano, J. D. M., 36, *38*
Alber, H. K., 8, *38*
Alberga, A., 237, 240, 248, *263*
Aldrich, T. B., 82, 86, *118*
Aldridge, R. R., 208, 209, *223*, *225*
Alexander, J. W., 128, *145*
Alexander, M., 74, *78*
Alloiteau, J. J., 45, *75*
Allsup, F. C., 104, *118*
Amenomori, Y., 51, *78*
Amos, J., 183, *197*
Anderson, A., 216, *227*
Andrada, J. A., 192, *195*
Antunes-Rodrigues, J., 96, *119*

Arai, Y., 51, 68, 72, 73, *75*
Archer, O. K., 123, 126, 135, *145*, *147*
Argue, H., 192, *196*
Arimura, A., 96, *115*
Armstrong, D. T., 102, *115*, *120*, 253 *263*
Arnason, B. G., 123, 127, 135, *147*
Arnaud, M., 262, *263*, *265*
Arvan, G., 141, *146*
Asanuma, Y., 123, 130, 137, 138, 139, 142, 144, *145*, *146*
Ason, E. K., 178, *195*
Astwood, E. B., 89, *117*
Atger, M., 252, 255, 256, 257, 258, *267*
Attramadal, A., 53, 62, 76, 233, 237, *263*, *268*, *269*
Auerbach, R., 124, *145*
August, C. S., 129, 131, 132, *145*
Aurbach, G. D., 165, *173*
Avanzino, G. L., 210, *223*
Avioli, L. V., 216, *224*
Avivi, P., 2, *38*
Awad, A. G., 176, 177, *197*
Axelrod, J., 62, 76, 237, *264*
Axman, M. C., 234, *264*
Aykent, Y. Y., 217, *226*

B

Bach, J.-F., 127, 137, 141, *145*
Badalamenti, G., 191, *197*

AUTHOR INDEX

Baggett, B., 62, *80*, 209, *225*, 236, 239, 268
Baird, C. E., 211, 221, *224*
Banerjee, A., 137, *146*
Banks, P., 27, *38*
Barbiroli, B., 231, 232, 263
Barclay, T. J., 133, *145*
Bardin, C. W., 252, 253, *264*
Bárdos, V., 51, 52, 53, 54, 55, 56, 77
Barer, R., 85, *115*
Barg, W. R., Jr., 154, *172*
Bargmann, W., 82, 88, *115*
Barker, K. L., 233, 235, *263*
Barnafi, L., 105, *116*
Barnea, A., 235, *263*
Barnett, J., 90, *120*
Barraclough, C. A., 42, 43, 45, 49, 52, 56, 57, 59, 61, *76*, 77
Barrett, S., 208, 209, *223*, *225*
Barry, J., 232, 233, *263*
Bartels, E. D., 180, *195*
Bartels, J., 201, *228*
Barton, R. W., 232, *263*
Bartsch, G. E., 178, *196*
Bashore, R. A., 108, *116*
Bastenie, P. A., 184, *195*
Battisto, J. R., 137, 138, 139, 141, 142, 144, *146*, *147*
Baulieu, E. E., 237, 240, 241, 243, 247, 248, 252, 255, 256, 257, 258, 261, *263*, *267*, *268*, *269*
Beale, D., 2, *39*
Beall, G. N., 189, 191, 192, *195*, *198*
Beard, J., 124, *145*
Beaulnes, A., 107, *119*
Beck, L., 201, *223*
Bedwani, J. R., 208, *223*
Beek, N., 95, *117*
Behrman, H. R., 215, *224*
Bejerano, A., 138, *149*
Beleslin, D., *116*
Bell, P. H., 154, *172*
Benedetti-Pichler, A. A., 8, *38*
Benhamou-Glynn, N., 191, *195*
Bennett, A., 218, 219, *224*
Benson, G. K., 102, *116*
Berde, B., 105, 107, *116*, *119*
Bergsma, D., 128, *145*

Bergström, S., 200, 201, 210, 214, 215, 220, 221, 222, *224*, *226*, *228*
Berkel, A. I., 132, *145*
Bern, H. A., 86, *116*
Berne, T., 237, *264*
Berson, S. A., 8, 9, 10, 11, *38*, *39*
Berti, F., 221, *224*
Berumen, F. O., 192, *195*
Bessada, R., 243, 247, *264*
Besser, G. M., 100, *116*, 183, *197*
Best, F. A., 208, 212, *227*
Best-Belpomme, M., 243, 247, *263*, *264*
Beziat, Y., 262, *263*
Biedl, A., 123, *145*
Biggart, J. D., 134, *145*
Billing, R. J., 231, 232, *263*
Binder, V., 182, *195*
Birge, S. J., 216, *224*
Bissett, G. W., 99, 111, *116*
Biswas, D. K., 243, *269*
Bitman, J., 231, *263*
Bittner, J. J., 48, *79*
Black, E., 184, *197*
Black, P. H., 132, *147*
Blackshawe, J. K., 108, *118*
Blair-Bell, W., 82, 83, 107, *116*
Blair-West, J. R., 204, 205, *225*
Blatchley, F. R., 207, 208, 215, *224*
Blattner, R., 125, *145*
Blecher, M., 221, *224*
Bliss, C. L., 31, *38*
Block, G. E., 238, 243, *266*
Block, M. H., 130, *149*
Bloom, F. E., 211, *225*
Bloom, G., 202, 206, *228*
Blumen, D., 107, *119*
Böhle, E., 222, *224*
Boeru, V., 134, *148*
Bogdanove, E. M., 53, *76*
Boggs, D. R., 129, *149*
Boissonas, R. A., 105, *116*
Bomskov, C., 134, *145*
Bond, G. C., 94, *118*
Bonjour, J.-P., 94, *116*, *119*
Bonnyns, M., 183, 184, 185, *195*
Borek, E., 232, *268*
Borlund, B., 202, *228*
Borth, R., 7, *38*
Bossert, H., 156, *172*

Bowers, C. Y., 96, *115*
Boyd, G. W., 93, *116*, 167, *172*
Boyd, N. R. H., 97, 99, 100, 106, 107, 109, 111, *116*, *117*
Bracci, C., 134, 135, *145*
Bradbury, J. T., 43, *76*
Bradley, P. B., 210, *223*, *224*
Bradley, T. R., 127, *148*
Bradshaw, M., 46, *76*
Braunsberg, H., 237, *263*
Brecher, G., 127, *148*
Brecher, P. I., 237, 243, 244, 246, 248, 249, 259, 260, 261, 262, *263*, *264*, *266*, *267*
Breckenridge, B., 202, *224*
Bresciani, F., 237, 241, 242, 243, 247, 248, 249, 250, *268*
Breslow, F., 88, *116*
Brewer, H. B., Jr., 152, 154, 158, *172*, *173*
Bricker, N. S., 216, *224*
Bridges, T. E., 93, *116*
Bridson, W., 31, *39*
Brobeck, J. R., 54, *80*
Brodie, A. H., 3, *38*
Bromwich, A. F., 111, *116*
Brooks, F. P., 105, *116*
Brooks, S. C., 236, *267*
Brostoff, J., 96, *116*
Brovetto, J., 99, 108, *116*
Browman, L. G., 45, *76*
Brown, B. L., 11, *38*
Brown, G. B., 217, *226*
Brown, J., 177, 178, 187, 188, 189, *195*, *197*
Brown, J. B., 208, *223*
Brown, W. T., 132, *146*
Brownell, G. L., 181, *198*
Brugger, M., 155, 156, 159, 160, *173*
Brunner, H., 105, *116*
Brush, M. G., 237, *264*
Bruton, O. C., 129, *145*
Bryson, M. J., 236, *269*
Buckton, K. E., 127, *145*
Bugbee, E. P., 82, 86, *118*
Bulbrook, R. D., 237, *264*
Bullock, F. D., 134, *149*
Burger, H. G., 37, *38*

Burke, G., 187, 191, 193, *195*, 207, *224*
Burnet, F. M., 124, 127, 129, *131*, *145*
Burton, A. M., 93, *116*
Bury, A. E., 167, 168, *172*
Bush, I. E., 248, *264*
Butcher, R. W., 211, 221, *224*
Byfield, P. G. H., 153, 154, 157, 167, *172*, *173*
Bygdeman, M., 213, 214, *224*, *227*, *228*
Byrnes, W. W., 55, *76*

C

Cabot, H. M., 99, 108, *116*
Cagnoni, M., 72, *76*
Calay, R., 184, *195*
Caldeyro-Barcia, R., 99, 108, *116*
Callantine, M. R., 237, 238, 253, 256, *264*, *268*
Cameron, E. C., 152, *172*
Cammarata, P. S., 206, 207, *226*
Cannan, R. K., 2, *38*
Carlson, L. A., 200, 201, 210, 220, 221, 222, *224*
Carmichael, H., 8, *38*
Carneiro, L., 177, 183, 184, 187, 188, 190, 191, *195*, *196*
Carpenter, M. P., 209, *224*
Carr, A. A., 216, 217, *224*
Carraro, A., 47, *76*
Catt, K. J., 37, *38*
Caviezel, F., 47, *76*
Cecil, H. C., 231, *263*
Cehovic, G., 202, *224*
Chabaud, J. P., 249, *264*
Chader, G. J., 244, 246, *267*
Chalkley, G. R., 239, 241, *266*
Chan, W. Y., 105, *116*
Chaperon, E. A., 143, *145*
Chard, T., 89, 90, 92, 97, 99, 100, 106, 107, 109, 111, *116*, *117*, *118*, *119*
Chauvet, J., 86, *115*
Chawla, R. C., 219, *224*
Cheney, B. A., 152, *172*
Cheng, K. W., 89, *116*
Cheng, S., 47, *76*
Chi, Y. M., 190, *196*
Chiaraviglio, E., 95, *116*

274 AUTHOR INDEX

Chien, J. R., 178, 184, 187, 191, *196*
Chopra, I. J., 177, 184, *195*
Chopra, U., 177, 184, *195*
Chow, B. P., 82, 86, *120*
Christensen, L. K., 182, *195*
Church, R. B., 232, 233, *264, 265*
Ciaccio, L. A., 253, *268*
Claman, H. N., 143, *145*
Clark, J., 243, 247, 248, 258, *264*
Clark, J. H., 134, *149*
Clark, M. B., 167, *172*
Clark, S. L., Jr., 125, 134, 138, *146*
Clarke, C. A., 180, *196*
Clemens, C. E., 237, *264*
Clemente, C. D., 94, *116*
Clements, F. W., 181, *195*
Cleveland, W. W., 132, *146*
Cleverley, J. D, 100, 101, *116*
Cobo, E., 108, 111, *116*
Coceani, F., 210, 218, *224, 228*
Coch, J. A., 99, 108, *116*
Cockcroft, D. W., 152, *172*
Coghlan, J. P., 204, 205, *225*
Cohen, S., 187, *195*
Cole, L. J., 139, *146*
Colucci, D. F., 154, *172*
Colucci, V., 237, 238, 239, *265*
Coninx, P., 204, *226*
Connolly, R. J., 181, *195*
Cooper, C. W., 163, 165, 168, *172*
Cooper, J. A., 8, 13, 31, *39*
Copp, D. H., 152, 154, 155, *172, 173*
Corcorran, N. L., 49, *78*
Cornette, J. C., 202, 209, 214, 215, *225, 227*
Cort, J. H., 114, *117*
Corvol, P. L., 255, 257, 258, *268*
Corwin, A. H., 8, *38*
Costa, E., 210, *228*
Cowan, D. M., 237, 241, *266*
Crawford, J. D., 221, *224*
Critchlow, B. V., 46, 51, 52, 53, *76, 79*
Cross, A. M., 128, 139, *148*
Cross, B. A., 94, 104, *117, 118*
Crowley, L. G., 237, *264*
Crowshaw, K., 200, 217, 218, *226*
Croxatto, H., 105, *116, 117*
Cryer, R. J., 183, *197*

Csapo, A., 111, 113, *117*
Cuatrecasas, P., 249, *264*
Currie, A. R., 98, *117*

D

Dale, H. H., 82, 83, 107, *117*
Dallman, M. F., 96, *120*
Dalmasso, A. P., 123, 127, 131, 135, *146, 147*
Dameshek, W., 134, *149*
D'Angelo, S. A., 52, 76, 182, *195*
Daniel, A. R., 85, *117*
Daniel, P. M., 192, *195*
Daniels, E. G., 215, 217, *225, 226*
Dardenne, M., 127, 137, 141, *145*
Daume, E., 53, *78*
David, M. A., 51, *76*
Davidson, A. G. F., 152, *172*
Davidson, J. M., 51, *76*
Davidson, O. W., 233, 236, 240, 241, *268, 269*
Davidson, W. D., 189, *198*
Davies, C. M., 154, *172*
Davies, J. I., 221, *226*
Davis, B. B., 95, *117*
Davis, M. E., 237, *264*
Davis, W. E., Jr., 139, *146*
Dawson, B., *173*
DeAngelo, A. B., 235, *264*
Debackere, M., 103, 104, *117*
DeDella, C., 253, 255, 256, *266*
Deftos, L. J., 152, 154, 161, 163, 165, 167, 168, 169, 170, *172, 173*, 206, *225*
De Groot, J., 53, *79*
deGroot, L. J., 189, *197*
DeHertogh, R., 237, 248, *264*
de la Lastra, M., 105, *116*
Del Castillo, E. B., 181, *198*
Del Rio, A. E., 90, *120*
Demeester-Mirkine, N., 184, *195*
Demetriou, J. A., 237, *264*
Dempsey, E. W., 45, *76*
Denton, D. A., 204, 205, *225*
Denys, P., Jr., 135, 138, *146*
DeRubertis, F. R., 95, *117*
Desbarats-Schönbaum, M., 185, *198*
Desclin, L., 51, 54, 56, *76*

AUTHOR INDEX

DeSombre, E. R., 63, 78, 236, 237, 238, 239, 240, 241, 242, 243, 244, 246, 247, 249, 250, 259, 260, 261, 262, *264*, *265*, *266*, *267*
DeSomer, P., 135, 138, *146*
DeSousa, M. A. B., 127, *148*
Desphande, N., 237, *264*
Devlin, J., 206, 212, *225*
Dewhurst, K. E., 180, *195*
de Wied, D., 203, *225*
Dhariwal, A. P. S., 96, *119*, *120*
Dicara, L. V., 95, *119*
Dicker, S. E., 105, *117*
Dietrich, F. M., 127, 128, *146*
DiGeorge, A. M., 128, *146*
Ditlove, J., *117*
Doak, S. M. A., 128, 139, *148*
Döcke, F., 52, *76*
Dörner, G., 52, *76*
Donaldson, L. E., 102, *117*
Doniach, D., 191, 192, *195*
Donnelly, R. B., 62, *80*, 236, *268*
Donovan, A. J., 237, *264*
Donovan, B. T., 53, *76*, 207, 208, 215, *224*
Dorrington, J. H., 209, *225*
Dorrington, K. J., 177, 178, 182, 183, 184, 187, 188, 190, 191, *195*, *196*, *197*, *198*
Dougherty, T. F., 137, *146*
Douglas, W. W., 85, *119*, 205, *227*
Dousa, T., 114, *117*
Downes, J. C., 108, *118*
DuCharme, D. W., 209, *225*
Duchateau, G., 135, *147*
Duda, P., 211, *225*
Dudley, H. W., 82, 86, *117*
Dukor, P., 127, 128, *146*
Dumont, J. E., 206, *227*
Durbin, R. P., 220, *228*
du Vigneaud, V., 82, *117*
Dziobkowski, C., 154, *172*

E

Eagle, H., 137, *146*
East, J., 127, *148*
Edwards, C. R. W., 97, 109, 111, *116*
Edwards, W. G., Jr., 200, *225*
Egrin, C., 185, *198*

Eik-Nes, K. B., 209, *225*
Eilber, F. R., 129, *146*
Eisenberg, M. M., 219, *224*
Eisenfeld, A. J., 62, *76*, 237, *264*
Ekelund, L., 222, *224*
Ekins, R. P., 11, 12, 14, 23, 27, 31, 34, 36, 38, 183, *196*
Ekka, E., 237, 248, *264*
Eley, K. G., 219, *224*
Eliasson, R., 212, *228*
El Kabir, D. J., 180, 191, 192, *195*
Ellis, D. J., 248, *264*
Ellis, F., 237, *264*
Ely, F., 100, *117*
Embrey, M. P., 213, *225*
Endröczi, E., 53, *77*
Enestrom, W. W., 184, *196*
Engleman, K., 167, 168, *172*
Englert, M. E., 154, *172*
Engring, N. H., 184, *196*
Ensor, J. M., 178, 187, 188, 189, 190, *195*, *196*, *197*
Epstein, A. N., 94, 95, *117*
Erb, S. D., 139, *149*
Erdos, T., 241, 243, 246, 247, 263, *264*
Ernström, U., 125, *146*
Evans, A., 236, 240, 241, *269*
Everett, J. W., 45, 51, 52, 54, *76*, 77, 79, 80

F

Fabian, M., 91, 107, *117*
Fahey, J. L., 129, *149*
Faiman, C., *117*
Fain, J. N., 202, 203, *225*
Fajans, S. S., 182, *196*
Falk, R. J., 252, 253, *264*
Fantini, F., 72, *76*
Fawcett, C. P., 89, *117*
Fefer, A. G., 129, *146*
Feherty, P., 237, 243, 247, *264*, *266*
Fels, S. S., 43, *79*
Fencl, M. M., 233, *264*
Fendler, K., 53, *77*
Ferguson, J. F., 216, *226*
Ferguson, K. A., 189, *197*
Ferris, T. F., 111, *117*
Fichman, M. P., 216, 217, *225*

Fichtelius, K. E., 123, *146*
Field, J. B., 95, *117*, 189, 190, *196*, 202, 204, 206, *225*, *228*
Fielitz, C. A., 99, 108, *116*
Filler, R. M., 129, 131, *145*
Filshie, G. M., 213, 214, *226*
Finney, D. J., 8, *38*
Fisher, D. A., 177, 184, *195*
Fisher, J., 194, *197*
Fisher, R. A., 180, *197*
Fiske, V. M., 45, *77*
Fitz, A. E., 93, *116*
Fitzpatrick, R. J., 103, 107, 108, *117*
Fitzsimons, J. T., 94, 95, *117*
Fjellstrom, D., 104, *117*
Flack, J. D., 203, 204, *225*
Flament-Durand, J., 51, 52, 54, 56, *76*, *77*
Flerkó, B., 44, 45, 46, 47, 49, 50, 51, 52, 53, 54, 55, 56, 57, 58, 59, 62, 63, 64, 65, 66, 71, *77*, *79*, *80*
Flesher, J. W., 237, 238, 239, *264*, *265*
Florsheim, W. H., 49, *78*, 193, *196*
Flynn, P. D., 221, *224*
Fochi, M., 47, *76*
Fogel, B. J., 132, *146*
Folca, P. J., 238, *264*
Folley, S. J., 99, 100, 101, 102, 103, 107, *116*, *117*, *119*
Folman, Y., 236, *264*
Forbes, A. D., 207, 208, 212, *226*
Ford, C. E., 124, 125, *146*
Forsling, M. L., 91, 92, 93, 99, 100, 106, 107, 109, 111, *116*, *117*, *118*, *119*
Foster, G. V., 167, *172*
Fowler, R. H., 8, *38*
Fox, B., 103, *117*
Fox, C. A., 100, 101, 103, 104, *117*
Franchimont, P., 89, 91, 100, 103, 110, *117*, *118*
Frantz, A. G., 167, *173*
Fraps, R. M., 52, *79*
Fraschini, F., 51, 52, *76*, *79*
Frawley, T. F., 216, 217, *226*
Frei, E., 129, *149*
Freinkel, N., 180, *196*
Friedberg, S. L., 190, *196*
Friedleben, A., 126, *146*

Friedman, S. M., 68, *79*
Friedmann, C. A., 218, 219, *224*
Fries, J., 247, *263*, *264*
Friesen, H. G., 89, *116*, *117*
Fromageot, C., 84, *120*
Fujimoto, S., 217, 218, *225*
Funder, J. W., 204, 205, 208, 209, *223*, *225*
Furth, E. D., 178, *196*
Furth, J. J., 74, *78*, 126, 135, *146*

G

Gabrielsen, A. E., 123, 126, *146*
Gaddum, J. H., 7, *38*
Galante, L., 134, *146*, 153, 154, 157, *173*
Gans, R., 59, *80*
Garay, G. L., 202, *225*
Garcia, L. A., 90, *120*
Gardier, R. W., 95, *120*
Gardner, P. S., 134, *149*
Garry, R., 182, 183, *196*, *197*
Gaunt, R., 96, *119*
Gauthier, G. F., 152, *172*
Gelehrter, T. D., 251, *269*
Gepts, W., 51, 54, 56, *76*
Gerhardt, V. J., 43, 61, *79*
Gershon-Cohen, J., 43, *79*
Ghetti, A., 72, *76*
Giambattista, M., 85, *119*
Gibson, H. B., 181, *195*
Gibson, W. J., 223, *228*
Gilman, A. G., 190, *196*
Ginsburg, M., 88, 91, 99, 110, 111, *117*, *118*
Girard, J., 30, *38*
Glascock, R. F., 236, 238, *264*
Glew, M. E., 207, 208, *226*
Glick, S. M., 99, 108, *118*
Glynn, J. P., 129, *146*
Goding, J. R., 208, 209, *223*, *225*
Görlich, L., 260, *266*
Goetz, K. L., 94, *118*
Goldring, D., 138, *149*
Goldstein, A. L., 123, 130, 134, 136, 137, 138, 139, 140, 141, 142, 143, 144, *145*, *146*, *147*, *149*

Gonda, M., 218, 227
Good, B. F., 180, 189, 197, 198
Good, R. A., 123, 126, 127, 128, 129, 131, 134, 135, 144, 145, 146, 147, 148, 149
Goodall, A., 135, 148
Goodman, A. D., 167, 168, 172, 173
Goodwin, F. L., 105, 118
Goonan, S. R., 107, 119
Gorbman, A., 232, 265
Gorden, P., 111, 117
Gordon, J., 237, 240, 241, 246, 266
Gorski, J., 231, 232, 233, 234, 235, 238, 239, 241, 243, 246, 247, 248, 258, 260, 262, 263, 264, 265, 266, 267, 268, 269
Gorski, R. A., 43, 45, 48, 49, 52, 53, 56, 57, 59, 61, 71, 72, 73, 74, 75, 76, 77, 78
Gospodarowicz, D., 247, 264
Gougoutas, J. Z., 215, 217, 226
Gowans, J. L., 127, 147
Graf, M. W., 128, 147
Grand, M. J. H., 184, 197
Granner, D., 251, 269
Grant, J. K., 205, 225
Grantham, J., 215, 226
Green, C., 134, 149
Green, D. E., 184, 194, 196, 198
Green, R., 64, 65, 77
Greenblatt, R. B., 236, 238, 268
Greenman, D. L., 232, 265
Greenwood, F. C., 30, 38
Greep, R. O., 82, 86, 120, 215, 224
Greer, M. A., 45, 54, 77
Gregoire, C., 135, 147
Gresham, E. M., 105, 119
Griffith, D., 129, 148
Grimley, P. M., 206, 225
Grostic, M. F., 215, 217, 226
Grote, I. W., 82, 86, 118
Gudmundsson, T. V., 134, 146, 153, 154, 157, 173
Guha, A., 137, 138, 141, 143, 144, 145, 146
Guilleux, J. C., 262, 263
Gupta, G. N., 236, 237, 238, 239, 265
Gurpide, E., 236, 265
Gusdon, J. P., 110, 118

Gutknecht, G. D., 202, 207, 208, 209, 214, 215, 225, 227
Guttmann, St., 156, 157, 158, 159, 160, 172

H

Habener, J. F., 165, 167, 168, 172, 173
Hacker, B., 232, 265
Hähnel, R., 247, 265
Haessler, H. A., 221, 224
Hätzel, I., 236, 241, 243, 249, 266
Hagerman, D. D., 232, 266
Hahn, W. E., 232, 265
Halász, B., 45, 46, 49, 51, 52, 53, 77, 78, 79
Haldar, J., 116
Hale, H. B., 67, 68, 78
Hales, C. N., 3, 38
Halkerston, I. D. K., 231, 265
Hall, C. A., 92, 118
Hall, R., 180, 182, 183, 196, 197
Hall, W. J., 208, 212, 227
Hallenbeck, G. A., 133, 147
Haller, E. W., 85, 120
Ham, A. W., 125, 147
Hamilton, J. B., 73, 80
Hamilton, T. H., 231, 232, 233, 234, 241, 262, 265, 266, 269
Hammar, J. A., 123, 125, 147
Handler, J. S., 215, 226
Hansel, W., 102, 115, 120
Hansen, A. E., 129, 148
Hansen, A. M., 134, 149
Hansson, E., 210, 225
Hanstein, W. G., 193, 196
Harbo, J. N., 201, 223
Hardy, M. A., 137, 138, 139, 141, 142, 144, 146, 147, 148
Harris, G. W., 48, 59, 78, 103, 118, 180, 195
Hatefi, Y., 193, 196
Hatton, R., 52, 76
Haun, C. K., 102, 118
Hawker, R. W., 108, 118
Hayashi, S., 69, 78
Hays, R. L., 103, 118, 120
Hayward, J. N., 51, 78, 93, 118
Hechter, O., 231, 265

Hedge, G. A., 96, *120*
Heinrichs, W. L., 237, 238, 239, 242, *266, 269*
Heller, H., 85, *115*
Hemmingsen, A. M., 45, *78*
Hendrick, J. C., 89, *118*
Henze, K. G., 152, *172*
Herlant, M., 85, *118*
Hernreck, A. S., 94, *118*
Herrmann, W. L., 238, 239, 242, *266, 269*
Hershman, J. M., 183, *196*
Hertz, R., 55, *78*
Herzog, J. P., 215, *225*
Hess, M. W., 123, 126, *147*
Hetzel, B. S., 180, 184, 185, *196, 198*
Heyder, E., 154, *172*
Hieronimus, B., 236, *269*
Hill, C. S., 168, *173*
Hillarp, N. Å., 45, 55, *78*
Hilliard, J., 51, *78*
Hillier, K., 206, *226*
Hinman, J. W., 215, 217, *225, 226*
Hirsch, P. F., 152, *172*
Hoekstra, W. G., 236, *264*
Hoet, J. J., 237, 248, *264*
Hoffenberg, R., 184, *197*
Hoffer, B. J., 211, *225*
Hoffmann, M. J., 184, 185, *196*
Hohlweg, W., 53, *78*
Holderness, M., 182, 183, 185, *196*
Holinka, C., 62, *80*
Holland, R. C., 94, *118*
Hollenberg, M. D., *119*
Hollingsworth, S. A., 106, *116*
Holm, L. W., 113, *119*
Holmes, R. A., 148, *196*
Holmes, S. W., 210, 211, *225*
Hope, D. B., 87, 88, *118, 119, 120*
Hopkins, T. F., 102, *119*
Hoppenstein, J. M., 97, *118*
Horit, I., 125, *147*
Horn, G., 43, 61, *79*
Horton, E. W., 208, 210, 211, 216, 219, *223, 225*
Horvat, J., 135, *147*
Hough, A., 262, *263*
Hough, D., 262, *265*
Howard, C. H., 90, *120*

Howe, M. L., 137, 138, 143, 144, *146, 147*
Howeler-Coy, J. F., 181, *195*
Howel-Evans, W., 180, *196*
Howell, W. H., 82, *118*
Howland, B. G., 168, *173*
Hudson, C. N., 97, 109, 111, *116*
Huffman, E. W. D., 8, *38*
Hughes, A., 237, *265*
Huguenin, R., 156, 157, 158, 159, 160, *172*
Hunt, J. C., 200, *225*
Huntingford, P. J., 102, *118*
Hurst, D. J., 63, *78,* 239, 240, 241, 242, 243, 244, 247, 249, 259, *265*
Hurwitz, J., 74, *78*
Hynie, S., 221, *226*

I

Ifft, J. D., 51, *78*
Ikeda, M., 250, *264*
Illei, G., 55, *77*
Illei-Donhoffer, A., 51, 53, 62, 63, 64, 65, 66, *77*
Ingbar, S. H., 180, *196*
Inman, D. R., 237, 240, 241, *266*
Irvine, W. T., 237, 238, *263, 264*
Isakovic, K., 135, *147*
Itoiz, J., 181, *198*

J

Jackson, D. B., 106, *116*
Jacobsen, E. D., 220, *225*
Jacobsohn, D., 48, 69, *78*
Jacobson, H. I., 62, *78,* 236, 237, 238, 239, 243, 247, *264, 265, 266*
James, M. A. R., 92, 106, 109, *118*
James, V. H. T., 96, *116,* 237, *263*
Janeway, C. A., 129, 131, *145*
Jankovic, B. D., 123, 127, 135, *147*
Janowitz, H. D., 218, *227*
Jaquenoud, P. A., 156, *172*
Jayasena, K., 88, 91, 110, 111, *117, 118*
Jensen, E. V., 62, 63, *78,* 236, 237, 238, 239, 240, 241, 242, 243, 244, 245, 246, 247, 249, 250, 259, 260, 261, 262, *264, 265, 266, 267*

AUTHOR INDEX

Jessup, R., 203, 204, 210, *225*, *227*
Jessup, S. J., 210, 223, *226*, *228*
Joel, P. B., 232, *266*
Johansson, H., 237, *266*
Johansson, R., 64, *80*
Johnson, D. C., 45, 48, *79*
Johnson, D. E., 177, 184, *195*
Johnson, J. A., 94, *118*
Johnson, M. W., 129, *147*
Johnston, H. H., 215, *225*
Johnston, P. J., 134, *149*
Jones, A. E., 187, 188, *197*
Jones, C. W., 106, *118*
Jones, J. J., 91, 106, 107, *117*, *120*
Jones, R. C., 7, *38*
Jones, R. L., 216, *225*
Jones, V. E., 133, *148*
Joseph, S. A., 49, *80*
Jütting, G., 236, *266*
Jung, I., 240, *263*
Jungblut, P. W., 63, 78, 236, 237, 238, 239, 240, 241, 242, 243, 244, 246, 247, 249, 259, 260, *265*, *266*
Jungmann, R. A., 204, *226*

K

Kagan, A., 99, 108, *118*
Kahn, I., 243, *269*
Kahnt, F. W., 153, 154, 157, *173*
Kahwanago, I., 237, 238, *266*
Kaiser, H., 7, *38*
Kakiuchi, S., 211, *225*
Kaltenbach, C. C., 208, 209, *223*, *225*
Kamber, B., 155, 156, 159, 160, *173*
Kamm, C., 82, 86, *118*
Kaneko, T., 189, 190, *196*, 202, 204, 206, *225*, *226*
Kanematsu, S., 51, *78*
Kannegiesser, H., 217, *226*
Kaplan, H. S., 129, 133, *145*, *147*
Karim, S. M. M., 206, 212, 214, *225*, *226*, *227*, *228*
Karsznia, R., 238, 239, *269*
Kataoka, K., 210, *226*
Kato, J., 51, 53, 62, 78, 237, *266*
Katzenellenbogen, B. S., 235, *266*
Katzman, P. A., 251, *267*

Kawashima, S., 70, *78*
Kawashima, T., 63, 78, 239, 240, 241, 242, 243, 244, 246, 249, 259, 260, *265*
Kay, H. E. M., 132, *145*, *146*
Kellie, A. E., 237, 243, 247, *264*, *266*
Kendall-Taylor, P., 189, 190, *196*, *197*
Kennedy, P. C., 113, *119*
Kennedy, T. H., 182, 187, *195*
Keston, A. S., 2, *38*
Keutmann, H. T., 152, 153, 154, 155, 160, 161, 165, 166, 170, 171, *172*, *173*
Kigawa, T., 51, *78*
Kihlstrom, J. E., 104, *117*
Kikuyama, S., 67, 68, 70, *78*
Kilborn, J. R., 183, *197*
Kim, U. H., 248, 249, *269*
Kimura, T., 69, *80*
Kindred, J. E. A., 125, 130, *147*
Kincl, F. A., 72, *78*
King, E. R., 253, *263*
King, R. J. B., 63, 64, 78, *80*, 237, 239, 240, 241, 242, 243, 246, 247, 256, *264*, *266*, *268*
Kipnis, D. M., 36, *39*
Kirk, P. L., 8, *38*
Kirkham, J. P., 114, *120*
Kirton, K. T., 207, 208, 212, *226*
Kitau, M. J., 99, *116*
Kitchin, A. H., 105, 107, *117*, *118*
Kitchin, F. D., 180, *196*
Kite, J. H., Jr., 192, *195*, *196*
Klahr, S., 216, *224*
Klainer, L. M., 190, *196*
Kleeman, C. R., 105, 106, *119*
Klein, J. J., 136, *147*
Klein, L. A., 107, *119*
Knaggs, G. S., 99, 100, 101, 103, 104, 107, *117*, *118*
Knigge, K. M., 49, *80*
Knight, R. A., 96, *119*
Knouff, R. A., 124, *145*
Knowles, F. G. W., 86, *116*
Kobayashi, F., 51, 73, 74, *78*
Kobayashi, Takashi, 51, *78*
Kobayashi, Takuro, 51, *78*
Köves, K., 51, 53, 78, *79*
Kohler, P. O., 250, 251, 252, 254, *267*

Koneff, A. A., 54, *80*
Konzett, H., 107, *118*
Korenman, S. G., 241, 242, 243, 247, 250, 251, 252, 254, *266*, *267*
Korolkiewicz, Z., 221, *227*
Kotani, M., 125, *147*
Kotin, P., 237, *264*
Kovács, K., 48, 56, *79*
Krane, S. M., 170, 171, 172, *173*
Krarup, N. B., 45, *78*
Krass, M. E., 103, *118*
Kravatz, A. S., 52, *76*
Kreici, M. E., 53, *79*
Krishna, G., 221, *226*
Kriss, J. P., 178, 182, 183, 184, 185, 187, 190, 191, 194, *196*, *198*
Krook, L., 166, *173*
Krüger, J., *147*
Kubista, T. P., 133, *147*
Kueh, Y., 152, *172*
Kukherjee, T., 213, *224*
Kumaresan, P., 99, 108, *118*
Kunze, H., 201, *228*
Kurcz, M., 43, 48, 53, 61, *79*
Kurihara, H., 185, *197*
Kurtzman, N. A., 215, *227*
Kuschinsky, G., 105, *116*
Kushinsky, S., 237, *264*
Kusomoto, H., 184, *198*
Kuss, E., 236, *266*
Kwon, S. U., 213, *224*, *228*
Kyncl, J., 85, *118*
Kyser, K. A., 237, 238, 240, 243, *266*

L

Labarca, E., 105, *117*
La Bella, F. S., 103, *118*
Ladosky, W., 68, *79*
Landon, J., 89, 90, 96, 99, 106, 107, 109, 111, *116*, *119*
Laragh, J. H., 105, 114, *118*, *120*
Lashof, T. W., 8, *38*
Laster, L., 220, *227*
Lauler, D. P., 215, *225*
Laurell, G., 123, *146*
Lauson, H. D., 91, *118*
LaVia, M. F., 130, *149*

Law, L. W., 129, 132, 133, 134, 137, 138, 139, 140, 144, *147*
Lawton, N. F., 183, *196*
Leach, B. E., 215, 217, *225*, *226*
Leathem, J. H., 43, *76*
Leckband, E., 140, *147*
Lederis, K., 85, *115*
Ledingham, J. G. G., 105, *118*
Lee, C., 237, 243, 247, *266*
Lee, J., 111, *116*
Lee, J. B., 167, *173*, 200, 215, 216, 217, 218, *226*
Lee, M. R., 161, *172*, *173*
Lee, S., 253, *268*
Lees, P., 104, *118*
Legros, J. J., 89, 91, 103, 110, *117*, *118*
Lehmeyer, J. E., 202, *226*
Leier, D. J., 204, *226*
Lejeune-Lenain, C. H. D., 36, *38*
Lemahieu, M. A., 234, *267*
Lemarchand-Béraud, T., 182, *196*
Lentati, R. L., 221, *224*, *227*
Lepkovsky, S., 54, *80*
Lequin, R. M., 155, *173*
Leskowitz, S., 133, *148*
Leveque, T. F., 85, *119*
Levey, G. S., 189, 190, *196*
Levey, R. H., 132, 134, *145*, *147*
Levine, N., 141, *147*
Levine, R., 219, *228*
Levine, S., 48, 59, *78*
Levy, R. P., 178, *196*
Lewald, J. E., 28, *39*
Lewis, G. P., 201, *226*
Lewis, U. J., 187, 188, *197*, 202, *224*
Leyten, R., 135, 138, *146*
Li, M., 47, *76*
Liao, S., 232, *263*
Liberti, P., 191, *197*
Lichardus, B., 114, *117*
Lieberman, S., 243, *269*
Liggins, G. C., 113, *119*
Lilly, F., 140, 141, 143, *146*, *147*, *149*
Lipman, L. M., 184, *196*
Lipschütz, A., 55, *79*
Lisk, R. D., 51, 56, 62, 64, 70, *79*, 237, 253, *266*, *268*
Litman, G. W., 194, *198*

AUTHOR INDEX

Little, J. R., 127, *148*
Littlejohn, M., 53, *79*
Lloyd, C. W., 85, *119*
Lloyd, S., 105, *117*
Lobsenz, I. L., 192, *195*
Lockett, M. F., 217, 218, *225*
Lonigro, A. J., 200, 216, 217, 218, *226*
Lowe, I. P., 202, 206, *228*
Luttge, W. G., 64, 65, 77
Lutwak, L., 166, *173*

M

McCann, S. M., 45, 51, 52, *79, 80*, 96, *119, 120*, 202, 204, *228*, 260, *266*
McCarthy, B. J., 232, 233, *264*
McClure, R. D., 123, 126, 135, *148*
McConnell, R. B., 180, *196*
McCoy, J. L., 129, *146*
McCracken, J. A., 207, 208, *226*
McCullagh, E. P., 182, *196*
Macdonald, I., 237, *264*
McDonald, I. R., 94, *119*
McEntee, E., 166, *173*
McGarry, J., 216, *227*
McGiff, J. C., 200, 216, 217, 218, *226*
MacGillivray, M. H., 133, *148*
McGuire, J. L., 62, 64, 70, *79*, 237, 253, 255, 256, *266*
McGuire, W. L., 178, *196*, 250, 251, 252, 254, *266, 267*
Macho, L., 205, *226*
MacIntyre, I., 134, *146*, 153, 154, 157, *173*
McKenna, J. M., 133, *145*
McKenzie, I. M., 176, 177, 178, 181, 182, 183, 184, 186, 187, 188, 189, 190, 191, *197*
McKeown, T., 114, *119*
MacLeod, R. M., 202, *226*
McNeilly, A. S., 99, 100, 103, 106, 107, 109, 111, *116, 119*
McPherson, A., 211, *225*
Macurdy, L. B., 8, *38*
Maderspach, K., 43, 61, *79*
Mahesh, V. B., 236, 238, *268*
Maibach, H. I., 129, *147*

Maier, R., 153, 154, 157, 159, 160, *173*, 201, 205, *226*
Main, I. H. M., 211, 219, *225*
Major, P. W., 177, 178, 182, 183, 184, 185, 186, *197*
Malamy, M., 74, *78*
Maluin, R. L., 94, *119*
Malvin, R. L., 94, *116*
Manabe, Y., 104, *119*
Mandelbrote, B. M., 179, 180, *195, 198*
Maqueo, M., 72, *78*
Margoulies, M., 204, *226*
Markee, J. E., 52, *79*
Markowsky, B., 129, 131, *145*
Marks, L. J., 107, *119*
Marmorston, J., 123, *148*
Marsh, J. M., 209, *226*
Marshall, A. H. E., 127, *148*
Martin, D., Jr., 251, *269*
Martin, L., 62, *79*, 236, *268*
Martin, L. C., 180, *197*
Martin, J. M., 202, *225*
Martin, M. J., 89, 90, 92, 93, *116, 119*
Martinez, C., 48, *79*, 123, 127, 131, 135, *146, 147, 149*
Martinez, M. M., 215, *227*
Martini, L., 47, 51, 52, *76, 79*
Massry, S. G., 105, 106, *119*
Matthews, E. W., 134, *146*
Matthews, J., 201, *226*
Maurer, H. R., 239, 241, *266*
Maximow, A. A., 123, 124, 130, *148*
May, B., 222, *224*
Mayer, G. P., 165, 167, 168, *172*
Mayol, R. F., 235, *266*
Mazer, R. S., 208, *226*
Means, A. R., 232, *266*
Medawar, P. B., 127, *148*
Meek, J. C., 187, 188, *197*
Meites, J., 51, *79*, 102, *119*
Melin, P., 104, *117*
Melvin, K. E. W., 168, *173*
Mench, M. L., 231, *263*
Menon, T., 210, *228*
Merlino, N. S., 221, *224*
Mess, B., 51, 52, 53, 62, 63, 64, 65, 66, 77, *79*
Méšter, J., 243, 247, *266*

AUTHOR INDEX

Metcalf, D., 123, 125, 128, 130, 135, *148*
Meyer, R. K., 55, *76*, *78*
Meyer, U., 201, *228*
Michael, R. P., 53, 62, *79*, 237, *267*
Michelis, M. F., 95, *117*
Micklem, H. S., 124, *146*
Middleton, P. A., 250, 251, *267*
Midgley, A. R., 13, 31, 36, *38*
Miles, L. E. M., 3, *38*
Milgrom, E., 252, 255, 256, 257, 258, *267*
Milhaud, G., 154, *173*
Milkovic, K., 98, *119*
Milkovic, S., 98, *119*
Miller, J. F. A. P., 123, 126, 127, 128, 129, 130, 131, 132, 134, 135, 139, 143, *148*
Miller, N. E., 95, *119*
Miltenberger, F. W., 97, *118*
Milton, A. S., 211, *226*
Minaguchi, H., 51, *78*
Mirsky, I. A., 107, *119*
Mitchell, G. F., 143, *148*
Mittler, J. C., *79*
Mizuno, M., 51, *78*
Mobbs, B., 237, *267*
Mohla, S., 261, *267*
Mole, B. J., 208, 209, *223*, *225*
Monaco, A. P., 128, 141, *148*
Montgomery, R. G., 209, *225*
Moore, G., 90, *120*
Moore, W. W., 94, *118*, *120*
Morace, G., 72, *76*
Moran, W. H., 97, *118*
Morgan, M. S., 232, 234, *264*
Mori, T., 69, *79*, 194, *197*
Morris, C. J. O. R., 186, *197*
Morrison, E., 129, *149*
Morrison, G. H., 7, 8, *38*
Morrow, R. I., 239, *266*
Morton, D. L., 129, *146*
Moses, A. M., 85, *119*
Motta, M., 52, *79*
Mousseron-Canet, M., 262, *263*, *265*
Mouw, V., 94, *119*
Mozes, E., 187, *197*
Mreaňa, G., 134, *148*

Mudd, J. G., 217, *226*
Mueller, G. C., 231, 232, 233, 234, 235, 238, 248, 249, 262, *263*, *267*, *269*
Mützel, W., 236, *269*
Muirhead, E. E., 215, 217, *225*, *226*
Mukherjee, T., 213, *228*
Mulder, A. H., 203, *225*
Mulrow, P. J., 111, *117*
Munchow, O., 105, *116*
Munro, D. S., 177, 178, 182, 183, 184, 185, 186, 187, 188, 189, 190, 191, 192, 193, *195*, *196*, *197*, *198*
Munsick, R. A., 105, *119*, *120*
Munson, P. L., 152, 154, *172*, 203, *227*
Murray, J. G., 219, *224*
Murray, T. M., 165, 167, 168, *172*, *173*
Musliner, T. A., 244, 246, *267*

N

Nabarro, J. D. N., 183, *196*
Nabseth, D. C., 107, *119*
Nagareda, C. S., 96, *119*
Nagasawa, J., 85, *119*
Nagy, E., 59, 60, 61, *79*
Nahimias, A. J., 129, *148*
Nakamoto, A., 135, *148*
Nakao, K., 93, *120*
Nallar, R., 96, *119*
Neer, R. M., 170, 171, *172*, *173*
Neher, R., 153, 154, 157, *173*
Nelson, J. C., 184, *196*
Nelson, N. J., 231, *264*
Nestel, P., 220, *228*
Neumann, H. G., 237, 238, 239, *265*
Neve, P., 206, *227*
Newman, G. B., 12, 23, 27, *38*
Nezamis, J. E., 219, *227*
Ng, K. K. F., 200, 216, 217, 218, *226*
Niall, H. D., 152, 154, 155, 161, 165, *173*
Nicholson, W. E., 100, *116*
Nicolette, J. A., 231, 234, *265*
Niemi, M., 64, *80*
Niswender, G. D., 13, 31, 36, *38*
Noguchi, A., 185, *197*
Nola, E., 249, 250, *268*
Nossal, G. J. V., 130, *148*

Noteboom, W. D., 234, 265
Notides, A. C., 243, 247, 260, 265, 267
Noumura, T., 68, 79
Nowinski, W. W., 134, 148
Numata, M., 241, 242, 243, 244, 245, 246, 249, 260, 261, 262, 264, 266
Nunn, A. C., 215, 227
Nutting, E. F., 206, 207, 226

O

Ochi, Y., 189, 197
Odell, W. D., 182, 197
O'Dor, R. D., 160, 173
Oerther, F., 215, 227
Oliver, G., 82, 119
Olivry, G., 86, 115
Olsson, K., 94, 119
O'Malley, B. W., 250, 251, 252, 253, 254, 255, 256, 257, 258, 260, 266, 267, 268
Onaya, T., 206, 207, 226
O'Riordan, J. L. H., 12, 23, 38
Orloff, J., 215, 226
Ormston, B. J., 183, 197
Oro, L., 222, 224
Orosz, A., 48, 79
Orth, D. N., 100, 116
Osoba, D., 123, 126, 127, 130, 132, 133, 134, 148
Ott, I., 82, 83, 100, 119
Owen, S. G., 180, 196

P

Pace-Asciak, C., 210, 218, 224, 228
Pack, B. A., 236, 267
Page, A. R., 129, 148
Pakula, S., 246, 267
Palka, Y. S., 51, 79
Palkovic, M., 205, 226
Palmer, E., 129, 148
Panisset, J. C., 107, 119
Paoletti, R., 221, 222, 224, 227
Papermaster, B. W., 123, 147
Pappenheimer, A. M., 126, 148
Park, E. A., 123, 126, 135, 148
Parker, C., 36, 39

Parkes, C. O., 160, 173
Parlow, A. F., 45, 46, 79
Parrott, D. M. W., 127, 148
Parsons, J. A., 152, 153, 154, 160, 173
Paschkis, K. E., 43, 79
Pasquina, A., 248, 263
Pastan, I., 189, 190, 196
Pasteels, J. L., 51, 79
Patel, R. C., 212, 226
Paton, D. N., 135, 148
Paul, R., 154, 172
Paul, W. E., 182, 197
Peacock, M., 165, 173
Pearse, A. G. E., 152, 173
Peart, W. S., 93, 116
Peeters, G., 103, 104, 117
Peng, T. C., 203, 227
Perinetti, H., 181, 198
Perks, A. M., 97, 120
Perla, D., 123, 148
Perrier, C. V., 220, 227
Peters, G., 105, 116
Petersen, W. E., 100, 101, 117, 119
Peterson, R. D. A., 129, 148
Peterson, R. E., 2, 38
Petrusz, P., 44, 57, 58, 59, 60, 61, 71, 77, 79
Pfaff, D. W., 237, 267
Pfeiffer, C. A., 42, 48, 79
Pharriss, B. B., 202, 207, 208, 209, 212, 214, 215, 225, 226, 227
Phillips, C., 219, 228
Phillips, J. P., 219, 227
Phillipsson, L., 123, 146
Phillis, J. W., 211, 227
Piacsek, B. E., 51, 79
Pickering, B. T., 87, 106, 118, 119
Pickford, M., 94, 105, 107, 115, 116, 117, 118
Pickles, V. R., 103, 118, 208, 212, 214, 227
Pierce, J. C., 123, 126, 135, 145, 147
Pike, J. E., 215, 217, 221, 224, 226
Pike, M. C., 127, 145
Pimstone, B. L., 184, 197
Pinchera, A., 183, 184, 185, 191, 197
Pinchera, M. G., 183, 184, 185, 197
Piper, P. J., 216, 227

Pittman, J. A., 183, *196*
Piyasena, R., 27, *38*
Pleshakov, V., 178, 182, 183, 184, 185, 187, 191, *196*
Pless, J., 156, 157, 158, 159, 160, *172*
Pliska, V., 114, *117*
Plomteux, G., 204, *226*
Podratz, K. C., 251, *267*
Poisner, A. M., 205, *227*
Polak, R. L., *116*
Pollard, A. A., 201, *223*
Pope, G. S., 236, *264*
Portanova, R., 84, *119*
Porter, R. R., 187, *195*
Posiero, J. J., 108, *116*
Posillico, J., 178, *196*
Potop, I., 134, *148*
Potts, J. T., Jr., 152, 153, 154, 155, 160, 161, 163, 165, 166, 167, 168, 169, 170, 171, *172, 173*
Powell, A. E., 89, *117*
Powell, D., 165, 167, 168, *172, 173*
Powers, R. S., 167, *173*
Pratt, O. E., 192, *195*
Preddie, E. C., 88, *119*
Pryor, J. S., 91, 107, *117*
Puca, G. A., 237, 241, 242, 243, 247, 248, 249, 250, *264, 268*
Puglisi, L., 222, *227*
Pupp, L., 45, 46, 49, 52, *78*
Purkerson, M., 216, *224*
Purves, H. D., 176, 177, 180, *195*

Q

Quilligan, E. J., 102, *120*
Quint, J., 137, 138, 139, 141, 142, 144, *146, 147, 148*

R

Rabson, A. S., 206, *225*
Radford, H. M., 51, *77*
Rall, T. W., 190, *196*, 210, 211, *225, 228*
Ralph, C. L., 52, *79*
Ram, J. S., *38*

Ramirez, V. D., 51, *79*
Ramwell, P. W., 200, 201, 203, 204, 205, 207, 208, 210, 212, 215, 219, 220, 221, 222, 223, *225, 226, 227, 228*
Rao, B. R., 241, 242, 253, 254, 255, 256, 257, 258, *266, 268, 269*
Ratcliffe, J. G., 96, *119*
Rathbun, M., 178, *196*
Rauch, R., *119*
Raulais, D., 154, *173*
Rayford, P. L., 8, 13, 31, *39*
Raynaud, J. P., 247, *263*
Raynaud-Jammet, C., 261, *268*
Rebar, R. W., 13, 31, 36, *38*
Rector, F. C., 215, *227*
Reddi, A. H., 231, *269*
Reeder, G. L., 239, *266*
Reel, J. R., 253, 256, *268*
Rees, R. J. W., 129, *148*
Reisfeld, R. A., 154, *172*
Réthelyi, M., 52, *79*
Reuter, L. A., 253, *268*
Reynolds, C. W., 182, *196*
Riggs, D. S., 181, *198*
Ringold, H. J., 248, *264*
Riniker, B., 153, 154, 155, 156, 157, 159, 160, 171, *172, 173*
Rittel, W., 153, 154, 155, 156, 159, 160, *173*
Ro'Ane, J. R., 221, *224*
Robert, A., 219, *227*
Roberts, G., 216, *227*
Roberts, J. S., 107, *119*
Roberts, S., 135, *148*
Roberts, V. S., 108, *118*
Robertson, D. M., 237, 243, 247, *264, 266*
Robison, G. A., 263, *269*
Rocha e Silva, M., 95, *119*
Rochefort, H., 241, 243, *268*
Rodbard, D., 8, 13, 16, 28, 31, *39*
Rodesch, F., 206, *227*
Rogers, A. W., *268*
Rohdenburg, J., 134, *149*
Roitt, I. M., 191, 192, *195*
Rolls, B. J., 94, 95, *117*
Ronan, R., 154, *172*
Rosas, R., 109, *116*
Rose, N. R., 192, *195, 196*

AUTHOR INDEX

Rose, S., 127, *148*
Rosen, F. S., 128, 129, 131, 132, *145, 149*
Rosenberg, D., 184, *197*
Rosenberg, I. N., 207, *223*
Rosenberg, M., 95, *119*
Rosenblum, A. L., 182, 183, 185, *187, 196*
Rosenfeld, G. C., 260, *266*
Ross, G. T., 8, 13, 31, *39*
Roth, J., 107, *119*, 190, *196*
Roth, L. J., 240, 243, *265, 269*
Roth-Brandel, U., 213, 214, *227, 228*
Rothchild, I., 102, *120*
Rothen, A., 82, 86, *120*
Row, V. V., 185, *198*
Rowe, W. P., 132, *147*
Rowlands, D. T., 130, *149*
Rowntree, L. G., 134, *149*
Roy, S., 236, 238, *268*
Rudick, J., 218, *227*
Rudinger, J., 85, *118*
Rudman, D., 90, *120*
Russell, P. S., 128, 129, *148, 149*
Russell, S. M., 96, *120*
Ruth, R. F., 124, *149*
Ruyford, P. L., 31, *39*
Ryden, J., 110, *120*

S

Saameli, K., 108, *120*
Sachs, H., 83, 84, 85, 89, *117, 119, 120*
Sadowski, J., 105, *120*
Saffran, M., 87, 88, 102, *119, 120*
Saha, N. N., 237, 238, 239, *265*
Saito, T., 93, *120*
Salmon, S. E., 129, *147*
Salsbury, C., 129, *148*
Samols, E., 14, *38*
Samuels, G. M. R., 210, *224*
Samuels, H. H., 251, *269*
Samuelsson, B., 201, 210, *225, 227*
Sandberg, G., 125, *146*
Sander, S., 237, *268*
Sandler, M., 206, *227, 228*
Sandrin, E., 156, 157, 158, 159, 160, *172*
Sanel, F. T., 124, 125, 134, 138, *149*
Sapori, M. L., 243, *269*

Sato, S., 185, *197*
Sauer, R., 154, 155, *173*
Saunders, W. G., 105, *120*
Savard, K., 209, *226*
Sawyer, C. H., 51, 52, *76, 77, 78, 79, 80*, 94, *118*
Sawyer, W. H., 102, 105, *116, 118*
Scaramuzzi, R. J., 207, 208, *226*
Scatchard, G., 34, *39*
Schäfer, E. A., 82, *119*
Schally, A. V., 96, *115*
Schapiro, S., 59, *79*
Scharrer, E., 82, *115*
Scher, W., 231, *268*
Schjeide, O. A., 232, *265*
Schlueter, R. J., 152, 153, 154, 160, *172, 173*
Schneebeli, G. L., 137, *146*
Schneider, H. P. G., 202, 204, *228*
Schoen, H. C., 53, *76*
Schönbaum, E., 176, 177, 185, *197, 198*
Scholes, G. B., 219, *224*
Schrader, W. T., 255, 257, 258, *266*
Schrier, R. W., 106, *120*
Schultze, R. G., 216, *224*
Schulz, R. A., 85, *119*
Schuster, E., 82, 83, *120*
Scoggins, B. A., 204, 205, *225*
Scott, J. C., 82, 83, 100, *119*
Scott, J. S., 185, *197*
Scott, T. W., 189, *197*
Sealey, J. E., 114, *120*
Searles, H. F., 45, *76*
Sedlakova, E., 114, *117*
Segal, S. J., 45, 48, 79, 231, 232, 233, 236, 240, 241, 243, *268, 269*
Segar, W. E., 94, *118, 120*
Seiki, K., 125, *147*
Sela, M., 187, *197*
Seldin, D. W., 215, *227*
Sellars, E. A., 176, 177, *197*
Sellman, J. C., 215, *227*
Selye, H., 68, *79*
Sgherzi, A. M., 31, 34, *38*
Sharard, A., 193, *197*
Share, L., 95, 107, *119*
Sharma, O. K., 232, *268*
Sharp, G., 182, 183, 185, *196*

Shaw, J. E., 200, 201, 204, 205, 210, 215, 219, 220, 221, 222, 223, *224*, *227*, *228*
Shaw, R. K., 129, *149*, 178, *196*
Shay, H., 43, 79
Sheppard, P. M., 180, *196*
Sherman, J. D., 134, *149*
Sherman, M. R., 252, 253, 254, 255, 256, 257, 258, 260, *267*, *268*
Shih, Y., 237, 256, *264*, *268*
Shio, H., 223, *228*
Shiplacoff, D., 237, 238, 239, *265*
Shishiba, Y., 178, 189, *197*, *198*
Shorter, R. G., 133, *147*
Shyamala, G., 239, 243, 247, 260, *265*, *268*, *269*
Sica, V., 249, 250, *268*
Sieber, P., 156, *173*
Siggins, G. R., 211, *225*
Silbert, D., 184, *197*
Silver, T. M., 201, *223*
Silverstone, J. T., 94, *116*
Simpson, M. E., 54, *80*
Simpson, S. A., 2, *38*
Singer, F. R., 165, 167, 168, *172*
Sirett, N. E., 180, *195*
Six, K. M., 203, *227*
Sjodin, K., 131, 135, *146*
Sjoholm, I., 110, *120*
Skermer, C., 37, *38*
Skogerboe, R. K., 7, 8, *38*
Sladovic, L., 134, *145*
Slater, F. D., 136, 137, *146*
Slater, J. D. H., 27, *38*
Small, M., 138, *149*
Smart, G. A., 180, *196*
Smellie, R. M. S., 231, 232, *263*
Smith, B. R., 183, 187, 188, 192, 193, *197*, *198*
Smith, D. E., 234, 243, *260*, *265*, *268*
Smith, E. R., 51, *76*
Smith, G. N., 208, 212, *227*
Smith, M. W., 91, 99, 114, *118*, *120*
Smith, R. E., *266*, *268*
Smith, S., 237, 238, 239, 241, 242, 243, 244, 246, 249, 250, 261, *264*, *265*, *266*
Smith, S. W., 88, *120*
Snedeker, E. H., 154, *172*
Snyder, N. J., 184, 194, *196*, *198*

Sölna, J., 233, *269*
Solomon, D. H., 177, 178, 184, 189, 191, 192, 194, *195*, *196*, *197*, *198*, 206, 207, *226*
Somlyo, A. P., 97, 113, *120*
Somlyo, A. V., 97, 113, *120*
Spaziani, E., 231, *268*
Specker, H., 7, *38*
Spelsberg, T. C., 255, 257, 258, 260, *267*, *268*
Speroff, L., 207, 208, 212, *228*
Staehelin, M., 159, 160, *173*, 201, 205, *226*
Stanbury, J. B., 183, 184, 185, *197*
Stanton, M. F., 140, *147*
State, D., 139, 141, *147*
Steggles, A. W., 239, 242, 243, 246, 247, 255, 256, 257, 258, 260, *266*, *267*, *268*
Steinberg, D., 220, 221, *228*
Steiner, A. G., 167, *173*
Steiner, A. L., 36, *39*
Sternik-Sagalara, K., 105, *120*
Stewart, J. C., 181, *195*
Stone, G. M., 62, 78, 79, 236, 239, *268*
Strahilevitch, M., 138, *149*
Strand, J. C., 200, 216, 217, 218, *226*
Strong, C. G., 200, *225*
Stumpf, W. E., 51, 53, *80*, 237, 240, 241, 243, 244, 246, 255, 260, *265*, *269*
Stutman, O., 129, 131, 134, 144, *149*
Sunshine, P., 184, *198*
Sutherland, E. W., 190, *196*, 210, 221, *224*, *228*, 263, *269*
Sutin, J., 94, *116*
Suzuki, T., 241, 242, 243, 244, 246, 249, 261, *265*, *266*
Swanson, H. E., 43, 44, 45, 59, 72, *80*
Sweat, M. L., 236, *269*
Szed, C., 129, *149*
Szego, C. M., 231, 266, *268*, *269*
Szentágothai, J., 49, *80*
Szreder, I., 105, *120*

T

Tait, J. F., 2, 3, *38*
Takabatake, Y., 84, *120*
Takasugi, N., 67, 68, 69, 70, 71, *80*

AUTHOR INDEX

Takewaki, K., 59, 68, 70, *80*
Takken, A., 102, *117*
Takman, B. H., 215, 217, *226*
Taleisnik, S., 45, *80*, 95, *116*
Talwar, G. P., 236, 240, 241, 243, *269*
Tampion, W., 11, *38*
Tashjian, A. H. J., 167, 168, *173*
Tata, J. R., 232, 234, 262, *265*
Taub, R. N., 134, *149*
Taylor, R. B., 128, *149*
Taylor, R. W., 237, *264*
Tebecis, A. K., 211, *227*
Tejasen, T., 51, *80*
Teng, C. S., 232, 233, 241, *269*
Terasawa, W., 52, *80*
Terenius, L., 236, 237, 239, *266*, *269*
Terragno, N. A., 200, 216, 217, 218, *226*
Thayer, S. A., 235, *266*
Theobald, G. W., 98, 108, 110, *120*
Thomas, G. H., *268*
Thomas, P. J., 88, 91, *118*
Thompson, C. J., 219, *225*
Thompson, E. B., 251, *269*
Thomson, W. B., 105, *120*
Thorén, L., 237, *266*
Thorn, N. A., 91, 93, 104, 114, *116*, *120*
Thun, K. J., 236, *266*
Tiboldi, T., 48, *79*
Tima, L., 44, 45, 46, 47, 52, 71, 77, 78, *80*
Timiras, P., 62, *80*
Ting, R. C., 133, 140, *147*
Toft, D. O., 241, 243, 246, 247, 252, 253, 254, 255, 256, 257, 258, 260, *265*, *267*, *269*
Tomkins, G. M., 251, *269*
Traber, D. L., 95, *120*
Trachewsky, D., 232, *269*
Trainin, N., 132, 134, 138, *147*, *149*
Trank, J. W., 94, *118*
Travis, R. H., 95, *120*
Tregear, G. W., 37, *38*, 165, *173*
Trench, C. A. H., 134, *149*
Triplett, R. F., 143, *145*
Truong, H., 248, *269*

Trussell, R. R., 212, *226*
Tse, A., 134, *146*
Tuohimaa, P., 64, *80*
Turnbull, A. C., 216, *227*
Turner, C. D., 67, 69, *80*
Tuyttens, N., 103, 104, *117*
Tyan, M. L., 139, *146*

U

Udenfriend, S., 2, *38*
Uhlarik, S., 49, 52, *78*
Uhr, J. W., 128, *147*
Ui, H., 233, 238, *269*
Unhjem, O., 233, *269*
Usardi, M. M., 221, 222, *224*, *227*
Utiger, R. D., 36, *39*, 182, 183, 185, 192, *195*, *196*, *198*
Uttenthal, L. S., 87, *120*
Utz, J. P., 129, *149*

V

Valtin, H., 96, *119*
van Demark, N. L., 103, *118*, *120*
Vander, A. J., 94, *119*, 215, *228*
Vanderheyden, I., 237, 248, *264*
VanderLaan, W. P., 187, 188, *197*, 202, *224*
van der Werff ten Bosch, J. J., 43, 44, 45, 46, 53, 59, 72, 76, *80*
Van Dewark, S. D., 256, *268*
van Dyke, D. C., 54, *80*
van Dyke, H. B., 82, 86, 87, 98, *117*, *120*
Vane, J. R., 216, 218, 219, *224*, *227*
Vanhaelst, L., 183, 185, *195*
Vanotti, A., 182, *196*
van Rees, G. P., 45, 46, 59, *80*
Vaughan, M., 220, 221, *228*
Verney, E. B., 93, *120*
Verroust, P. J., 106, *120*
Versteeg, D. H. G., 203, *225*
Vértes, M., 64, *80*
Vidor, G. I., 181, *195*
Vigersky, R., 259, *263*
Villee, C. A., 53, 62, 78, 233, 237, 244, 246, *264*, *266*, *267*

Vincent, J. D., 93, *118*
Vizsolyi, E., 97, *120*
Vivian, S. R., 103, *118*
Vogt, M., 84, *120*
Vogt, W., 201, *228*
Voloschin, L., 49, *80*
Volpé, R., 185, *198*
Volta, F., 218, *224*
Vonderhaar, B. K., 248, 249, *269*
von Euler, U. S., 212, *228*
von Gaudecker, B., 88, *115*
Von Kolliken, R. A., 124, *149*
von Konschegg, A., 82, 83, *120*
Vorherr, H., 105, 106, *119*

W

Wada, K., 233, *268*
Wagner, J. W., 48, *77*
Wagner, R., 260, *266*
Waksman, B. H., 123, 127, 135, *147*
Walker, F. C., 134, *149*
Walker, J. M., 99, *116*
Walker, W., 90, *120*
Wall, J. R., 180, *198*
Walmsley, C. F., 107, 108, *117*, *118*
Warren, J. C., 233, *263*
Waters, M. F. R., 129, *148*
Watson, J. W., 134, *149*
Way, L., 220, *228*
Waynforth, H. B., 237, *264*
Weddell, A. G. M., 129, *148*
Weeks, J. R., 200, 201, 206, 207, 208, 209, 210, 220, 221, *224*, *225*, *228*
Weiss, B., 210, 221, *226*, *228*
Weissman, I. L., 130, 133, *145*, *149*
Welch, M., 236, *265*
Wendlandt, S., 211, *226*
Wenzel, M., 236, *269*
Whalen, R. E., 64, 65, *77*
Wheeler, M., 99, 108, *118*
White, A., 123, 130, 134, 135, 136, 137, 138, 139, 140, 141, 142, 143, 144, *145*, *146*, *147*, *148*, *149*
White, R. G., 127, *148*
Whitehead, J. K., 2, 38, *39*
Widnell, C. C., 232, 234, 262, *265*
Wiener, M., 237, *264*

Wiest, W. G., 253, 254, 255, 256, 257, 258, *268*, *269*
Wilber, J. F., 182, *197*
Wilkes, B., 133, *145*
Wilks, J. W., 102, *120*
Willems, C., 206, *227*
Willems, H., 156, *172*
Williams, E. D., 134, *146*
Williams, E. D., 206, *227*, *228*
Williams-Ashman, H. G., 231, *269*
Williamson, A. M., 178, 189, *197*
Williamson, Sr., 200, 217, 218, *226*
Wilson, A. L., 7, *39*
Wilson, D. W., 219, *228*
Wilson, R. D., 95, *120*
Winnick, R. E., 84, *120*
Winnick, T., 84, *120*
Wiqvist, N., 213, 214, *224*, *227*, *228*
Wiseman, B., 209, *224*
Witter, A., 203, *225*
Wittkower, E. D., 179, *198*
Wolf, B., 139, *149*
Wolf, G., 95, *119*
Wolfe, L. S., 210, 218, *224*, *228*
Wollman, A. L., 73, *80*
Wolstencroft, J. H., 210, *223*
Wolthuis, O. L., 45, 46, *80*
Wong, E. T., 194, *198*
Wong, F. M., 134, *149*
Wood, E. C., 111, 113, *117*
Wood, M. L., 128, *148*
Woodhan, J., 100, *116*
Woodhouse, N. J. Y., 134, *146*
Woolley, D., 62, *80*
Wotiz, H. H., 237, 248, 259, *263*
Wren, T. R., 231, *263*
Wright, P. A., 208, *226*
Wright, P. M., 219, *225*
Wright, R. D., 204, 205, *225*
Wuu, T. C., 87, *120*
Wyllie, J. H., 216, 219, *224*, *227*
Wyngarden, L. J., 207, 208, 209, *227*
Wyss, R. H., 238, 239, 242, *269*

Y

Yalow, R. S., 8, 9, 10, 11, 38, *39*
Yamashita, A., 125, *147*

Yates, F. E., 96, *120*
Yates, K. M., 268
Yazaki, I., 48, 57, *80*
Yoshida, D., 129, *148*
Yoshida, S., 93, *120*
Yoshinaga, K., 215, *224*
Young, R. B., 236, *269*
Yrarrazaval, S., 52, *76*
Yunis, E. J., 131, 134, 144, *149*

Z

Zehnder, K., 156, 157, 158, 159, 160, *172*
Zehr, J. E., 94, *118*
Zimmering, P. E., 243, *269*
Zisblatt, M., 140, 141, 143, *146, 147, 149*
Zor, U., 189, 190, *196*, 202, 204, 206, *225, 228*
Zuber, H., 153, 154, *173*

SUBJECT INDEX

A

Abortion, therapeutic, with prostaglandins, 213–214
ACTH
  prostaglandin effects on release of, 203–205
  vasopressin as releasing factor for, 95–96
Actinomycin D, in blockage of androgen sterilization, 73–74
Adrenal gland, prostaglandin effects on, 203–205
Androgen
  in induction of polyfollicular ovary syndrome, 42–45
    age and dosage effects on, 43–45
    mechanism of action, 62–67, 71–74
    neonatal treatment of, in reduction of estradiol-binding capacity, 63–67
Androgen-sterilized rat, 42–48
  polyfollicular ovary syndrome (POS) induction in, 42–43
Ataxia-telangiectasia, as immunological disease, 129

B

Barbiturates, in blockage of androgen sterilization, 73
Bruton sex-linked agammaglobulinemia, thymic malfunction and, 128–129

C

Calcitonin(s), 151–173
  chemistry of, 152–161
  in fish, 167
  in humans, 167–169
  isolation of, 152–153
    problems in, 153–154
  from salmon, increased potency of, 160–161
  secretion of
    control, 161–163
    dietary calcium in, 165–167
    gastrointestinal factors and, 165
  sequence determination in, 154–155
  structure and function in, 156–161
    constant and variable regions, 156–157
    specific residues and biological activity, 157–158
  synthetic
    biological activity of, 158–160
    preparation, 156
  therapeutic uses of, 169–172
Cancer, see Tumors
Carbohydrate metabolism, prostaglandin effects on, 220–222
Central nervous system (CNS)
  prostaglandin activity and, 210–212
  steroid hormone differentiation in, 41–80

SUBJECT INDEX

Chlorpromazine, as protectant against steroid-induced sterility, 70–71
Corticotropin-releasing factor, vasopressin as, 95–96
Cyclic AMP
 LATS activity and, 190–191
 prostaglandins and, 222–223
 radioimmunoassay of, 36
Cyproterone acetate, in blockage of androgen sterilization, 73

D

Deoxycorticosterone, induction (neonatal) of sterility by, 68–69
DiGeorge syndrome, thymic malfunction and, 128

E

Epithelial secretory cells, of thymus gland, 125
Estradiol
 binding capacity for, of neural and nonneural target tissues, 63–67
 induction of polyfollicular ovarian syndrome by, 67–68, 71
 uptake and retention of, by hypothalamic areas, 62
Estrogen
 anestrous state produced by, 68
 binding by target tissues, 235–240
  cytosol dependence of nuclear binding, 244–246
 effects on cellular processes, 231–235
 induction of polyfollicular ovarian syndrome by, 67–68
 receptors, 235–250
  intracellular localization of, 240–244
  properties and purification of proteins of, 246–250
Exophthalmos-producing substance (EPS), relationship to TSH and LATS, 186

F

Fallopian tubes, prostaglandin effects on, 214–215
Fetus, circulating oxytocin in, 113–114

Fish, calcitonin studies on, 167
Follicle-stimulating hormone, secretion of, 74–75
 cyclic mechanism of, 51–53
 derangement mechanism, 56–61
 tonic mechanism of, 49–51

G

Gonadotropin(s)
 prostaglandin effects on, 207–209
 secretion of
  cyclic mechanism of, 51–53
  dual hypothalamic mechanism controlling, 48–53, 74
  tonic mechanism for, 49–51
Graves' disease, experimental analog of, 191–192
Growth hormone, prostaglandin effect on release of, 202–203

H

Hormones, saturation analysis of, 1–2, 37
Hypothalamus
 gonadotropin-secretion control in, 48–53
 oxytocin synthesis in, 83–85
 vasopressin synthesis in, 83–85

I

Immune disorders, thymic malfunction and, 128–130

J

Jod-Basedow phenomenon, in etiology of thyrotoxicosis, 181

K

Kidney, prostaglandin effects on, 215–218

L

Labor, see Parturition
Lactation, oxytocin role in, 100

Leukemia, immunological deficiency and, 129
Lipid metabolism, prostaglandin effects on, 220–222
Long-acting thyroid stimulator (LATS), 175–198
  absorption by thyroid extracts,
    future applications of, 193
    LATS dissociation after, 193
    partial purification of, 192–193
  altered time course in vitro and in vivo, 189–190
  assay methods for, 177–179
  chemical nature of, 186–189
  clinical importance of, 183–186
  clinical markers of, 184–186
    eye signs, 185–186
    neonatal thyrotoxicosis, 184–185
    pretibial myxedema, 184
    thyroid autoantibodies, 185
    TSH and EPS, 186
  concentration methods for, 187
  cyclic AMP and, 190–191
  discovery of, 177
  effects related to actions of TSH, 189–191
  with γG immunoglobulins, 186–187
  H and L chain of, 188–189
  nonpituitary origin of, evidence, 182–183
  proteolysis of, 187–188
  stimulation of thyroid by, evidence, 181–182
  in thyrotoxicosis, 176
    earlier theories of, 179–181
    thyroid function and, 183–184
Luteinizing hormone
  in rats with polyfollicular ovary syndrome, 45–48
    derangement mechanism, 56–61
  secretion of, 74–75
    cyclic mechanism of, 51–53
    tonic mechanism of, 49–51
Lymphocytes of thymus, origin of, 124–125
Lymphoid system, thymus role in development and function of, 125–128

M

Malignancy, see Tumors

N

Natriuretic hormone
  properties and release of, 114
  prostaglandins and, 215–218
Neurophysin, 86–93
  circulating type, 89–93
    measurement of, 89–90
    significance of, 90–93
  as precursor of oxytocin and vasopressin, 88
  properties of, 87–88

O

Osmoreceptors, control of vasopressin release by, 93–94
Ovarian hormones
  effects at subcellular level, 229–269
    biochemical significance of, 259–263
    estrogens, 231–250
    progestins, 250–263
Ovaries, prostaglandin effects on, 207–209
Oxytocin, 98–115
  circulating
    in labor, 109
    measurement, 98–100
    in umbilical blood, 111–112
  fetal release of, 111–114
  in lactation, 100–101
  miscellaneous functions of, 107
  neurophysin as precursor of, 88–89
  in parturition, 107–111
    in animals, 107
    in humans, 107–111
  radioimmunoassay of, 99–100
  release from posterior pituitary gland, 85–86, 115
  as a releasing factor, 101–103
  in salt and water metabolism, 104–107
  in sperm transport, 103–104
    in female, 103–104
    in male, 104
  synthesis in hypothalamus, 83–86

in tumors, 107
Ovulating hormone, in androgen-sterilized rats, 45–48

P

Paget's disease, calcitonin therapy of, 169–172
Pancreas, prostaglandin effects on, 218
Parturition
   oxytocin role in, 107–111
   prostaglandin initiation of, 212–214
Pituitary gland, ovulating hormone in, in androgen-sterilized rats, 45–48
Polyfollicular ovary syndrome (POS)
   androgen in, possible site of action, 48–61
   induction by neonatal estrogen administration, 67–68
   induction by testosterone, 42–45
   in rats with anterior hypothalamic lesions, 54–56
Posterior pituitary gland
   natriuretic hormone and, 114
   neurosecretion by, 83–86
   oxytocin release from, 85–86
   physiology of, 81–120
   prostaglandin effects on, 212–218
   vasopressin release from, 85–86
   in the fetus, 97–98
Progesterone, in neonatal induction of sterility, 71
Progestins
   effects at subcellular level, 250–258
      cytosol dependence of nuclear binding, 257
      early effects, 250–251
      receptor complexes, 254–257
      receptor interactions, 251–254
      receptor proteins, properties and purification, 258
Prostaglandins
   cyclic AMP and, 222
   effects on
      carbohydrate and lipid metabolism, 220–222
      fallopian tubes, 21–215
      kidney, 215–218
      posterior pituitary gland, 212–218
      uterus, 212–214
   endocrinological implications of, 199–228
   general description and activity of, 200–202
   interaction with exocrine hormones, 218–220
      pancreas, 218
      stomach, 218–220
   natriuretic effects of, 215–218
   neuroendocrinological actions of, 210–212
   structural formulas of, 200
   tropic hormone effects of, 202–209
      ACTH-adrenals, 203–205
      gonadotropin-ovaries, 207–209
      growth hormone, 202–203
      TSH-thyroid, 206–207

R

Reserpine, as protectant against steroid-induced sterility, 70

S

Salmon, calcitonin from, 160–161
Salt metabolism, oxytocin effects on, 104–107
Saturation analysis techniques, 1–39
   applications of, 4
   definitions in, 6–11
   basic concepts of, 1–39
   linearization of assay response curves, 30–31
   practical aspects of, 31–37
   precision of, 6, 10–11, 23–27
   principles of, 3–31
   reaction with reagent, 34–36
   sensitivity of, 6, 7–8
   separation of free and bound moieties in, 36–37
      measurement of hormone distribution, 37
   specificity of, 27–30
   theory of, 3–6
Secretory cells, in thymus epithelium, 125
Sperm transport, oxytocin role in,

103–104
Sterility, steroid-induced, protection against, 70–74
Steroid hormones
  differentian in CNS, 41–80
  in induction of polyfollicular ovary syndrome, possible mechanism of action, 69–70
  sterility induction by, protection against, 70–74
Stomach, prostaglandin effects on, 218–220

T

Testes, prostaglandin effects on, 209
Testosterone, in induction of polyfollicular ovary syndrome, 43–45
Thymosin, in development and functions of lymphoid tissue, 121–149
Thymus gland
  cellular function of, hypothesis of, 142–143
  embryonic development of, 123–124
  endocrine function of, 122, 131–142
    hypothesis for, 142–143
    thymic extracts, 134–142
    thymic grafts, 131–134
  lymphocytes of, origin, 124–125
  malfunction related to clinical disorders of, 128–130
  mechanism of action of, 130–142
  as progenitor of cells, 130–131
  thymectomy in studies of, 125–128
Thyroid gland, calcitonin from, 152
Thyroid-stimulating hormone (TSH)
  prostaglandin effects on, 206–207
  relationship to LATS and exophthalmos-producing substance (EPS), 186, 189–191
Thyroid stimulator, long-acting, see Long-acting thyroid stimulator

Thyrotoxicosis
  genetic factors of, 180
  Jod-Basedow phenomenon in, 181
  LATS in, 176, 179–183
  neonatal, LATS in, 184–185
  psychosomatic theory of, 179–180
  toxic adenoma in, 181
Tumors
  immunological deficiency and, 129
  oxytocin in, 107

U

Umbilical circulation, oxytocin in, 111–113
Uterus, prostaglandin effects on, 212–214

V

Vasopressin, 93–98
  as corticotropin-releasing factor, 95–96
  neurophysin as precursor of, 88–89
  release by posterior pituitary gland, 85–86, 115
    control, 93–95
    of fetus during parturition, 97–98
    relation to higher levels of brain, 95
  synthesis in hypothalamus, 83–85
Vitamin B_{12}, saturation analysis of, 30, 31
Volume receptors, control of vasopressin release by, 94–95

W

Wasting disease, 131
  neonatal thymectomy and, 126–127
Water metabolism, oxytocin effects on, 104–107